OXFORD MEDICAL PUBLICATIONS

Psychopharmacology:
Recent Advances and Future Prospects

BRITISH ASSOCIATION
FOR PSYCHOPHARMACOLOGY MONOGRAPHS

Psychopharmacology:
Recent Advances and Future Prospects

BRITISH ASSOCIATION
FOR PSYCHOPHARMACOLOGY
MONOGRAPH
No. 6

EDITED BY

SUSAN D. IVERSEN
Director of Behavioural Pharmacology
Merck Sharp & Dohme Research Laboratories
Harlow, Essex

Oxford New York Tokyo
OXFORD UNIVERSITY PRESS
1985

Oxford University Press, Walton Street, Oxford OX2 6DP
Oxford New York Toronto
Delhi Bombay Calcutta Madras Karachi
Kuala Lumpur Singapore Hong Kong Tokyo
Nairobi Dar es Salaam Cape Town
Melbourne Auckland
and associated companies in
Beirut Berlin Ibadan Nicosia

Oxford is a trade mark of Oxford University Press

British Library Cataloguing in Publication Data

Psychopharmacology: recent advances and future
prospects.— (A British Association for
Psychopharmacology monograph; no. 6) — Oxford
medical publications)
1. Psychopharmacology
I. Iversen, Susan D.   II. Series
615'.78   RC483
ISBN 0-19-261478-9

Library of Congress Cataloging in Publication Data
Main entry under title:
Psychopharmacology: recent advances and future prospects.
(British Association for Psychopharmacology monograph;
no. 6) (Oxford medical publications)
Bibliography
Includes index.
1. Psychopharmacology— Congresses. I. Iversen,
Susan D., 1940-   II. Series.   III. Series: Oxford
medical publications.
RC483.P7783   1985   615'.78   85-3091
ISBN 0-19-261478-9

Set by Joshua Associates Ltd, Oxford
Printed in Great Britain by
St Edmundsbury Press,
Bury St. Edmunds, Suffolk.

Preface

The tenth anniversary of the British Association of Psychopharmacology was celebrated in Guernsey on 4–7 April 1984. It was decided that the occasion should be marked by a meeting that was special both in venue and in scientific content. Psychopharmacology as a discipline continues its rapid growth drawing scientists from many disciplines in their quest to unravel the mode of action of drugs on brain function both in health and disease.

We elected to undertake a broad review of the whole subject, in the belief that so many advances have been made in the past few years that it should be possible to devise a stimulating meeting and useful reference volume to mark our tenth anniversary.

Five topics were selected for review, and these illustrate well the state of the art and focus on a number of fundamental issues in psychopharmacology.

The President, Gene Paykel organized a review of current research on anti-depressants. A wide range of effective antidepressants exist, most of which inhibit the re-uptake of noradrenaline or serotonin in brain. Dr Pinder reminded us that more than 150 compounds, mainly using these mechanisms are in various stages of development by the pharmaceutical companies. A few atypical anti-depressants of uncertain neuropharmacological mechanisms are available, but major breakthroughs in the treatment of depression seem unlikely until more is known of the aetiology and neuropharmacological basis of the disorder. Clinicians repeat that anti-depressant drugs with a more rapid onset of action than existing agents would be valuable. It is notable that there are few animal tests modelling the behavioural features of depression which respond reliably and selectively to antidepressant drugs. However, in view of the slow onset of action of these drugs, it is surprising that behavioural pharmacologists rarely study chronic dosage regimes in animals.

Turning to the second topic, the minor tranquillizers, the major break-through afforded by the discovery of the endogenous benzodiazepine receptor can begin to be appreciated. When specific receptors for a class of drug molecules can be described and studied, rapid advances can be made in medicinal chemistry to design novel ligands. In the case of the benzodiazepines this approach had led both to the discovery of a range of non-benzodiazepine agonist ligands and the introduction of a novel pharmacological concept — that of the 'inverse agonist'. Assuming the benzodiazepines to be full agonists, a number of partial agonists and antagonists have been described which fulfil conventional pharmacological criteria. Most interesting, however, are a range of compounds which act on the same receptors but possess pharmacological effects opposite to those of the benzodiazepines. These have been termed 'inverse agonists'. Within the partial agonists compounds may be found which have some but not all the effects of the classic benzodiazepines. If this proves to be the case, anxiolytics or anti-convulsants without sedative effects or muscle relaxant properties may be developed.

The topic 'Psychopharmacology of cognition' reflects an area of enormous clinical importance, the dementias, where no effective medication exists at present. Accordingly, the lectures reflected recent advances in our understanding of the chemical pathology associated with profound cognitive dysfunction seen in dementia of Alzheimer's type AD. The degeneration of the forebrain acetylcholine system in AD is now well documented and for this reason there is considerable interest in the possibility of using cholinergic agents in the treatment of senile dementia. Basic cholinergic pharmacology in the CNS will now no doubt receive renewed attention, long overdue. Animal models of cognitive disorders will play an important role in the evaluation of potentially important new cerebroactive drugs. A wide range of behavioural tests are available from experimental neuropsychology to assess attention, perception, learning, and memory in rodents and in primates.

In the fourth session, 'Schizophrenia' was the focus of attention, and evidence relating to the aetiology, genetic basis, and neurochemical dysfunction in this disorder was discussed. An important principle emerged which would apply equally to depression or anxiety states — notably that inferring a neurochemical basis for a neuropsychiatric condition on the basis of the mechanisms of action of the drugs it responds to, may be misleading. Efficacious neuroleptics block dopamine receptors, but the evidence for heightened endogenous dopamine activity in schizophrenia is still highly contentious. Changes in post synaptic dopamine receptors may be secondary to other neurochemical changes in the brains of schizophrenic patients. Since a wide range of other monoamine transmitters and neuropeptides are known to interact functionally with the striatal and limbic dopamine pathways, this is a strong possibility. Furthermore, drugs which selectively modify these chemical pathways, for example antagonists of the neuropeptides substance P or neurotensin, could modify dopaminergic function as effectively as dopamine-receptor-blocking agents. It is clearly difficult to interpret neurochemical results on post-mortem brain tissue from drug treated patients, but such studies are of great importance in all neuropsychiatric conditions and hopefully will lead to a greater understanding of the primary neurochemical changes underlying these illnesses.

In the final symposium fundamental aspects of human psychopharmacology were discussed in a range of papers defining the effect of stimulant drugs on human performance. Inevitably, the issue of addiction was raised, since many of the psychostimulants which have beneficial effects in small doses, lead to detrimental effects when taken in larger doses and almost invariably to addiction. It was an appropriate finale to a review of modern psychopharmacology to be reminded that psychoactive drugs may improve brain function or restore dysfunction, but may also be instruments of self-destruction.

Harlow, Essex   S. D. I.
November 1984

Contents

Contributors

C. A. BLOXHAM, *Department of Pathology, Newcastle General Hospital, Westgate Road, Newcastle upon Tyne, NE4 6DE, UK.*

L. G. BROOKES, *Upjohn Limited, Fleming Way, Crawley, West Sussex, RH10 2NJ, UK.*

J. M. CANDY, *MRC Neuroendocrinology Unit, Newcastle General Hospital, Westgate Road, Newcastle upon Tyne, NE4 6BE, UK.*

J. S. CHADDHA, *Department of Endocrinology, Medical College of Georgia, Augusta, Georgia 30912, USA.*

A. W. CLARE, *Professor of Psychological Medicine, Department of Psychological Medicine, St Bartholomew's Medical College, London, UK.*

A. COPPEN, *MRC Neuropsychiatry Research Laboratory, West Park Hospital, Epsom, KT19 8PB, UK.*

J. CRAWLEY, *Division of Radioisotopes, MRS Clinical Research Centre, Watford Road, Harrow, Middlesex, HA1 3UJ, UK.*

A. J. CROSS, *Division of Radioisotopes, MRC Clinical Research Centre, Watford Road, Harrow, Middlesex, HA1 3UJ, UK.*

T. J. CROW, *Division of Psychiatry, MRC Clinical Research Centre, Watford Road, Harrow, Middlesex, HA1 3UJ, UK.*

D. CURSON, *Medical Director, Bowden House Clinic, Harrow-on-the-Hill, Middlesex, UK.*

A. DARRAGH, *Institute of Clinical Pharmacology, P.O. Box 469, 1, James's Street, Dublin, 8, Republic of Ireland.*

B. M. DAVIS, *Departments of Psychiatry and Medicine, Mt. Sinai School of Medicine, 100th St. & 5th Avenue, New York, NY 10029, USA.*

K. L. DAVIS, *Departments of Psychiatry and Pharmacology, Mt. Sinai School of Medicine, 100th St. & 5th Avenue, New York, NY 10029, USA.*

R. DOROW, *Research Laboratories of Schering AG, Pharmaceutical Research, Neuroendocrinology and Neuropsychopharmacology, Postfach 65 03 11, D–100 Berlin 65, Federal Republic of Germany.*

J. A. EDWARDSON, *MRC Neuroendocrinology Unit, Newcastle General Hospital, Westgate Road, Newcastle upon Tyne, NE4 6BE, UK.*

E. GOODALL, *Academic Unit of Human Psychopharmacology, Medical College of St Bartholomew's Hospital, London, EC1, UK.*

R. B. GREENBLATT, *Department of Endocrinology, Medical College of Georgia, Augusta, Georgia 30912, USA.*

A. N, GRIFFITHS, *Department of Pharmacology and Therapeutics, University of Wales College of Medicine, Heath Park, Cardiff, CF4 4XN, UK.*

V. HAROUTUNIAN, *Department of Psychiatry, Mt. Sinai School of Medicine, 100th St. & 5th Avenue, New York, NY 10029, USA.*

R. HARTNOLL, *University College Hospital (National Temperance Hospital), Drug Dependence Clinic, 122 Hampstead Road, London NW1 2LT, UK.*

T. B. HORVATH, *Department of Psychiatry, Mt. Sinai School of Medicine, 100th St. & 5th Avenue, New York, NY 10029, USA.*

L. I. IVERSEN, *Neuroscience Research Centre, Merck Sharp and Dohme Research Laboratories, Eastwick Road, Terlings Park, Harlow, Essex, CM20 2QR, UK.*

S. D. IVERSEN, *Merck Sharp and Dohme Limited, Neuroscience Research Centre, Eastwick Road, Terlings Park, Harlow Essex, CM20 2QR, UK.*

C. A. JOHNS, *Department of Psychiatry, Mt. Sinai School of Medicine, 100th St. & 5th Avenue, New York, NY 10029, USA.*

E. C. JOHNSTONE, *Division of Psychiatry, MRC Clinical Research Centre, Watford Road, Harrow, Middlesex, HA1 3UJ, UK.*

M. KENNY, *Institute of Clinical Pharmacology, P.O. Box 469, 1, James's Street, Dublin, 8, Republic of Ireland.*

B. E. LEONARD, *Pharmacology Department, University College, Galway, Republic of Ireland.*

R. LEWIS, *University College Hospital (National Temperance Hospital), Drug Dependence Clinic, 122 Hampstead Road, London NW1 2LT, UK.*

M. MITCHESON, *University College Hospital (National Temperance Hospital), Drug Dependence Clinic, 122 Hampstead Road, London NW1 2LT, UK.*

R. C. MOHS, *Department of Psychiatry, Mt. Sinai School of Medicine, 100th St. & 5th Avenue, New York, NY 10029, USA.*

C. H. NEZHAT, *Department of Endocrinology, Medical College of Georgia, Augusta, Georgia 30912, USA.*

E. S. PAYKEL, *Professor of Psychiatry, St. George's Hospital Medical School, London, SW17 0RE, UK.*

E. K. PERRY, *Department of Pathology, Newcastle General Hospital, Westgate Road, Newcastle upon Tyne, NE4 6BE, UK.*

R. H. PERRY, *MRC Neuroendocrinology Unit, Newcastle General Hospital, Westgate Road, Newcastle upon Tyne, NE4 6BE, UK.*

R. M. PINDER, *Scientific Development Group, Organon International B.V., P.O. Box 20, 5340 BH Oss, The Netherlands.*

M. POULTER, *Division of Psychiatry, MRC Clinical Research Centre, Watford Road, Harrow, Middlesex, HA1 3UJ, UK.*

A. E. OAKLEY, *MRC Neuroendocrinology Unit, Newcastle General Hospital, Westgate Road, Newcastle upon Tyne, NE4 6BE, UK.*

S. R. OLDLAND, *Division of Radioisotopes, MRC Clinical Research Centre, Watford Road, Harrow, Middlesex, HA1 3UJ, UK.*

F. OWEN, *Division of Psychiatry, MRC Clinical Research Centre, Watford Road, Harrow, Middlesex, HA1 3UJ, UK.*

A. RICHENS, *Department of Pharmacology and Therapeutics, University of Wales College of Medicine, Heath Park, Cardiff, CF4 4XN, UK.*

T. W. ROBBINS, *Department of Experimental Psychology, University of Cambridge, Downing Street, Cambridge, CB2 3EB, UK.*

M. ROSSOR, *Department of Neurology, King's College Hospital, Denmark Hill, London SE5 9RS, UK.*

M. A. H. RUSSELL, *Addiction Research Unit, Institute of Psychiatry, London, SE5, UK.*

F. SCHULSINGER, *Psychologisk Institut, Kommunehospitalet, Copenhagen, Denmark.*

T. SILVERSTONE, *Academic Unit of Human Psychopharmacology, Medical College of St Bartholomew's Hospital, London, EC1, UK.*

A. Z. TERAN, *Department of Endocrinology, Medical College of Georgia, August, Georgia 30912, USA.*

P. J. TYRER, *Mapperley Hospital, Portchester Road, Nottingham, NG3 6AA, UK.*

N. VEAL, *Division of Radioisotopes, MRC Clinical Research Centre, Watford Road, Harrow, Middlesex, HA1 3UJ, UK.*

R. J. WEST, *Addiction Research Unit, Institute of Psychiatry, London, SE5, UK.*

K. WOOD, *MRC Neuropsychiatry Research Laboratory, West Park Hospital, Epsom, KT19 8PB, UK.*

G. D. ZANELLI, *Division of Radioisotopes, MRC Clinical Research Centre, Watford Road, Harrow, Middlesex, HA1 3UJ, UK.*

PART 1
Affective disorders

1

How effective are antidepressants?

E. S. PAYKEL

This chapter will survey the efficacy and place of antidepressants in the treatment of depression. I will range widely, but cannot be comprehensive. Space will not permit all the evidence, much of it from recent reviews (Paykel and Coppen 1979; Paykel 1982), on which the conclusions are based.

Akiskal and McKinney (1975) in an attempted synthesis, presented ten possible models of depression, ranging from the biological to the existential. These remind us that depressive disorder may be a final common pathway for multiple causes. It should not be expected that treatment would be limited only to the physical modality. A properly balanced presentation would allot full space to social and environmental measures, to psychotherapeutic and to behavioural approaches. These are beyond my mandate, but I will touch on controlled trials of psychotherapy and of cognitive therapy, to consider their place in relation to antidepressants.

Also, the term 'depression' covers a range of severity and other qualities from normal mood to severe psychotic illness. Recent prevalence figures for mild clinical disorder in women are around 5-10 per cent. Most see their general practitioners within the same year although they may not be diagnosed. Perhaps 90 per cent of depressives are treated in general practice, but almost all the evidence on treatment efficacy comes from psychiatric out-patients or in-patients. In a recent study (Sireling, Paykel, Freeling, Rao, and Patel, in press) we found that among antidepressant-treated patients in general practice only a half satisfied the Research Diagnostic Criteria for major depression, and only a third scored 17 or more on the Hamilton Depression Scale, both common inclusion criteria for psychiatric out-patient drug trials. More studies are needed of effectiveness and indications for treatments in such mild depressives.

In classification, the bipolar–unipolar division is obviously of value. However, most affective disorders are unipolar and here a broad separation into endogenous (or psychotic) and neurotic is still useful in treatment choice. The recent evidence is clear that symptom pattern is only very weakly related to absence or presence of stress, and it appears to be symptom pattern and severity rather than absence of precipitant stress which is associated with response to physical treatments (Paykel 1982; Paykel 1979).

ECT

Electroconvulsive therapy is still the touchstone physical treatment for severe depression against which all the other treatments must be measured. There have been five recent British double-blind controlled trials against simulated ECT with anaesthesia. The Knowle study found ECT only very weakly superior to placebo treatment. The Northwick Park study found effects that were clearly significant but not very strong. However, the Edinburgh, Sutton, and Leicester studies (Brandon, Cowley, McDonald, Neville, Palmer, and Wellstood-Eason, 1984), all found strong and conclusive effects. It is possible that the close care given to all patients in these difficult studies might mask greater differences in routine treatment. The study which showed the weakest effects employed unilateral brief pulse ECT. Robin and de Tiserra (1982) found brief pulse less effective than sine wave or high-energy pulse applications, and unilateral non-dominant ECT tends on average to be a little less effective than bilateral ECT (D'Elia and Raotma 1975).

With regard to who responds, eight predictor studies have shown that patients at the psychotic or endogenous extreme do better than neurotic depressives (Paykel 1979). Only two studies have failed to do so. The Northwick Park study found the best response in deluded depressives.

TRICYCLIC ANTIDEPRESSANTS

The tricylics have now been available for 25 years. They are well-studied drugs and there is no doubt of their overall superiority to placebo. Ten years ago Morris and Beck (1974) reviewed trials of the six tricyclics then available in the USA. There were 93 studies, of which 62 showed drugs superior to placebo and 31 failed to do so. This is far in excess of chance expectation of 5 per cent significance.

We do have the problem of the negative studies. Some are due to small samples, particularly with the variability in outcome common in depression, some to unresponsive subjects, low doses, or short treatment periods. Undoubtedly part of the problem also lies in limited efficacy. The spontaneous outcome of depression is often quite good, with added non-specific treatment effects from support and hospital admission. The element which the drugs add is on average limited, although it is very marked in some patients. The proportion of the total variance in antidepressant trials which is attributable to drug effects it is often quite low, around 10 per cent. Put another way, an additional 20–30 per cent of recoveries occur above those which might occur without the drug.

On the basis of early studies it has been claimed that endogenous depressives respond better than neurotic depressives to tricyclics. However, the evidence is not very clear-cut, even in the earlier studies (Paykel 1979). In recent years there have been many American reports that depressives with delusions do badly with tricyclics and much better with ECT. Rao and Coppen (1979) found the best response to amitriptyline in the middle range of the Newcastle Scale rather than at the most endogenous extreme. A number of studies have shown tricyclics superior to placebo in out-patient neurotic depressives, anxiety states (Paykel 1979), phobic and obsessional neuroses (Marks 1983). In Morris and Beck (1974) out-patient studies tended more to give positive results than did in-patient studies. Probably the best response is in depressions of moderate severity and endogenous symptoms, with quite a good response in neurotic depressives and poor response in many severe psychotic depressives, one endogenous group.

Regarding pharmacokinetics, although blood levels suggest linear or curvilinear relationships with response under carefully controlled conditions, the relationships are weak and therapeutic monitoring is of limited practical value, mainly in the elderly or resistant cases. The most striking clinical fact is the increasing divergence between the American practice of pushing doses up to 300 mg daily in in-patients when response does not occur, and our relative caution in this country.

NEWER DRUGS

There are at present 17 antidepressants of tricyclic structure, related pharmacology, or apparently having similar clinical effects, available on the UK market, and several others have appeared and have been withdrawn. This is many more than in the USA. Pharmacologically, the majority are still amine reuptake inhibitors, selective or non-selective to varying degrees. An older drug which has only minor use, iprindole, and two more important newer drugs, mianserin and trazodone, have rather different or obscure actions.

To consider the place of the newer drugs we need to identify the disadvantages of the older ones. The tricyclics, although the mainstay of antidepressant treatment have a number of limitations. The first is the overall efficacy. Second, improvement is delayed. In trials drug–placebo differences do not appear until about three weeks and are often not impressive until six weeks. Third, there are side-effects and toxicity. Fourth, we need drugs which are clinically more selective, particularly for the depressives who do not respond well to current treatment. Fifth, one would like to see drugs which are pharmacologically different, since they are more likely to be different clinically.

To what extent do the newer drugs meet these desiderata? The first two can be dismissed rapidly. There is no convincing evidence that any of the newer drugs is more efficacious or acts more quickly than the old. Differences in pharmacology have so far also proved disappointing. Most of the newer drugs are reuptake inhibitors, although they may be more selective. Equally disappointing are clinical differences. The drugs which do have different pharmacology do not seem to have clinical effects which are much different; something which is quite remarkable in the view of the different proposed modes of action or selective effects on different neurotransmitters. It is probably too early to be a convinced sceptic here, since the data available for the most recent drugs are still sparse. There are, for instance, some suggestions that the effects of the selective serotonin reuptake inhibitors zimelidine and fluvoxamine are less on retarded depression and more on anxiety (Aberg-Wisted 1982; Norton *et al.*, in press). This would be in keeping with the evidence that clomipramine is superior to nortriptyline in obsessional disorders (Thoren, Asberg, Cronholm, Jornestedt, and Traskman 1980). However, the main difference in clinical profile is the greater sedative effect of some of the old drugs, sometimes desirable, sometimes unwanted.

One is forced back on toxicity. The common unwanted tricyclic anticholinergic and sedative effects are usually at the level of minor irritants but do limit doses in general practice, and major bladder problems can occur. Cardiotoxicity is mainly a problem in those with previous cardiac disorders, or in overdoses. The tricyclics have become an important cause of suicide (Crome and Newman 1979). The newer drugs do clearly produce less anticholinergic effects and cardiotoxicity. The advantages are not all one-sided: mianserin causes considerable sedation and can cause agranulocytosis; the selective serotonin uptake inhibitors produce nausea, and zimelidine produced worse. The newer drugs are expensive and their efficacy rests on a less solid base. I would emphasize the importance of comparisons with placebo. It is difficult to show drug effects in depression, and dangerous to depend on absence of significant difference from a standard drug unless superiority to placebo has also been demonstrated in the same sample. As clinical experience increases and costs fall, I think that we will see a swing towards the newer drugs, but we should be clear that the advantage is a relatively small one.

MONOAMINE OXIDASE INHIBITORS

The MAO inhibitors have a smaller place in therapeutics than the tricyclic antidepressants partly because of interactions, partly because of doubts over efficacy which arose when several large in-patient controlled trials simultaneously found a tricyclic superior to placebo but an MAO inhibitor ineffective. Phenelzine has been the best-studied drug. Among thirteen published controlled comparisons with placebo, four have been negative, three doubtfully positive and six positive (Paykel 1979; Paykel *et al.*, 1982*a*). All the negative studies were carried out on in-patients whereas five of the six positive studies were in out-patients, in keeping with the widely-held view that responders are likely to be more mildly ill atypical depressives (Paykel 1979).

Here too the picture is not clear-cut. The concept of atypical depression is imprecise, incorporating anxiety, reversed functional shift symptoms and other features of neurotic depression. In our study (Paykel, Rowan, Parker, and Bhat 1982*a*), although anxious depressives tended to do better on phenelzine than amitriptyline, the difference was very small. The evidence that tricyclics are effective in anxiety disorders has already been discussed. Even the conclusion that phenelzine is ineffective in severe depressives needs re-evaluation, since most were early studies with low doses and treatment periods by modern standards. Many clinicians believe that tranylcypromine is effective in severe depressives. Delineation of responsive subgroups on previous history of response, family history, or ultimately, on biochemistry, may have more to offer than does symptom picture.

A new and interesting generation of selective reversible MAO inhibitors is emerging, but it is too early to gauge their value. What is clear is that dosages of older MAO inhibitors have been too low in the past. There has been some disagreement as to the role of acetylator phenotype for hydrazine MAOIs, but three of eight studies have shown strong effects, and in our own study (Paykel, West, Roman, and Parker 1982*b*), even on a dose of 60–75 mg daily phenelzine was only strongly superior to placebo in slow acetylators, suggesting that fast acetylators need even larger doses.

OTHER DRUG TREATMENTS

Space will permit only brief *ex cathedra* statements regarding some other putative antidepressants. For tryptophan used alone, evidence has been remarkably scanty and based on very small samples (D'Elia, Hanson, and Raotma 1978). Confining attention to trials with the inadequate criterion of at least ten patients per treatment group, although some studies have suggested comparability to tricyclics, until recently there was no study showing superiority to placebo. In the nick of time the excellent study of Thomson, Rankin, Ashcroft, Yates, McQueen, and Cummings (1982) found both tryptophan and amitriptyline superior to placebo in general practice depressives. The evidence that tryptophan potentiates other treatments is much better and this may be its real therapeutic place. Three studies have shown potentiation of MAO inhibitors while one failed to do so. For potentiation of tricyclics the score is two studies positive and two negative. Two studies have failed to show potentiation of ECT.

Another drug used by general practitioners is flupenthixol. However, effects of thioxanthenes appear to be predominantly neuroleptic. Conclusive evidence of superiority to placebo in depression is lacking. Given the risk of tardive dyskinesia, I believe it to be much over-used, although neuroleptics do have a small place in the treatment of depression, at least as adjuncts.

In spite of the pharmacological dangers, MAO inhibitor tricyclic combinations have been used in resistant depressions fairly widely in this country. Marley and Wozniak (1983) have reviewed the evidence. It is clear that with careful use the interaction is not a major problem. Efficacy of the combination is still unclear. Two clinical trials have suggested that it is no better than the more effective single constituent, but neither study was in resistant depressives and most clinicians can cite patients who only improved when the combination was started.

LONG-TERM TREATMENT

It is difficult to get accurate figures regarding the long-term outcome of modern treatment of depression because there has not yet been time for sufficiently long-term and representative follow-up studies. Although most depressives improve fairly rapidly in acute treatment, a moderate proportion show incomplete remission with persisting symptoms and social disability. At least 20 per cent relapse within a year and at least 50 per cent have another episode later. Emphasis has been shifting towards these longer term problems.

Two different situations need to be distinguished: routine antidepressant continuation after acute treatment, and long-term maintenance. Four studies have now been published of the effects of early withdrawal within two months in patients responding to tricyclics versus continuation for six months to a year (Mindham, Howland, and Shepherd 1973; Paykel, DiMascio, Haskell, and Prussoff 1975; Coppen, Ghose, Montgomery, Rama Rao, Bailey, and Jorgensen 1978*a*; Stein, Rickels, and Weiss 1980). All found early withdrawal followed by a substantial relapse rate, varying from 29 per cent to 69 per cent, which was at least halved by continuation. It should be standard practice to recommend this where the response looks genuinely related to the drug.

There are also studies indicating the value of antidepressant continuation for six months after ECT (Paykel 1979). There is not yet clear-cut evidence that the same rules apply to MAO inhibitors but there are hints that they do.

For long-term maintenance, there are now eight controlled studies showing lithium superior to placebo in bipolars and seven in unipolars, without in either case a negative study of which I am aware (Paykel 1979; Coppen, Abou-Saleh, Milln, Bailey, Metcalfe, Burns, and Armond 1981; Kane, Quitkin, Rifkin, Ramos-Lorenz, Nayak, and Howard 1982; MRC 1981). The question remains as to the place of antidepressants in long-term maintenance. In bipolars, two controlled trials have found tricyclics no better than placebo and inferior to lithium partly because of increased mania (Prien, Klett, and Caffey 1973; Kane *et al.* 1982). In unipolars, the evidence is more evenly split. Two studies have shown tricyclics superior to placebo and equal to lithium (Prien *et al.* 1973; MRC 1981) as opposed to one which found no superiority to placebo (Kane *et al.* 1982) and three finding inferiority to lithium (Kane *et al.* 1982; Coppen, Ghose, Rao, Bailey, and Peet 1978*a*; Coppen *et al.* 1981). One additional study (Bialos, Giller, Jatlow, Docherty, and Harkness 1982) showed a high rate of relapse following discontinuation of amitriptyline after long-term maintenance.

These studies may be a little too kind to lithium. Clinically, there are some bipolars who do not respond, although carbamazepine may be a better second choice than tricyclics. Many unipolars do well on tricyclic antidepressants and most psychiatrists have quite a number of patients on long-term tricyclics or MAO inhibitors. Most maintenance studies have in any case been in the more severe rather than milder depressives, in whom lithium may be of less value.

Lithium is not very impressive as an acute antidepressant, even in bipolars.

What is more striking is the potentiation of tricyclics and MAO inhibitors which sometimes occurs clinically (Nelson and Byck 1982; Montigny, Cournoyer, Morisette, Langlois, and Caille 1983). Overall, as fears of irreversible glomerular renal damage have receded, the use of lithium is likely to grow again.

PSYCHOTHERAPIES AND BEHAVIOURAL THERAPIES

There have now been a number of controlled trials of psychodynamic psycho-therapies in depressives, all funded by the Psychopharmacology Branch of the US National Institute of Mental Health and good examples of successful applica-tion of drug trial methodology. The first was our continuation study of ami-triptyline (Paykel *et al.* 1975) in which half the patients also received weekly individual psychotherapy from social workers and the other half once-monthly low contact. Psychotherapy had no effect on the relapse rate but there was a clear effect in improving social adjustment and interpersonal relationships. In similar studies, Friedman (1975) found that conjoint marital therapy improved marital relationships, but had only weak effects on symptoms compared with acute treatment with amitriptyline. Covi *et al.* (1974) found little effect from group therapy, but this study lacked social adjustment measures.

These studies suggested that psychotherapy was of value, but primarily for interpersonal relationships and social maladjustment, and that drugs were more effective for the symptoms of depression. The most recent study found a differ-ent pattern (DiMascio, Weissman, Prusoff, Neu, Zwilling, and Klerman 1979). Amitriptyline and individual psychotherapy both had effects in improving symptoms and approximately to the same extent, although the combination was the best treatment. The drug had more effect in endogenous depressions, the psychotherapy in situational depressions.

The last decade has also seen some interest in behavioural therapies. In two American studies and one British study, cognitive therapy appeared at least equal to tricyclic antidepressant treatment (Rush, Beck, Kovacs, and Hollen 1977; Murphy, Simons, Wetzel, and Lustman 1984; Blackburn, Bishop, Glen, Whalley, and Christie 1981) while in a second British study it was superior to 'usual' general practice treatment (Teasdale, Fennell, Hibbert, and Amies 1984). All the studies were in out-patients or in general practice.

These studies indicate that when rigorously evaluated, psychotherapeutic treatments have useful effects. It is not clear that the effects are specific, rather than the result of the supportive element in the greatly increased contact with patients. Resolving this will require a placebo for the time element in treatment, and comparisons of different psychotherapeutic modalities. Also uncertain is the effect in severe depression. There have been no studies of in-patients and in the earlier out-patient studies effects were relatively weak, although in general practice depressive effects of cognitive therapy and drug therapy appear com-parable.

COMPARISONS OF TREATMENT

Lastly, how do acute treatments rank in efficacy? For ECT vs. drug treatments there is considerable evidence favouring ECT. Among nine clinical trials comparing ECT with tricyclic antidepressants (Paykel 1979), six found ECT better overall, two studies found equal effects, and one study found the drug faster although ultimately of equal effect. For MAO inhibitors the predominance is even more marked, six studies favouring ECT and one study finding equal effects. However, these were all in-patient studies and findings in milder or more neurotic patients might be quite different.

Similar comparisons can be made for other treatments. In a recent paper (Quality Assurance Project 1983) effects of different antidepressant treatments were evaluated in relation to the standard deviation of pretreatment scores using the technique of meta-analysis. In this alternative approach to counting studies in order to aggregate the results of many different studies, 'effect sizes' are produced for each treatment.

In endogenous depressives, the 'effect size' in placebo control groups was 0.78. ECT more than doubled this non-specific improvement while tricyclic and newer antidepressants approximately doubled it. MAO inhibitors were minimally worse than placebo.

For neurotic depressives the pattern was different. The mean placebo 'effect size' was 1.07, larger than for endogenous depression, and specific treatment 'effect sizes' were smaller. Psychotherapy added an element equivalent to a little less than two-thirds of the non-specific improvement; tricyclics and newer antidepressants about a half, with sedatives and MAO inhibitors rather less and neuroleptics less still. The psychotherapy effect was almost certainly overstated since it occurred at an average of 20 weeks, while drug treatment effects were seen after four to eight weeks. I think that this synthesis also understated the effect of MAO inhibitors. The technique has a number of pitfalls in the way it pools studies but it illustrates the relative rankings of treatments and the importance of spontaneous remission and non-specific effects against even the most powerful specific treatments.

CONCLUSIONS

Depression is heterogeneous, spanning a range of severity, qualities, causes and treatment modalities. None of the treatments are as powerful as we tend to think; overall spontaneous improvement and non-specific treatment effects contribute a great deal.

The most powerful treatment for severe depression is still ECT. The tricyclic and related drugs come next. Although they are far the most widely-used treatments of depression their efficacy is only moderate. The newer drugs are small advances, worthwhile but not dramatic and clinically rather similar to the older drugs. MAO inhibitors have been underrated; they have a useful place which safer new drugs would much expand. In the longer term depression produces considerable morbidity, for which both lithium and the antidepressants produce useful effects, with a slowly expanding place for the former. Psychodynamic psychotherapies and behavioural therapies produce definite effects which are probably smaller overall than those of the drugs, but they may be more important in the milder and more reactive depressions.

Critical evaluation mandates realism. We need new drugs of radically different classes: as different as lithium from the tricyclics. However, pharmacotherapy of depression has come a long way in its quarter-century. It has focused attention on the neurotransmitter mechanisms underlying depression, even if all the answers are not in. It has produced treatments which, even if not miraculous, are effective and widely and easily available.

REFERENCES

Aberg-Wisted, A. C. (1982). A double-blind study of zimelidine, a serotonin reuptake inhibitor and desipramine, a noradrenaline uptake inhibitor in endogenous depression. 1. Clinical findings. *Acta psychiat. scand.* **66**, 50–65.

Akiskal, H. S. and McKinney, W. T. (1975). Overview of recent research in depression: integration of ten conceptual models into a comprehensive clinical frame. *Arch. gen. Psychiat.* **32**, 285–305.

Bialos, D., Giller, E., Jatlow, P., Docherty, J., and Harkness, L. (1982). Recurrence of depression after discontinuation of long-term amitriptyline treatment. *Am. J. Psychiat.* **139**, 325–9.

Blackburn, I. M., Bishop, S., Glen, A. I. M., Whalley, L. J., and Christie, J. E. (1981). The efficacy of cognitive therapy in depression: a treatment trial using cognitive therapy and pharmacotherapy each alone and in combination. *Br. J. Psychiat.* **139**, 181–9.

Brandon, S., Cowley, P., McDonald, C., Neville, P., Palmer, R., and Wellstood-Eason, S. (1984). Electroconvulsive therapy: results in depressive illness from the Leicestershire trial. *Br. med. J.* **288**, 22–5.

Coppen, A., Ghose, K., Rao, R., Bailey, J., and Peet, M. (1978*a*). Mianserin and lithium in the prophylaxis of depression. *Br. J. Psychiat.* **133**, 206–10.

——, ——, Montgomery, S., Rama Rao, V. A., Bailey, J., and Jorgensen, A. (1978*b*). Continuation therapy with amitriptyline in depression. *Br. J. Psychiat.* **133**, 28–33.

——, Abou-Saleh, M. T., Milln, P., Bailey, J., Metcalfe, M., Burns, B., and Armond, A. (1981). Lithium continuation therapy following electroconvulsive therapy. *Br. J. Psychiat.* **139**, 284–7.

Covi, L., Lipman, R. S., Derogatis, R., Smith, J. E., and Pattison, L. J. H. (1974). Drugs and group psychotherapy in neurotic depression. *Am. J. Psychiat.* **131**, 191–8.

Crome, P. and Newman, B. (1979). Fatal tricyclic antidepressant poisoning. *J. R. Soc. Med.* **72**, 649–53.

D'Elia, G. and Raotma, H. (1975). Is unilateral ECT less effective than bilateral ECT? *Br. J. Psychiat.* **30**, 667–74.

——, Hanson, L., and Raotma, H. (1978). L-tryptophan and 5-hydroxytryptophan in the treatment of depression. A review. *Acta psychiat. scand.* **57**, 239–52.

DiMascio, A., Weissman, M. M., Prusoff, B. A., Neu, C., Zwilling, M., and Klerman, G. L. (1979). Differential symptom reduction by drugs and psychotherapy in acute depression. *Arch. gen. Psychiat.* **36**, 1450–6.

Friedman, A. S. (1975). Interaction of drug therapy with marital therapy in depressive patients. *Arch. gen. Psychiat.* **32**, 619–37.

Kane, J. M., Quitkin, F. M., Rifkin, A., Ramos-Lorenzi, J. R., Nayak, D. D., and Howard, A. (1982). Lithium carbonate and imipramine in the prophylaxis of unipolar and bipolar II illness. *Arch. gen. Psychiat.* **39**, 1065–9.

Marks, I. (1983). Are there anticompulsive or antiphobic drugs? Review of the evidence. *Br. J. Psychiat.* **143**, 338–47.

Marley, E. and Wozniak, K. M. (1983). Clinical and experimental aspects of interactions between amine oxidase inhibitors and amine re-uptake inhibitors. *Psychol. Med.* **12**, 735–49.

Mindham, R. H. S., Howland, C., and Shepherd, M. (1973). An evaluation of continuation therapy with tricyclic antidepressants in depressive illness. *Psychol. Med.* **3**, 5–17.

Montigny, de C., Cournoyer, G., Morissette, R., Langlois, R., and Caille, G. (1983). Lithium carbonate addition in tricyclic antidepressant-resistant unipolar depression. *Arch. gen. Psychiat.* **40**, 1327–34.

Morris, J. B. and Beck, A. T. (1974). The efficacy of antidepressant drugs. *Arch. gen. psychiat.* **30**, 667–74.

MRC (1981). Continuation therapy with lithium and amitriptyline in unipolar depressive illness: a controlled clinical trial. *Psychol. Med.* **11**, 409–16.

Murphy, G. E., Simons, A. D., Wetzel, R. D., and Lustman, P. J. (1984). Cognitive therapy and pharmacotherapy. *Arch. gen. Psychiat.* **41**, 33–41.

Nelson, C. J. and Byck, R. (1982). Rapid response to lithium in phenelzine non-responders. *Br. J. Psychiat.* **141**, 85–6.

Norton, K. R. W., Sireling, L. I., Bhat, A. V. Rao, B. M., and Paykel, E. S. (1984). A double-blind comparison of fluvoxamine, imipramine and placebo in depressed patients. *J. affect. Discord.* **7**, 297–308.

Paykel, E. S. (1979). Predictors of treatment response. In *Psychopharmacology of affective disorders* (ed. E. S. Paykel and A. Coppen), pp. 193–220. Oxford University Press, Oxford.

— (ed.) (1982). *Handbook of affective disorders.* Churchill Livingstone, Edinburgh.

— and Coppen, A. (ed.) (1979). *Psychopharmacology of affective disorders.* Oxford University Press.

—, DiMascio, A., Haskell, D., and Prusoff, B. A. (1975). Effects of maintenance amitriptyline and psychotherapy on symptoms of depression. *Psychol. Med.* **5**, 67–77.

—, Rowan, P. R., Parker, R. R., and Bhat, A. V. (1982*a*). Response to phenelzine and amitriptyline in sub-types of neurotic depression. *Arch. gen. Psychiat.* **39**, 1041–9.

—, West, P. S., Rowan, P. R., and Parker, R. R. (1982*b*). Influence of acetylator phenotype on antidepressant effects of phenelzine. *Br. J. Psychiat.* **141**, 243–8.

Prien, R. F., Klett, C. J., and Caffey, E. M. (1973). Lithium carbonate and imipramine in prevention of affective disorder. *Arch. gen. Psychiat.* **29**, 420–25.

Quality Assurance Project. (1983). A treatment outline for depressive disorders. *Aust. N.Z. J. Psychiat.* **17**, 129–46.

Rao, V. A. R. and Coppen, A. (1979). Classification of depression and response to amitriptyline therapy. *Psychol. Med.* **19**, 321–5.

Robin, A. and De Tissera, S. (1982). A double-blind controlled comparison of therapeutic effects of low and high energy electroconvulsive therapies. *Br. J. Psychiat.* **141**, 357-66.

Rush, A. J., Beck, A. T., Kovacs, M., and Hollon, S. (1977). Comparative efficacy of cognitive therapy and pharmacotherapy in treatment of depressed outpatients. *Cognitive Ther. & Res.* **1**, 17-37.

Sireling, L. I., Paykel, E. S., Freeling, P. F., Rao, B. M., and Patel, S. (in press). Depression in general practice: case thresholds and diagnosis. *Brit. J. Psychiat.*

Stein, M. K., Rickels, K., and Weise, C. C. (1980). Maintenance therapy with amitriptyline: a controlled trial. *Am. J. Psychiat.* **137**, 370-1.

Teasdale, J. D., Fennell, M. J. V., Hibbert, G. A., and Amies, P. L. (1984). Cognitive therapy for major depressive disorder. *Br. J. Psychiat.* (in press).

Thomson, J., Rankin, H., Ashcroft, G. W., Yates, C. M., McQueen, J. K., and Cummings, S. W. (1982). The treatment of depression in general practice: a comparison of L-typtophan, amitriptyline, and a combination of L-tryptophan and amitriptyline with placebo. *Psychol. Med.* **12**, 741-51.

Thoren, P., Asberg, M., Cronholm, B., Jornestedt, L., and Traskman, L. (1980). Clomipramine treatment of obsessive-compulsives, I. A controlled trial. *Arch. gen. Psychiat.* **37**, 1281-5.

2

The biology of depressive illness: 5-HT and other matters

A. COPPEN AND K. WOOD

In considering the biology of depressive illness one must start by examining the epidemiology and natural history of the condition. Depressive illness is a disease of middle and old age; the median age for the onset of the first episode is 42 years. It is more common in women than in men. It is episodic in nature, often, but not always, occurring after no obvious situational disturbance in the patient's life, and is usually self-limiting. Patients usually spontaneously improve between 6 and 18 months after the onset of the illness. Although an immense amount of work has been devoted to the importance of life events and their role in the precipitation of an attack, far less effort has been devoted to explaining why patients recover, often without any dramatic change in their life situation (Angst 1981). Often, too, there seems to be a seasonal influence on the onset of depressive illness, which occurs most commonly in late spring with a second peak in the incidence of the illness in autumn (Eastwood and Peacocke 1976).

Investigations into the chemical pathology of depressive illness have been mainly centred around three areas: (a) endocrine disturbances, (b) electrolyte disturbances, and (c) neurotransmitters; 5-hydroxytryptamine (5-HT) noradrenaline and dopamine. Fashions change as to the most popular area of investigation. The 1950s and 1960s were the most active period for endocrine investigations although neuroendocrine investigations have recently been an area of intense investigation.

The interest in possible endocrine abnormalities was brought about by the fact that well-defined causes of certain cases of affective disorder were due to the over-activity or under-activity of the adrenal cortex (Coppen 1967; Brooksbank and Coppen 1967). Another well established cause of depressive illness is myxoedema which, if diagnosed early, is a most satisfying condition to treat (Checkley 1982). We can now detect under-activity of the thyroid using a sensitive test of thyroid-stimulating-hormone, and this abnormality now appears to be quite a common cause of the milder forms of depressive illness. The Dexamethasone Suppression Test, whatever its practical value, does reveal a profound neuroendocrine disorder in about 70 per cent of depressive cases (Carroll 1982; Coppen, Abou-Saleh, Milln, Metcalfe, Harwood, and Bailey 1983).

The study of electrolytes in depressive illness has been the subject of numerous investigations. We have demonstrated quite profound changes in the transport of sodium into the CSF (Coppen 1960) and a raised 'residual' sodium (i.e. mainly intracellular sodium) in depression (Coppen 1965). This appears to be a state-dependent abnormality. These findings have been replicated by Colt, Dunner, Wang, Ross, Pierson, and Fieve (1982) recently. If these whole-body changes in residual sodium also occur in the CNS, one would predict profound functional changes in neuronal functioning. In particular, the decreased activity of Na^+/K^+ATPase may be responsible for increased residual sodium and for decreased 5-HT uptake (Hesketh, Glen, and Reading 1977). Calcium, too, has a profound effect on the CNS. It has been known for several years that cases of hypo- and hyperparathyroidism are associated with severe affective disturbances. The new group of calcium channel blockers that can reduce intracellular sodium is a powerful tool in exploring the aetiological importance of changes in electrolytes in depression and mania.

The main impetus of the study of the monoamines comes from the development of antidepressants. The mode of action of antidepressant drugs is still largely unknown. Our own interest in the role of 5-HT was based on an observation (repeated several times) that tryptophan markedly and substantially potentiates the antidepressant action of a monoamine oxidase inhibitor (MAOI) (Coppen, Shaw, and Farrell 1963). Other interpretations of this data are possible, e.g. it may be other metabolites of tryptophan such as tryptamine that are active antidepressants. Evidence that increasing brain 5-HT improves depression raises the question – is depression a 5-HT deficiency disease?

The 1960s and 1970s saw a tremendous number of investigations into the concentration of monoamines in post-mortem brains of suicides and in the metabolites of these amines, 5HIAA, HVA, and MHPG in the CSF, either with or without the probenecid technique (van Praag 1982). We will not attempt to enumerate those investigations, but we think a cautious interpretation of the results is that there is evidence of a decrease in brain 5-HT and its metabolite 5HIAA in the brains of suicides, and evidence of a decrease in the concentration of 5HIAA (and HVA) both before and after the administration of probenecid in the CSF of depressive patients.

More recently, attention has moved to the study of the platelet. In the next chapter, we have presented some of the evidence that the platelet is a useful and practical model of the neurone to study in patients, although it cannot be too often emphasized that the platelet data must be interpreted with great caution.

There seems to be a useful consensus emerging about certain abnormalities in the platelet of depressives, which if present in the neurone could have important functional consequences. There is evidence that the active transport of 5-HT by the platelets of depressive patients is impaired (Tuomisto and Tukiainen 1976; Coppen, Swade, and Wood 1978). This impairment is apparently a trait characteristic and is present after clinical recovery. Also we have found a very marked seasonal variation both in depressive and in normal subjects. The V_{max} is decreased in the summer months as compared to the winter months (Swade and Coppen 1980).

What is the consequence of this impaired transport of 5-HT? As far as the platelet is concerned, there is evidence that 5-HT concentrations are markedly decreased in the platelet of patients suffering from depressive illness (Coppen, Turner, Rowsell and Padgham 1976). If an analogous process occurs in the 5-HT neurones then one would predict a reduced store of 5-HT, which may have important functional consequences producing some of the features of depressive illness. We have no direct evidence of 5-HT transport systems in the neurone of depressive patients but we have evidence that the 5-HT concentration in the brains of suicides is decreased.

Closely associated with the site of the 5-HT transport system is the imipramine binding site. Post-mortem studies of suicides have revealed a decreased density of imipramine binding sites in these brains (Perry, Marshall, Blessed, Tomlinson, and Perry 1983). Thus there is evidence that the abnormalities that have been revealed in the platelet may be relevant to the neurones of those patients.

Of particular interest to the assessment of the aetiological importance of the abnormality is the observation that lithium salts, which profoundly reduce the recurrence of both depressive and manic episodes (Coppen, Noguera, Bailey, Burns, Swani, Hare, Gardner, and Maggs 1971), normalize the reduced 5-HT uptake in these patients (Coppen, Swade, and Wood 1980).

What would be the effect of reduced 5-HT availability on the 5-HT receptors? There is a report of an increased 5-HT$_2$ receptor density in the brains of suicides (Stanley and Mann 1983) that would be consistent with a transmitter deficiency. We have examined 5-HT receptor activity by studying the 5-HT-induced aggregation of platelets (unpublished observations). We could not find any abnormality in drug-free depressive patients but we did find increased 5-HT receptor sensitivity in recovered patients on long-term lithium. This would suggest that, in addition to increasing 5-HT uptake, lithium enhances serotonergic transmission by increasing its receptor sensitivity.

5-Hydroxytryptamine is derived from tryptophan via a process of hydroxylation of tryptophan to form 5-hydroxytryptophan (5-HTP) and the decarboxylation of 5-HTP to form 5-HT. The hydroxylation of tryptophan is regarded as the rate-limiting process in the formation of 5-HT. These processes probably occur, within the CNS, in serotonergic neurones where tryptophan is selectively taken up. Brain tryptophan as an essential amino acid is derived from the diet. Blood tryptophan occurs in two forms, (1) tryptophan which is bound to plasma proteins and (2) free or unbound tryptophan which usually accounts for some 10 per cent of the total tryptophan. It is generally held that it is the free tryptophan which is available for transport into the central nervous system. The position is complicated by the fact that tryptophan has to compete with certain other amino acids for transport into the CNS. The concentration of plasma tryptophan and other amino acids in depressive patients has been the object of much study. Some, but not all, investigators have found a decrease in the amount of free tryptophan or the ratio of free tryptophan to the other amino acids sharing the same transport system (Coppen, Eccleston, and Peet 1973; Møller, Kirk, and Flemming 1976; Peet, Moody, Worrall, Walter, and Naylor 1976). Some of the confusion may be resolved by our observation of the seasonal variations in the concentration of free tryptophan in both depressive and normal subjects. We have found two distinct troughs in the concentration of free trypto-phan in the spring and autumn in depressive patients. This is in contrast to normal subjects, who show peaks in the plasma tryptophan at these times (Swade and Coppen 1980). Seasonal variation in tryptophan have now been reported by many groups. It is tempting to relate these seasonal variations to the seasonal incidence of depressive illness.

Another variate that may be of relevance is the well-documented evidence of an association between depression and decreased plasma folate levels, par-ticularly in view of the fact that folate deficiency can decrease 5-HT synthesis (Botez, Young, Bachevalier, and Garthier 1979). We have found an interesting association between plasma folate levels and morbidity in patients maintained on long-term lithium. We have found the one year morbidity of patients with plasma folate concentrations of more than 8 ng/ml to be half that of patients with a plasma folate of less than 8 ng/ml. It should be noted that the cut-off point is not one that would be considered to be indicative of folate deficiency. It has been suggested that folate may be concerned with tetrahydro biopterin synthesis (Leeming, Harpey, Brown, and Blair 1982). Tetrahydro biopterin is a co-enzyme in the hydroxylation of tryptophan, and we have some evidence that the urinary excretion of total biopterin is reduced in depressive patients (Blair and Coppen, unpublished observations).

There is evidence that, in addition to the weakness of 5-HT transport, there may be deficiencies in the supply of the precursor and in the formation of 5-HT. Although there is ample evidence that tryptophan markedly potentiates the antidepressant action of a MAOI, there is increasing evidence that trypto-phan is an effective antidepressant, especially in doses of 3 g a day which would be expected to interfere less with the transport of other important amino acids than did the earlier higher doses (Thomson, Rankin, Aschroft, Yates, McQueen, and Cummings 1982).

The study of the interactions of hormonal factors with the central nervous system is still at an early stage. The dexamethasone suppression test, for example, reveals a profound neuroendocrine abnormality in a high proportion of patients with depressive illness (Coppen *et al.* 1983). The periodic abnormality still persists in spite of successful prophylactic treatment by lithium of patients with recurrent depression. We have found that approximately one-third of patients attending the lithium clinic have an abnormal test result. Repeated one year later, we found that a proportion of patients with an abnormal result became normal and vice versa. It is probable that the elucidation of the underlying abnormality of this test may throw considerable light on mechanisms responsible for the illness. However, the seasonal variations in some of the variants we have described may in part explain why patients both relapse and recover from illness as their biochemical state becomes more or less favourable for normal affective state.

One endocrine factor that has found to be associated with affective changes is the thyroid. Recent work by Atterwell (1981) has shown that thyroid function can profoundly effect 5-HT-mediated responses in animals. Some years ago, Prange, Wilson, and Rabon (1969) showed that the antidepressant action of tricyclics could be enhanced by giving small doses of T_3 concomitantly with imipramine, a finding that has been replicated recently (Goodwin, Prange, Post, Muscettola, and Lipton 1982). More recently, we have found marked differences in response in patients on long-term therapy between those with a TSH of 5 mμ/l or below and those with a TSH of above 5 mμ/l. The affective morbidity was twice as high in the group with a moderately raised TSH, which may be indicative of mild hypothyroid condition. Certainly over the years we have found administration of 20 or 40 μg of T_3 useful in managing certain patients who seem otherwise poor responders to lithium and other antidepressive medication.

It should be realized that the patients who are vulnerable to depressive illness may be affected by a wide variety of different factors in areas where we can usefully intervene. Certainly, our data suggests that thyroid function and folic acid state are two important areas which should be assessed and corrected if found lacking. Slowly a picture is emerging that will make the management of affective disorders a more rational and satisfying exercise. In particular, we should look to see how environmental, seasonal factors can interact in vulnerable individuals to produce the picture of depressive illness that we find in our everyday practice.

REFERENCES

Angst, J. (1981). Clinical indications for a prophylactic treatment of depression. *Adv. biol. Psychiat.* 7, 218–29.

Atterwell, C. K. (1981). Effect of acute and chronic T_3 administration to rats on central 5-HT and dopamine mediated behavioural responses and related brain biochemistry. *Neuropharmacology* 20, 131–44.

Botez, M. I., Young, S. M., Bachevalier, J., and Gauthier, S. (1979). Folate deficiency and decreased brain 5-hydroxytryptamine synthesis in man and rat. *Nature, Lond.* 278, 182–3.

Brooksbank, B. W. L. and Coppen, A. (1967). Plasma 11-hydroxycorticosteroids in affective disorders. *Br. J. Psychiat.* 113, 395–404.

Carroll, B. J. (1982). The dexamethasone suppression test for melancholia. *Br J. Psychiat.* 140, 292–304.

Checkley, S. (1982). Endocrine changes in psychiatric illness. *Clin. Neuroendocrin.* 11, 266–82.

Colt, E., Dunner, D., Wang, J., Ross, D. C., Pierson, R. N., and Fieve, R. R.

(1982). Body composition in affective disorders before, during and after lithium carbonate therapy. *Arch. gen. Psychiat.* **39**, 577–81.

Coppen, A. (1960). Rate of entry of ^{24}Na from blood to cerebrospinal fluid in depression. *Proc. R. Soc. Med.*

— (1965). Mineral metabolism in affective disorders. *Br. J. Psychiat.* **111**, 1133–42.

— (1967). Biochemistry of affective disorders. *Br. J. Psychiat.* **113**, 1237–64.

—, Eccleston, E. G., and Peet, M. (1973). Total and free tryptophan concentration in the plasma of depressive patients. *Lancet* ii, 60–3.

—, Shaw, D. M., and Farrell, J. P. (1963). Potentiation of the antidepressive effect of monoamine oxidase inhibitor by tryptophan. *Lancet* ii, 1178–80.

—, Swade, C., and Wood, K. (1978). Platelet 5-hydroytryptamine accumulation in depressive illness. *Clinical chim. Acta* **87**, 165–8.

—, —, and — (1980). Lithium restores abnormal platelet 5-HT transport in patients with affective disorders. *Br. J. Psychiat.* **136**, 235–8.

—, Turner, P., Rowsell, A. R., and Padgham, C. (1976). 5-hydroxytryptamine (5-HT) in the whole-blood of patients with depressive illness. *Post-grad. med. J.* **52**, 156–8.

—, Abou-Saleh, M., Milln, P., Metcalfe, M., Harwood, J., and Bailey, J. (1983). Dexamethasone suppression test in depression and other psychiatric illness. *Br. J. Psychiat.* **142**, 498–504.

—, Noguera, R., Bailey, J., Burns, B. H., Swani, M. S., Hare, E. H., Gardner, R., and Maggs, R. (1971). Prophylactic lithium in affective disorders: Controlled trial. *Lancet* ii, 275–9.

Eastwood, M. R. and Peacocke, J. (1976). Seasonal patterns of suicide, depression and electroconvulsive therapy. *Br. J. Psychiat.* **129**, 472–5.

Goodwin, F. K., Prange, A. J. Jr., Post, R. M., Muscettola, G., and Lipton, M. A. (1982). Potentiation of antidepressant effects by L-triiodothyronine in tricyclic nonresponders. *Am. J. Psychiat.* **139**, 34–8.

Hesketh, J. E., Glen, A. I. M., and Reading, H. W. (1977). Membrane ATPase activities in depressive illness. *J. Neurochem.* **28**, 1401–2.

Leeming, R. J., Harpey, J.-P., Brown, S. M., and Blair, J. A. (1982). Tetrahydrofolate and hydroxocobolamin in the management of dihydropteridine reductase deficiency. *J. ment. Defic. Res.* **26**, 21–5.

Møller, S. E., Kirk, L., and Fremming, K. H. (1976). Plasma amino acids as an index for subgroups in manic depressive psychosis: correlation to effect of tryptophan. *Psychopharmacology* **49**, 205–13.

Peet, M., Moody, J. P., Worrall, E. P., Walker, P., and Naylor, G. J. (1976). Plasma tryptophan concentration in depressive illness and mania. *Br. J. Psychiat.* **128**, 255–8.

Perry. E. K., Marshall, E. F., Blessed, G., Tomlinson, B. E., and Perry, R. H. (1983). Decreased imipramine binding in the brains of patients with depressive illness. *Br. J. Psychiat.* **142**, 188–92.

Prange, A. J. Jr., Wilson, I. C., and Rabon, A. M. (1969). Enhancement of imipramine antidepressant activity by thyroid hormone. *Am. J. Psychiat.* **126**, 457–69.

Stanley, M. and Mann, J. J. (1983). Increased serotonin$_2$ binding sites in frontal cortex of suicide victims. *Lancet* i, 214–16.

Swade, C. and Coppen, A. (1980). Seasonal variations in biochemical factors related to depressive illness. *J. affect. Dis.* **2**, 249–55.

Thomson, J., Rankin, H., Ashcroft, G. W., Yates, C. M., McQueen, J. K., and Cummings, S. W. (1982). The treatment of depression in general practice –

a comparison of L-tryptophan and amitriptyline with placebo. *Psychol. Med.*
12, 741–51.
Tuomisto, J. and Tukiainen, E. (1976). Decreased uptake of 5-hydroxytrypt-
amine in blood platelets from depressed patients. *Nature Lond.* **262**, 596–8.
van Praag, H. M. (1982). Neurotransmitters and CNS disease: depression. *Lancet*
ii, 1259–64.

3

Platelet transport and receptor sites in depressive illness

KEITH WOOD AND ALEC COPPEN

In order to establish the underlying pathology of depressive illness several lines of investigation have been made. Some investigators have established the pharmacological actions of antidepressive treatments in laboratory animals and extrapolated their findings to therapeutic modes of action of these treatments in depressed patients. Others have made a more direct approach by studying the depressed patient. This latter approach is inherently difficult.

The last decade has seen the movement away from measurements of amines and their metabolites in the brains, CSF, and urine of depressed patients to other areas of investigation. One such line of investigation was brought about by the synthesis of potent and selective radio-labelled ligands with high specific activity that enabled the labelling and hence quantification of receptor binding sites. The second line of investigation was brought about by the finding that blood platelets possess monoamine oxidase (MAO) activity, an active transport process for 5-hydroxytryptamine (5-HT) and the presence of binding sites for α- and β-adrenoceptor ligands, 5-HT ligands and, ^{3}H-imipramine: all of which are of potential interest to biological psychiatry.

Although such platelet studies are relatively easy to carry out, and there is the added advantage of making serial measurements (e.g. before, during, and after antidepressant treatments) using the ethically justifiable procedure of routine venepuncture, the fundamental problem of such studies is whether the platelet mirrors and parallels CNS activity.

For many years it was thought that the therapeutic mode of action of the tricyclic antidepressants was the inhibition of uptake of released 5-HT or noradrenaline (NA). However, Vetulani, Sulser, and their colleagues (Vetulani, Stawartz, Dingell, and Sulser 1976) suggested an alternative therapeutic mechanism of action of these drugs. They found that chronic antidepressant therapy results in the 'downregulation' or desensitization of the activity of central postsynaptic β-adrenoceptors. According to their hypothesis, chronic antidepressant treatment results in the normalization of the activity of these receptors with consequent attenuation of depressive symptoms.

The principal mechanism governing the release of NA into the synaptic cleft involves α-adrenoceptors located presynaptically on the nerve terminal (Stärke

1977). Activation of these receptors by the endogenous agonist results in the reduced release of NA. According to Crews and Smith (1978), chronic anti-depressant treatment causes subsensitivity of presynaptic adrenoceptors, which leads to the enhanced release of NA. Supersensitivity of these presynaptic receptors during a depressive illness, which would reduce the amount of NA released into the synaptic cleft, would induce supersensitivity of the post-synaptic receptors. Attenuation of the activity of the presynaptic receptor by chronic antidepressant treatment would tend to normalize the activity of the postsynaptic receptor and amelioration of the symptoms of the illness would occur. While there is broad agreement that chronic antidepressant treatment attenuates both pre- and postsynaptic adrenergic receptors in rat brain, the findings from platelet studies in depressed patients are not so consistent.

PLATELET α-ADRENOCEPTORS AND ASSOCIATED BINDING SITES

Newman, Williams, Bishopric, and Lefkowitz (1978) demonstrated, using ^{3}H-dihydroergocryptine (DHE) as ligand, that α-adrenoceptors were present on the surface of blood platelets. We (Wood and Coppen 1980, 1981) were there-fore able to compare the binding of DHE to platelets of depressed patients with the binding of DHE to platelets of normal controls. No significant differ-ence could be detected in the value of Kd between depressed patients and controls. There were, however, significantly fewer binding sites on intact platelets of depressed patients when compared with the controls. García-Sevilla, Zis, Hollingsworth, Greden, and Smith (1981), however, using ^{3}H-clonidine as ligand, found that the number of binding sites was increased in depressed patients when compared with a control group. The availability of newer ^{3}H-antagonists which were much more selective for the α_2-adrenoceptor binding site (the majority, if not all, of the sites on human platelets are of the α_2 sub-type) allowed other investigators to pursue this problem. Diaguji, Meltzer, Tong, U'Pritchard, Young, and Kravitz (1981) and Stahl, Lemoine, Ciaranello, and Berger (1983), using ^{3}H-yohimbine, and Pimoule, Briley, Gay, Loo, Sechter, Zarifian, Raisman, and Langer (1983), using ^{3}H-rauwolscine, could detect no difference in the number of platelet α_2-adrenoceptor binding sites between controls and depressed patients. Leonard's group (Healy, Carney, and Leonard 1983), using DHE as their ligand, have shown that the number of binding sites was increased during a depressive illness. A comparison of these studies is shown in Table 3.1. Of the six published studies, no two have been conducted under identical conditions. For example, we (Wood and Coppen 1981) studied only females, while Stahl *et al.* (1983) studied only males: both groups studied the binding characteristics of intact platelets rather than platelet membrane prepara-tions. All the other studies used membrane preparations and a selection of male and female patients and controls. García-Sevilla's investigation was the only one conducted with an agonist (clonidine), all the others used antagonists or

TABLE 3.1. *Characteristics of studies that have compared platelet α-adrenoceptor binding in controls and depressed patients*

	Diagnostic description of patients	Preparation of platelets used in incubations	[3H]-ligand	Ligand in excess to determine specific binding
Wood and Coppen (1981)	Primary depressive illness: females	Intact	DHE (dihydroergocryptine)	phentolamine
García-Sevilla *et al.* (1981)	Major depressive disorder: males and females	Membranes	clonidine	clonidine
Daiguji *et al.* (1981)	Major depressive illness: males and females	Membranes	yohimbine	noradrenaline
Pimoule *et al.* (1983)	Endogenous or reactive depression: males and females	Membranes	rauwolscine	phentolamine
Healy *et al.* (1983)	Primary diagnosis of depression: males and females	Membranes	DHE	yohimbine
Stahl *et al.* (1983)	Major depressive disorder: males	Intact	yohimbine	phentolamine

ligands with mixed agonist/antagonist properties.

Since chronic antidepressant treatment causes subsensitivity of presynaptic adrenoceptors in rat brain (Crews and Smith 1978), and if the platelet model parallels the CNS, one should expect that platelet adrenoceptors are similarly affected during antidepressant treatment. García-Sevilla *et al.* (1981), in a small group of patients, reported that chronic treatment of depressed patients with amitriptyline or imipramine resulted in a significant reduction in the number of clonidine binding sites. Similarly, Healy *et al.* (1983) reported a significant reduction in the number of platelet adrenergic binding sites after either amitriptyline or trazadone treatment. Moreover, this reduction was observed only in those patients who responded clinically to treatment. Pimoule *et al.* (1983), on the other hand, failed to detect a significant change in the number of ^{3}H-rauwolscine binding sites during amitriptyline or chlorimipramine treatment, and Stahl *et al.* (1983) came to a similar conclusion using ^{3}H-yohimbine as ligand.

García-Sevilla *et al.* (1981) also reported that short-term treatment with lithium decreased the number of platelet binding sites, whereas we (Wood and Coppen 1983) found that patients receiving long-term (mean duration of treatment = 5.7 years) prophylactic lithium treatment had a similar number of adrenergic binding sites to drug-free depressed patients. We concluded that lithium treatment with remission from a depressive illness is not associated with a change toward normal of α_2-adrenoceptor density and therefore represents a trait in patients prone to depressive illness.

Arguments as to the validity of each investigators' results have been varied. It has been argued that studies using intact platelets are more physiological than studies carried out with membrane preparations but have the disadvantage of a higher degree of non-specific binding than incubations carried out with membranes. Arguments could be put forward as to the validity of using agonists rather than antagonists and vice versa to label binding sites. From the above it would appear that there is little overall agreement about the status of platelet α_2-adrenoceptors during depressive illness and their subsequent change during treatment.

It must be emphasized that binding studies do have their limitations. While it is true that one can quantitate the number of receptor binding sites, they may not be coupled to the complete receptor system. Since human platelet α_2-adrenoceptors regulate basal- and prostaglandin-stimulated adenylate cyclase activity and platelet aggregation, one may determine the activity and sensitivity of the α-adrenoceptors using either of the above assay systems. For example, we have studied NA- and adrenaline-induced platelet aggregation in depressed patients and controls in an attempt to determine whether there is an overall reduction in the α_2-adrenoceptor mediated response (Wood, Swade, and Coppen 1984*a*). The results of this investigation, using NA as agonist, indicated that platelet α-adrenoceptors are subsensitive in depressed patients when compared with normal controls: no such difference was noted when adrenaline was used as the agonist. These results therefore parallel our previous (Wood and Coppen 1981) binding studies. It is difficult to reconcile the different findings between NA and adrenaline, but, as Elliot and Grahame-Smith (1982) concluded on the basis of antagonist inhibition studies, '^{3}H-DHE binds to the α_2 adrenoceptor of intact platelets which is responsible for NA-induced platelet aggregation'. It is noteworthy therefore, that the abnormality of the aggregatory responses in depressed patients in our study was only seen with NA and not seen with adrenaline.

García-Sevilla, García-Vallejo, and Guimon (1983) also carried out platelet aggregation experiments. Their results, using adrenaline as agonist, indicate that platelets from patients with a major depressive disorder have an enhanced platelet aggregatory response. These authors also reported that the inhibition of this response by yohimbine in depressed patients was no different from that obtained in normal controls, and they stressed that this result was consistent with antagonist binding studies which demonstrated the absence of changes in platelet α_2-adrenoceptor density (Pimoule *et al.* 1983, Diaguji *et al.* 1981, Stahl *et al.* 1983). García-Sevilla *et al* (1983) concluded that the aggregation experiments conducted in their laboratory paralleled their previous ^{3}H-clonidine binding studies, and put forward the view that the enhanced effects of adrenaline on platelet aggregation and the unchanged inhibition by yohimbine, together with other binding data (Daiguji *et al.* 1981, inter alia), suggested that depression might be related to a dysfunction of the high-affinity state of the α_2-adrenoceptor, which preferentially recognizes agonists and mediates physiological responses.

The question inevitably arises as to whether the platelet α-adrenoceptor binding site is equivalent to the pre- or postsynaptic position of the α_2-adrenoceptor in the CNS. Surgical or chemical denervation of noradrenergic neurones have been used to establish the localization of release-modulatory α_2-adrenoceptors. Noradrenergic denervation has been found to increase, or failed to decrease, the specific binding of ^{3}H-clonidine (U'Prichard and Snyder 1979). These results have been interpreted as evidence for the predominantly postsynaptic localization of α_2-adrenoceptors in the CNS.

The difficulty of extrapolating from the platelet to the CNS now becomes evident. Experimental evidence from Healy *et al.* (1983) and García-Sevilla *et al.* (1981) of attenuation of supersensitive presynaptic α_2-adrenoceptors by chronic antidepressant treatment is difficult to reconcile with the predominant postsynaptic localization of α_2-adrenoceptors.

Our findings (Wood and Coppen 1981) of a decreased sensitivity of α_2-adrenoceptors are consistent with the neuroendocrine results of Matussek, Ackenheil, Hippius, Müller, Schröder, Schultes, and Wasilewski (1980), amongst others, who have shown that the secretion of growth hormone following the administration of clonidine is reduced in depressed patients when compared with normal controls. This clonidine-growth hormone response is probably mediated by a postsynaptic α_2-adrenoceptor. The results, taken as a whole, indicate the difficulties of extrapolating from the platelet to the discrete anatomical localization of CNS α_2-adrenoceptors.

LYMPHOCYTE β-ADRENOCEPTOR BINDING SITES

Studies of β-adrenoceptor activity in depressed patients have also yielded inconsistent results. For example, Pandey *et al.* (1979) have shown that the isoprenaline-stimulated increase in adenylate cyclase activity in the leucocytes of depressed patients is lower than in controls which suggests a subsensitivity of the β-adrenoceptor. Extein, Tallman, Smith, and Goodwin (1979) also found that isoprenaline-stimulated cAMP production in lymphocytes was decreased in manic and depressed patients. They also measured the binding of ^{3}H-dihydro-alprenolol to lymphocytes and found that specific binding was decreased in depressed and manic patients when compared to normal controls and euthymic patients. These results, therefore, suggest decreased lymphocyte β-receptor functioning during a depressive illness. Neither desipramine nor lithium treatment was associated with a change in ^{3}H-dihydroalprenolol binding or isoprenaline-stimulated cAMP production. Healy *et al.* (1983), also using ^{3}H-dihydroalprenolol as ligand, found that the density of lymphocyte binding sites (B_{max}) was significantly greater when compared with a normal control group and was significantly attenuated in those patients who therapeutically responded to either amitriptyline or trazadone treatment.

Are there any explanations for these inconsistencies? Undoubtedly one of the problems is the heterogeneity of white blood cells. Is the abnormality present in all leucocytes (Pandey, Dysken, Carter, and Davis 1979) or in lymphocytes (Healy *et al.* 1983)? Is the abnormality present for example, in both the T and B lymphocytes? Do depressed patients have abnormal populations of T and B lymphocytes? Although platelet investigations have been criticized on the basis that the majority of investigations have been carried out on 'crude platelet populations', i.e. platelets derived from platelet-rich-plasma and which may not therefore be representative of the total platelet population, the argument against using white cells is perhaps greater. Lymphocytes proliferate during chronic infection and they also have, unlike the platelet, great variability in their half-life, and comparisons between depressed patients and controls may be a reflection of general lymphocyte function rather than discrete changes in β-adrenoceptor activity. It has also been established that an intensive physical training programme in young adults leads to a decreased lymphocyte β-adrenoceptor density (Butler, Kelly, O'Malley, and Pidgeon 1983). The changes in β-receptor density found in depressed patients and its change during clinical recovery may reflect changes in physical activity rather than be a marker of depressive illness.

PLATELET 5-HT RECEPTORS

Two distinct 5-HT receptors have been identified in mammalian brain on the basis of radioligand binding (see Peroutka and Snyder 1980). The binding to 5-HT$_1$, receptors, which are labelled by ^{3}H-5-HT and ^{3}H-LSD, is regulated by guanine nucleotides. Binding to 5-HT$_2$ receptors occurs with ^{3}H-spiperone, ^{3}H-mianserin and ^{3}H-LSD. These latter receptors are not affected by guanine nucleotides but are sensitive to chronic antidepressant treatment and mediate the behavioural syndrome following central 5-HT stimulation (Peroutka and Snyder 1982). A significant decrease in the number of 5-HT$_2$ binding sites occurs after one week of antidepressant treatment and is maximal after 3–6 weeks of chronic treatment (Peroutka and Snyder 1980). Since this decrease is observed at clinically effective doses, alterations in 5-HT receptors may have important implications for the aetiology and treatment of depressive illness. In a clinical context, it has been reported (Stanley and Mann 1983) that there is a significantly greater number of 5-HT$_2$, but not 5-HT$_1$, receptors in the frontal cortex of suicide victims when compared with a control group. One is therefore tempted to speculate that antidepressants may exert their therapeutic effect by reducing and hence restoring the number of 5-HT$_2$ receptors to normal levels.

Although radioligand binding experiments are possible, no such investigations to the knowledge of the authors, have been carried out in patients suffering from a major depressive disorder. Healy *et al.* (1983) have used an aggregation technique to monitor the responsiveness of platelet 5-HT receptors in patients with a depressive illness and the change in the sensitivity of these receptors during antidepressant treatment. These authors reported that platelet 5-HT receptor responsiveness was reduced in depressed patients (when compared to a control group) and increased in those patients who responded clinically to antidepressant treatment. On the contrary, our aggregation data (Wood, Abou-Saleh, and Coppen 1984*b*) suggested that the functional activity of platelet 5-HT$_2$ receptor system was normal during a depressive illness.

These studies again indicate the variability of results obtained by different investigators when using platelets from controls and depressed patients. There would also appear to be a discrepancy between the action of antidepressants on platelet 5-HT$_2$ receptor sites and on central 5-HT$_2$ receptor sites. This may be due to the fact that platelet receptors cannot be described in the same terms as central receptors. By analogy with such receptors, the platelet 5-HT$_2$ site should have a high affinity for ^{3}H-spiperone; but Schäcter and Grahame-Smith (1982) failed to reveal a binding site for spiperone in the intact human platelet.

PLATELET ^{3}H-IMIPRAMINE BINDING SITES

High-affinity ^{3}H-imipramine binding sites have been detected on human platelets and in brain and they appear to be associated with the 5-HT uptake system. As Langer, Zarifian, Briley, Raisman, and Sechter (1981) have pointed out, this binding site fulfils many of the criteria to be expected of a specific site of drug action or a pharmacological receptor and this topic is therefore included in this chapter. It has been demonstrated that patients with a major depressive disorder have significantly fewer ^{3}H-imipramine binding sites on their platelets than normal controls (Briley, Langer, Raisman, Sechter, and Zarifian 1980).

Until the exact association of this ^{3}H-imipramine binding site with the 5-HT uptake site is established it seems a little premature to discuss in detail the findings of ^{3}H-imipramine binding in depression. Rather we will discuss the associated platelet 5-HT uptake process whose abnormality is well established in patients with a depressive illness.

PLATELET 5-HT UPTAKE

Decreased 5-HT uptake by blood platelets of depressed patients has been reported by several groups and seems to be one of the most consistently found abnormalities in biological psychiatry (Tuomisto and Tukiainen 1976; Coppen *et al.* 1978; Healy *et al.* 1983). It does not appear that this abnormality is specific for depressive illness since a decrease in 5-HT uptake has been observed in other disorders such as schizophrenia (Rotman, Modai, Munitz, and Wijsenbeek 1979; Giret, Launay, Loo, Dreux, Benyacoub, and Zarifian 1980) and in cirrhotic and hypertensive patients (Ahtee, L. Pentikäinen, P. Pentikäinen, and M. Paasonen 1974). The uptake of 5-HT is reduced in drug-free depressed patients and this abnormality is still present even when the patients have recovered (and are drug-free) from their depressive illness (Coppen *et al.* 1978).

It was assumed that one of the therapeutic modes of action of tricyclic antidepressant drugs was the inhibition of 5-HT uptake into serotonergic neurones within the CNS. However, upon looking at the change in platelet 5-HT uptake characteristics in depressed patients undergoing treatment with monoamine reuptake inhibitors (Wood, Swade, and Coppen 1982), it was noticed that these patients clinically improved if there was a smaller rather than a larger degree of uptake inhibition.

Whilst examining the effect of various antidepressants and putative antidepressants on the uptake of 5-HT *in vitro*, it was noted that amitriptyline and desipramine, amongst others, at equivalent therapeutic concentrations, i.e. 0.1–0.01 μmol/l actually stimulated the uptake of 5-HT into platelets of normal controls. These experiments *in vitro* were complemented by studies *ex vivo*. Eleven depressed patients were treated with 150 mg of amitriptyline for four weeks. Platelet 5-HT uptake characteristics were determined at baseline, i.e. the day before administration of amitriptyline and then after four weeks of treatment. Analysis of the results indicated that the eleven patients could be classified into two distinct groups, i.e. those who had an inhibition of platelet 5-HT uptake and those who had a stimulation of uptake. Stimulation of uptake could not be accounted for by low plasma levels of amitriptyline nor of its metabolite nortriptyline. Of the seven patients who had an inhibition of uptake none improved by more than 50 per cent on the Hamilton Rating Scale, whereas of the four patients who had stimulation of uptake, three attained at least 50 per cent improvement based on their Hamilton Rating Scale Score. Therapeutic improvement may, therefore, be related to a facilitation of uptake rather than inhibition. Healy *et al.* (1983) also demonstrated increased platelet 5-HT uptake (indicated by an increase in V_{max}) during successful treatment with either amitriptyline or trazadone.

What other evidence is available that would substantiate our claim that therapeutic improvement is associated with a facilitation, rather than inhibition, of platelet 5-HT uptake? The net effect of 5-HT uptake should be mirrored by the content of 5-HT in platelets. Coppen, Turner, Rowsell, and Padgham (1976) found that whole blood 5-HT was significantly reduced in drug-free depressed patients and therefore concurs with the uptake data. Upon recovery from the depressive illness, the 5-HT content increased and approached that of normal controls. However, Coppen *et al.* (1978) found that drug-free recovered patients still had abnormally low transport rates and, therefore, does not concur with the platelet 5-HT content data. How does one explain an increase in platelet 5-HT content after administration of a 5-HT uptake inhibitor? Mück-Šeler, Deanović, Jamnicky, Jakupćević, and Mihovilović (1983) have shown in a series of moderately to severely depressed patients that maprotiline treatment results in an increase in platelet 5-HT content with a corresponding decrease in the severity of their depressive symptoms. This increase in platelet 5-HT content is consistent with the facilitation of 5-HT uptake by maprotiline.

CONCLUSIONS

Do the results of possible facilitation of 5-HT-uptake affect any of the current hypotheses of affective disorder? The amine deficiency hypothesis has been criticized since it does not explain the discrepancy between the time-course of the biochemical and pharmacological effects which are elicited by antidepressant drugs within minutes or hours and their therapeutic action to become evident, which requires treatment for weeks (Vetulani *et al.* 1976). Vetulani and his colleagues put forward a new possible common mechanism of action of antidepressant treatments which involved a reduction in the sensitivity of the noradrenergic cAMP generating system in the limbic forebrain. Criticism of this newer hypothesis could be levelled at the desirability of having a common mechanism of action on antidepressant treatments. For example, would one prescribe a MAO inhibitor to a highly endogenously depressed patient or prescribe ECT for a reactive patient?

Uptake inhibition would not seem to be the explanation of antidepressant treatment since inhibition would occur after a relatively short interval after administration of the drug. If facilitation of 5-HT uptake occurs one could envisage a time-lag before clinical efficacy becomes apparent, since the build-up of depleted stores of 5-HT would occur only after a substantial period of time.

This adaptation of the deficiency hypothesis and the possible mechanism of action of certain antidepressive treatments has been put forward on the basis of experiments conducted *in vitro* and *ex vivo* on human platelets from normal controls and depressed patients; not from animal studies. We are not happy to extrapolate findings from binding and receptor sites on human platelets to those in the CNS. If 'downregulation' and desensitization occur in the CNS then it is due to discrete changes in the levels of endogenous agonists in the micro-environment of the synapse: no such micro-environment is associated with the platelet. The discrepancy in the results from the platelet receptor systems in depression and their change during antidepressant treatment illustrates this case.

The platelet 5-HT uptake process of platelets which may not be under such influence by endogenous agonists may be a more reliable indicator of CNS function. This advantage together with the finding of the facilitation of uptake by certain antidepressive treatments may lead to the development of other more effective antidepressants.

ACKNOWLEDGEMENTS

We gratefully acknowledge the assistance of our colleagues over many years. We are particularly indebted to the patients and the controls for their willing co-operation during the course of these studies. We wish to express our thanks to the Medical Research Council and Astra Pharmaceuticals for financial assistance during the course of these studies. We are grateful to Drs D. Clive Williams and Orla Phillips, Trinity College, Dublin, for many helpful discussions concerning the 5-HT uptake results.

REFERENCES

Ahtee, L., Pentikäinen, L., Pentikäinen, P., and Paasonen, M. (1974). 5-Hydroxytryptamine in blood platelets of cirrhotic and hypertensive patients. *Experientia* **30**, 1328–9.

Briley, M. S., Langer, S. Z., Raisman, R., Sechter, D., and Zarifian, E. (1980). Tritiated imipramine binding sites are decreased in platelets of untreated depressed patients. *Science* **209**, 303–5.

Butler, J., Kelly, J. G., O'Malley, K., and Pidgeon, F. (1983). β-Adrenoceptor adaptation to acute exercise. *J. Physiol.* **344**, 113–17.

Coppen, A., Swade, C., and Wood, K. (1978). Platelet 5-hydroxytryptamine accumulation in depressive illness. *Clinica chim. Acta* **87**, 165–8.

—, Turner, P., Rowsell, A. R., and Padgham, C. (1976). 5-Hydroxytryptamine in the whole-blood of patients with depressive illness. *Post-grad. med. J.* **52**, 156–8.

Crews, F. T. and Smith, C. B. (1978). Potentiation of responses to field stimulation of isolated left atria during chronic antidepressant administration. *J. Pharmac. exp. Ther.* **215**, 143–9.

Daiguji, M., Meltzer, H. Y., Tong, C., U'Prichard, D. C., Young, M., and Kravitz,

H. (1981). α₂-Adrenergic receptors in platelet membranes of depressed patients: no change in number or ³H-yohimbine affinity. *Life Sci.* **29**, 2059-64.

Elliot, J. M. and Grahame-Smith, D. G. (1982). The binding characteristics of ³H-dihydroergocryptine on intact human platelets. *Br. J. Pharmac.* **76**, 121-30.

Extein, I., Tallman, J., Smith, C. C., and Goodwin, F. K. (1979). Changes in lymphocyte beta-adrenergic receptors in depression and mania. *Psychiat. Res.* **1**, 191-7.

García-Sevilla, J. A., García-Vallejo, P., and Guimon, J. (1983). Enhanced α₂-adrenoceptor-mediated platelet aggregation in patients with major depressive disorder. *Eur. J. Pharmac.* **94**, 359-60.

—, Zis, A. P., Hollingsworth, P. J., Greden, J. F., and Smith, C. B. (1981). Platelet α₂-adrenergic receptors in major depressive disorder. *Arch. gen. Psychiat.* **38**, 1327-33.

Giret, M., Launay, J. M., Loo, H., Dreux, C., Benyacoub, A., and Zarifian, E. (1980). Modifications of biochemical parameters in blood platelets of schizophrenic and depressive patients. *Neuropsychobiology* **6**, 290-6.

Healy, D., Carney, P. A., and Leonard, B. E. (1983). Monoamine-related markers of depression: changes following treatment. *J. Psychiat. Res.* **17**, 251-60.

Langer, S. Z., Zarifian, E., Briley, M., Raisman, R., and Sechter, D. (1981). High-affinity binding of ³H imipramine in brain and platelets and its relevance to the biochemistry of affective disorders. *Life Sci.* **29**, 211-20.

Matussek, N., Ackenheil, M., Hippius, H., Müller, F., Schröder, H-Th., Schultes, H., and Wasilewski, B. (1980). Effect of clonidine on growth hormone release in psychiatric patients and controls. *Psychiat. Res.* **2**, 25-36.

Mück-Šeler, D., Deanović, Z., Jamnicky, B., Jakupćević, M., and Mihovilović, M. (1983). Maprotiline in the treatment of endogenous depression: comparison of therapeutic effect with serotonin level in blood platelets. *Psychopharmacology* **79**, 262-5.

Newman, K. D., Williams, L. T., Bishopric, N. H., and Lefkowitz, R. J. (1978). Identification of α-adrenergic receptors in human platelets by ³H-dihydroergocryptine binding. *J. clin. Invest.* **61**, 395-402.

Pandey, G. N., Dysken, M. W., Garter, D. L., and Davis, J. M. (1979). Beta-adrenergic receptor function in affective illness. *Am. J. Psychiat.* **136** 675-8.

Peroutka, S. J. and Snyder, S. H. (1980). Long-term antidepressant treatment decreased spiroperidol-labelled serotonin receptor binding. *Science* **210**, 88-90.

— and — (1982). Recognition of multiple serotonin receptor sites. In *Serotonin in biological psychiatry: Advances in biochemical psychopharmacology*, vol. 34 (ed. B. T. Ho, J. C. Schoolar, and E. Usdin, pp. 155-72. Raven Press, New York.

Pimoule, C., Briley, M. S., Gay, C., Loo, H., Sechter, D., Zarifian, E., Raisman, R., and Langer, S. Z. (1983). ³H-Rauwolscine binding in platelets from depressed patients and healthy volunteers. *Psychopharmacology* **79**, 308-12.

Rotman, A., Modai, I., Munitz, H., and Wijsenbeek, H. (1979). Active uptake of serotonin by blood platelets of schizophrenic patients. *FEBS Lett.* **101**, 134-6.

Schächter, M. and Grahame-Smith, D. G. (1982). 5-Hydroxytryptamine and the platelet: specific binding and uptake. In *5-Hydroxytryptamine in peripheral reactions* (ed. F. De Clerk and P. M. Vanhoutte), pp. 83-94. Raven Press, New York.

Stahl, S. M., Lemoine, P. M., Ciaranello, R. D., and Berger, P. A. (1983). Platelet alpha₂-adrenergic receptor sensitivity in major depressive disorder. *Psychiat. Res.* **10**, 157–64.

Stanley, M. and Mann, J. J. (1983). Increased serotonin-2 binding sites in frontal cortex of suicide victims. *Lancet* i, 214–16.

Stärke, K. (1977). Regulation of noradrenaline release by pre-synaptic receptor systems. *Rev. Physiol. Biochem. & Pharmac.* **77**, 1–124.

Tuomisto, J. and Tukiainen, E. (1976). Decreased uptake of 5-hydroxytryptamine in blood platelets from depressed patients. *Nature, Lond.* **262**, 596–98.

U'Prichard, D. C. and Snyder, S. H. (1979). Distinct α-adrenergic receptors differentiated by binding and physiological relationships. *Life Sci.* **24**, 79–82.

Vetulani, J., Stawarz, R. J., Dingell, J. V., and Sulser, F. (1976). A possible common mechanism of action of antidepressant treatments. *Naunyn-Schmiedeberg's Arch. Pharmac.* **293**, 109–14.

Wood, K. and Coppen, A. (1980). Hormonal influences on α-adrenoceptors – preliminary results. In *The menopause and postmenopause* (ed. N. Pasetto, R. Paoletti, and J. L. Ambrus), pp. 55–61. MTP Press Ltd., Lancaster.

— and — (1981). Platelet alpha-adrenoceptor sensitivity in depressive illness. *Adv. Biol. Psychiat.* **7**, 85–9.

— and — (1983). Prophylactic lithium treatment of patients with affective disorders is associated with decreased platelet ³H-dihydroergocryptine binding. *J. affect. Disord.* **5** 253–8.

—, Swade, C. C., and Coppen, A. (1982). Zimelidine: a pharmacokinetic and pharmacodynamic study in depressive illness. *Br. J. clin. Pract.*, suppl. **19**, 42–7.

—, —, and — (1984a). Platelet α-adrenergic receptors in depression: ligand binding and aggregation studies. *Acta pharmac. & tox.* (in press).

—, —, Abou-Saleh, M., and Coppen, A. (1984b). Peripheral serotonergic receptor sensitivity in depressive illness. *J. affect. Disord.* (in press).

4

Animal models of depression and the detection of antidepressants

B. E. LEONARD

Although the neuroanatomical and neurochemical composition of the human and sub-human brain is basically similar, there is no convincing evidence to suggest that even the most developed non-human primate suffers from an identifiable mental illness. To paraphrase Roth and Kerr (1970), the depressive state is probably peculiar to *Homo sapiens*. Thus the state of the mood and cognitive function, as exemplified by feelings of guilt, worthlessness, pessimism, are unlikely to be present in an animal species that does not have a well-defined concept of self-esteem or of the future. Other features of the depression syndrome such as apathy, loss of appetite and libido, and impaired attention and memory, might be simulated in animals following the appropriate behavioural manipulation. This has led several investigators to study changes in behaviour and brain neurotransmission that may be linked to reward and punishment.

Despite the advances which have been made in the development of animal models of depression in recent years, most of those routinely used by research laboratories in the pharmaceutical industry have remained surprisingly inept at accurately predicting clinically effective antidepressants, and in generating new hypotheses of the pathophysiology of depression. Thus, almost every significant advance in antidepressant drug treatment, from the discovery of iproniazid and imipramine to the second generation antidepressants such as mianserin, has resulted either from astute clinical observation or serendipity.

Hitherto, most animal models which have been used for the selection of putative antidepressants have been based on the simple amine deficiency theory, which postulates that depression arises as a result of a deficiency in biogenic amine neurotransmitters in the synaptic cleft. Thus, it has been assumed that antidepressants 'work' by blocking the reuptake or intraneuronal metabolism of biogenic amine neurotransmitters, generally assumed to be noradrenaline and serotonin. As the ability of monoamine oxidase inhibitors and tricyclic antidepressants to antagonize the hypothermia and behavioural depression caused by acute reserpine treatment provided a useful model for the detection of imipramine and iproniazid-like drugs, a plethora of antidepressants has been developed which have similar pharmacological and toxicological profiles to the parent compounds. The more recent findings of Sulser, Vetulani, and Mobley

(1978) on changes in the sensitivity of β-adrenoceptors following chronic anti-depressant treatment of ECS, and the changes in the sensitivity of serotonin type 2 receptors and α 2-adrenoceptors following chronic antidepressant treatment (Peroutka and Snyder 1980; Smith, Hollingsworth, García-Sevilla, and Zis 1983) has led to the amine theory being modified to take into account the adaptation of receptors which appear to correlate with the onset of the anti-depressant response. Whether such changes in receptor density are causally related to the therapeutic action of the antidepressants is unproven, but at least this measure serves to detect all known antidepressants irrespective of their structure or acute effects on one or more neurotransmitter systems.

The purpose of the following short review is to describe some of the animal models of depression which have been developed. This article is not intended to be fully comprehensive, and those interested in the biochemical models in which the effects of chronic antidepressant treatments on adrenergic or sero-tonergic receptors have been studied are referred to studies of Sulser *et al.* (1978), Peroutka and Snyder (1980), and Smith *et al.* (1983).

DEVELOPMENTAL MODELS OF DEPRESSION

Bowlby (1960) observed that the removal of children from their mothers induced depressive symptoms that were characterized by hyperactivity followed by despair and withdrawal. Harlow (1958) has shown that a similar behaviour could be elicited by the removal of the infant monkey from its mother. Despite the promising nature of the earlier studies, Kaufman (1974) has shown that far greater changes in infant behaviour occur in monkeys reared by their mothers in relative isolation from other monkeys than occurs in response to separation from the natural mother. The relationship between such events as isolation from the mother in childhood and the onset of depression in the adult is still an unresolved question, and the behaviour of the monkey following prolonged isolation from its mother probably bears a closer resemblance to psychotic behavior than depression (McKinney, Young, Suomi, and Davis 1973).

LEARNED HELPLESSNESS MODELS

Seligman (1975) developed a model of learned helplessness which mimics some of the main features of depression, particularly of the kind that are precipitated by unfavourable environmental events. Dogs exposed to an unavoidable elec-trical shock were subsequently found to be unable to learn to avoid an aversive stimulus, and remained motionless and 'helpless' in such a situation. Studies by Glazer and Weiss (1976) using the rat also showed that this species could exhibit 'behavioural despair'. These investigators analysed the changes elicited by unavoidable shock and showed that the relatively short-term stress (as shown by freezing behaviour, increased sympatho-adrenal activity, etc.) carry over into the learning phase, which may account for the initial immobility. These investigators then showed that the persistent inability of the animal to respond is confined to the learned immobility that has been acquired during the unavoidable shock situation. Thus the 'learned helplessness' behaviour does not generalize to other types of behaviour that had been learned in the absence of the shock. Such findings have led to a serious reappraisal of the relevance of this model to depression.

Even though the relevance of the 'learned helplessness' model to depression may be questioned, the usefulness of short-term immobility to stress may provide a useful model for the detection of antidepressant drugs. The method developed by Porsolt, Anton, Blavet, and Jalfre (1978) involves placing rodents individually into a water-filled glass cylinder from which they cannot escape. After a few minutes of vigorous swimming and attempted escape, the animals remain quiet, only making movements sufficient to keep their heads above the water. Exposure to the same environment 24 h later shows that the animals have 'learned' not to try to escape from the container and therefore they remain immobile. Porsolt *et al.* (1978) used this model as a test for antidepressant activity. They showed that both 'standard' tricyclic antidepressants such as amitriptyline and imipramine, and atypical antidepressants such as mianserin and iprindole, increase the time in which the animals struggle to escape from the container on being placed in it on the second occasion. Clearly, drugs that caused marked sedation or reduce the muscle tone will produce 'false positives' in such a test situation, but Porsolt *et al.* (1978) did show that low doses of anxiolytics and neuroleptics were ineffective in this test. Despite the widespread use of the Porsolt 'learned immobility' test as a screening method for antidepressants, a critical evaluation of the test by O'Neill and Valentino (1982)

TABLE 4.1. *Effects of nomifensin and trazodone on the duration of immobility in the learned helplessness test*

| Treatment | Administration of drugs: | |
	Acute (1 day)	Chronic (14 days)
Controls (saline)	252.4 ± 11.4	259.0 ± 9.4
Nomifensin (5 mg/kg)	124.6 ± 24.0†	110.2 ± 14.2†
Trazodone (50 mg/kg)	261.4 ± 10.8	215.7 ± 9.4*

All values expressed as the duration of immobility (seconds) following 5 min immersion in the container of water at 25 °C. Each group consisted of 10 rats (♂, 250 g).
Values expressed as mean ± SEM.
* $p < 0.05$.
† $p < 0.001$ vs. appropriate controls.
In the chronically treated trazodone group, dose administered was (2×50 mg/kg daily).
See Górka, Earley, and Leonard (1984) for details.

suggests that it suffers from the same fundamental problems as the original Seligman (1975) model. Thus, it was shown that rodents exhibit 'behavioural despair' independently of their ability to escape from the cylinder of water and that the phenomenon did not generalize to a shock escape task. O'Neill and Valentino (1982) therefore conclude that the immobility may reflect either an adaptive response to the particular situation, physical fatigue, or a combination of these factors. Such criticisms, together with the observation of Wallach and Hedley (1979) that such psychotropic drugs as caffeine, antihistamines, and pentobarbital also reverse the 'behavioural despair' behaviour, suggest that such a model is an inadequate representation of depression and of limited value in the detection of antidepressant drugs.

RESERPINE-INDUCED 'DEPRESSION'

The serendipitous discovery that imipramine reversed the symptoms of ptosis and hypothermia induced in rodents by reserpine pretreatment, led to the development of the reserpine reversal test as a model for the detection of antidepressants. As a result of the almost universal use of this test by the pharmaceutical industry, a plethora of tricyclic antidepressants were discovered over the past two decades, all of which have a qualitatively similar pharmacological and therapeutic profile to imipramine. Such drugs are assumed to reverse the reserpine-induced symptoms by elevating the intersynaptic concentrations of biogenic amines, largely as a result of the drugs impeding the reuptake of biogenic amines from the synaptic cleft. Monoamine oxidase inhibitors also reversed the acute effects of reserpine primarily by blocking the intraneuronal catabolism of the biogenic amines.

The very success of the reserpine antagonism test in the development of a variety of both tricyclic antidepressants, such as desipramine, clomipramine, dothiepin, doxepin, and some of the newer antidepressants which lack the tricyclic structure (for example, nomifensin, maprotiline, viloxazine, zimelidine, and citalopram), has restricted the development of other animal models of depression. Furthermore, as both the conventional reserpine antagonism test and the 'learned helplessness' test of Porsolt *et al.* (1978) could select tricyclic antidepressants after their acute administration, the development of animal models which enabled antidepressants to be selected only following their chronic administration was also hampered. Thus atypical antidepressants such as iprindole, mianserin, salbutamol, and flupenthixol, which did not affect the amine reuptake mechanism and were therefore inactive in reserpine-antagonism tests, were only discovered to be antidepressants following their clinical assessment, often for other psychiatric and non-psychiatric conditions. Such findings stressed the need to develop new animal models that did not rely on a specific structure or acute biochemical profile involving an inhibition of amine reputake.

It is against this background that Jancsár and Leonard (1983*a*) examined the acute and chronic effects of two novel antidepressants on the exploratory

TABLE 4.2. *Changes in the exploratory activity of rats in the 'open field' apparatus, following the chronic administration of reserpine alone or in combination with mianserin*

Group	Drug (dose)	Ambulation (squares crossed)	Rearing (number)	Grooming (number)	Defaecation (No. faeces)
Control	Saline	73.5 ± 1.8	7.5 ± 0.9	1.5 ± 0.6	0.7 ± 0.4
Reserpine	0.1 mg/kg × 14 days	$104.6 \pm 9.2*$	$2.3 \pm 0.4*$	$0.3 \pm 0.3*$	1.3 ± 0.5
Mianserin	5.0 mg/kg × 14 days	73.0 ± 1.6	5.5 ± 1.2	2.0 ± 0.7	1.3 ± 0.5
Reserpine + Mianserin	0.1 mg/kg × 14 days 5.0 mg/kg × 14 days	$78.2 \pm 1.7\dagger$	$6.2 \pm 0.8\dagger$	$3.5 \pm 0.8\dagger$	1.0 ± 0.5

Each value represents the mean ± SEM of 10 rats (♂, 250 g). Behaviour assessed in 'open field' for 3 min.
* $p < 0.01$ vs. saline.
† $p < 0.05$ vs. reserpine alone. See Jancsár and Leonard (1983a) for details.

behaviour of rats which had been treated acutely or chronically with reserpine. Vetulani, Stawarz, Dingell, and Sulser (1976) had shown that chronic administration of reserpine induces a hyperactivity of the adenylate cyclase coupled to the β-adrenoceptor in the cortex of the rat brain. As chronically administered antidepressants were shown by these investigators to decrease the activity of this receptor complex, we postulated that both the behavioural and biochemical effects of reserpine could be antagonized by chronically administered antidepressants, irrespective of the acute pharmacological profile of the antidepressant. The results of the study by Jancsár and Leonard (1983*a*) showed that, as anticipated, acutely-administered mianserin did not antagonize the hyperactivity and reduced rearing behaviour of the chronically reserpinized rats when they were placed in a stressful novel environment such as the 'open field' apparatus. Following their administration for 14 days, however, mianserin significantly attenuated the hyperactivity and reversed the increased rearing scores of the reserpinized animals.

The results of this study suggest that although the acutely reserpinized rodent model of depression is of limited value in the detection of antidepressant activity, the chronically reserpinized animal may offer the possibility for selecting drugs that differ in their pharmacological profile from the tricyclic antidepressants.

MURICIDAL RAT MODEL OF DEPRESSION

Lesions of the olfactory bulbs increases the incidence of mouse-killing behaviour in strains of rat that would not normally exhibit this behaviour (Vergnes and Karli 1963). Increased irritability has also been shown to occur when specific serotonin neurotoxins, such as 5,7-dihydroxytripytamine, are injected bilaterally into the olfactory bulbs (Cairncross, Cox, Forster, and Wren 1979), a situation that may explain the enhanced muricidal behaviour in rats which have been surgically bulbectomized. Several investigators have shown that a defect in brain serotonin function is associated with muricidal behaviour. Thus, administration of the tryptophan hydroxylase inhibitor, parachlorophenylalanine (Sheard 1969), and the administration of serotonin neurotoxins (Vergnes and Kempf 1982), have been shown to induce muricidal behaviour. Conversely, drugs facilitating central serotonergic neurotransmission attenuate muricidal behaviour. Antidepressant drugs, which are specific serotonin-uptake inhibitors following their acute administration, for example, fluoxetine (Gibbons and Glusman 1978), the serotonin agonists quipazine and 5-hydroxytryptophan (Bocknik and Kulkarni 1974), and the releasing agent fenfluramine (Gibbons and Glusman 1978), all antagonize spontaneous or neurotoxin-induced muricidal behaviour. As such tricyclic antidepressants as imipramine, desipramine, and amitriptyline also attenuate muricidal behaviour (Eisenstein, Iorid, and Clody 1982), the effects of drugs on such behaviour has been used as a rapid screening test for potential antidepressants. However, it is now well established that many centrally acting drugs which do not have antidepressant activity in man also show positive 'antidepressant' activity in this test. Besides fenfluramine, amphetamine, and antihistamines, have, for example, been shown to be active in the muricidal rat model (see Einsenstein *et al.* 1982). Thus, from these experimental studies it may be concluded that the muricidal rat model may be useful for defining the effects of a centrally acting drug on serotonin metabolism but cannot be used as a reliable model for the detection of antidepressants.

OLFACTORY BULBECTOMY MODEL OF DEPRESSION

The main advantage of this model over all other models described is that it will selectively detect antidepressant activity only following the chronic administration of the drug. Furthermore, the time taken for the activity of the antidepressant to become established, and the daily dose necessary for the drug to exhibit activity, approximates to that found therapeutically. A critical evaluation of the neuroanatomical, neurophysiological, neuropharmacological, and behavioural aspects of this model have been given elsewhere (Leonard and

TABLE 4.3. *Effect of some psychotropic drugs on the behaviour of the olfactory bulbectomized rat in the 'open field' apparatus*

Exp. No.	Treatment			Ambulation (squares crossed)	Rearing (No.)
1.	Sham	+	saline	89.1 ± 11.3	12.2 ± 2.4
	Sham	+	nomifensin (3 mg/kg)	68.0 ± 9.3	7.3 ± 2.1
	OB	+	saline	132.0 ± 4.1*	20.6 ± 2.8*
	OB	+	nomifensin (3 mg/kg)	97.5 ± 6.6‡	24.1 ± 3.9*
2.	Sham	+	saline	91.5 ± 5.5	14.3 ± 1.5
	Sham	+	mianserin (5 mg/kg)	74.3 ± 8.9	14.6 ± 1.6
	OB	+	saline	130.6 ± 9.6*	26.5 ± 1.8*
	OB	+	mianserin (5 mg/kg)	106.4 ± 9.2‡	20.4 ± 1.0*
3.	Sham	+	saline	85.2 ± 2.7	7.0 ± 1.3
	Sham	+	reserpine (0.1 mg/kg)	115.3 ± 8.4*	9.2 ± 1.7
	OB	+	saline	166.8 ± 6.7†	27.6 ± 2.2†
	OB	+	reserpine (0.1 mg/kg)	174.1 ± 7.9†	28.8 ± 2.6†

* $p < 0.05$.
† $p < 0.01$ vs. sham + saline.
‡ $p < 0.05$ vs. OB + saline.
Each group consisted of 10 rats ($\delta \backsim 250$ g); results expressed as mean SEM.

Observations made for 3 min; no consistent changes found in grooming behaviour or in defaecation scores, and therefore values not included. See Jancsár and Leonard (1983*b*) for details.

Tuite 1981; Jancsár and Leonard 1983*b*). Detailed studies of the chronic effects of both tricyclic antidepressants (for example, amitriptyline, imipramine, desipramine) and non-tricyclic antidepressants such as mianserin, nomifensin, zimelidine, salbutamol, and E-flupenthixol, have been shown to be active in attenuating the hyperactivity shown by bilaterally bulbectomized rats when placed in the stressful, novel enviroment of the 'open field' apparatus (Jancsár and Leonard, 1980, 1981, 1983*b*). Detailed studies by Cairncross *et al.* (1979) and by Van Riezen, Schnieden, and Wren (1977) have shown that deficits in passive avoidance learning by bulbectomized rats may be antagonized by the chronic administration of antidepressants; neuroleptics, anxiolytics, sedative-hypnotics, and centrally-acting anticholinergic drugs are inactive in this test. Furthermore, following their acute administration, all antidepressants so far examined have failed to show activity.

Studies by Jancsár and Leonard (1984) of the turnover of the biogenic amine neurotransmitters, and GABA, in different regions of the brain following bilateral bulbectomy, have shown that the turnover of both noradrenaline and serotonin was decreased, GABA was increased, while that of dopamine was decreased in the midbrain only. These effects were particularly pronounced in the amygdaloid cortex, an area of the limbic system that contain projections from both the, main and accessory olfactory bulbs. Preliminary studies show that chronic antidepressant administration largely normalizes the effects of bulbectomy on the turnover of biogenic amines. It has also been shown that the α_1-adrenoceptor density is increased, while that of the β-adrenoceptor density is slightly decreased in this brain region, as assessed by tritiated ligand binding techniques. Whether these changes in adrenoceptor activity are causally or coincidentally related to the behavioural effects of chronic antidepressant treatment cannot be ascertained.

Besides the various types of antidepressants shown to be active in the bulb-ectomy model, drugs facilitating GABAergic transmission, such as gamma vinyl GABA and baclofen, and serotonergic agonists (for example, methysergide), have also been shown to be active. As these drugs have not been tested for their possible antidepressant activity in adequately controlled clinical trails, it is not possible to state whether or not there are 'false positives' in the bulbectomy model. Nevertheless, preliminary results suggest that some GABA agonists may have antidepressant activity (Lloyd, Morselli, Depoortere, Founier, Zivkovic, Scatton, Broekkamp, Worms, and Bartholini 1983). Of the established anti-depressants, trazodone, a serotonin uptake inhibitor with some serotonin receptor agonist properties, does not appear to be active in this model.

From these studies, it may be concluded that the olfactory bulbectomy model of depression is probably the most useful so far developed for the detection of potential antidepressants, and for evaluating the possible mechanism of action of antidepressants on the physiological and biochemical mechanisms that appear to be deranged following the selective surgical lesion to the olfactory bulbs which form part of the limbic system in the rodent.

THE APOMORPHINE ANTAGONISM MODEL FOR THE DETECTION OF ANTIDEPRESSANTS

Interest in the possible involvement of the dopaminergic system in the mode of action of antidepressants has arisen from the observation that many antidepressants inhibit the reuptake of tritiated dopamine into synaptosomes from the rat brain (Randrup and Braestrup 1977). Furthermore, Serra, Argiolas, Fadda, and Gessa (1979) showed that chronic mianserin or amitriptyline treatment prevents the hypomotility of rats that are subsequently injected with a low (0.05 mg/kg) acute dose of apomorphine. These findings have been extended by Chiodo and Antelman (1980), who showed that the ability of apomorphine to selectively depress the spontaneous electrical activity of dopaminergic neurons in the zone compacta of the substantia nigra was attenuated following the chronic administration of tricyclic antidepressants or iprindole. It can be concluded from such studies that prolonged antidepressant treatment results in a subsensitivity of dopamine autoreceptors.

An investigation of the effects of chronic treatment (14 days) of rats with citalopram, nomifensin, salbutamol, E-flupenthixol, and sulpiride in antagonizing the hypomotility induced by the acute administration of apomorphine has been summarized elsewhere (Hasan and Leonard 1983). In this study, it was shown that those drugs with proven antidepressant activity attenuate the hypomotility of apomorphine, whereas those lacking such activity (e.g. reserpine) do not.

Like the bulbectomy model, the apomorphine antagonism model only appears to select antidepressants following their chronic administration, and irrespective of their structure or presumed acute effects on one or more neurotransmitter systems.

CONCLUSIONS

There is no evidence that the developmental models of depression in primates or dogs have given the researcher any insight into the pathogenesis of depression or in elucidating the mode of action of antidepressant drugs. The 'learned helplessness' model of Porsolt *et al.* (1978) has the advantage of enabling some types of antidepressants to be detected after their acute administration, an advantage which it shares with the reserpine antagonism of muricidal rat models. However, all three models lack specificity and are of little value in clarifying the mode of action of antidepressants.

The three models of depression which enable antidepressants to be selected only following their chronic administration, may be of more value to the researcher in that the duration of treatment necessary is similar to that needed for the therapeutic activity to become apparent in depressed patients. Whether such models in general, or the bulbectomized rat model in particular, will be of any value in the elucidation of the mode of action of antidepressants and/or in the pathogenesis of depression must await further investigation.

ACKNOWLEDGEMENTS

I wish to express my gratitude to the numerous present and past postgraduate students of this Department who have been largely responsible for the evaluation of many of the models of depression outlined in this review.

REFERENCES

Bocknik, S. E. and Kulkarni, A. S. (1974). Effect of a decarboxylate inhibitor (Ro. 4-4602) on 5-HTP induced murcide blockade in rats. *Neuropharmac.* **13**, 279-87.

Bowlby, J. (1960). Grief and mourning in infancy and early childhood. *Psychoanal. Stud. Child.* **15**, 9-52.

Cairncross, K. D., Cox, B., Forster, C., and Wren, A. F. (1979). Olfactory projection system, drugs and behaviour: a review. *Psychoneuroendocrin.* **4**, 253-73.

Chiodo, L. A. and Antelman, S. M. (1980). Tricyclia antidepressants induce subsensitivity of pre-synaptic dopamine autoreceptors. *Eur. J. Pharmac.* **64**, 203-4.

Einsenstein, N., Iorid, L. C., and Clody, D. E. (1982). Role of serotonin in the blockade of muricidal behaviour by tricyclic antidepressants. *Pharmac. Biochem. & Behav.* **17**, 847-9.

Gibbons, J. L. and Glusman, M. (1978). Effects of quipazine, fluoxetine and fenfluramine on murcide in rats. *Fed. Proc. Fedn Am. Socs exp. Biol.* **39**, 257.

Glazer, H. I. and Weiss, J. M. (1976). Long-term interference effect. An alternative to 'learned helplessness'. *J. exp. Psychol. Anim. Behav. Processes* **2**, 202-13.

Górka, Z., Earley, B., and Leonard, B. E. (1984). Effect of bilateral olfactory bulbectomy in the rat, alone or in combination with antidepressants, on the learned immobility model of depression. *Neuropsychobiol.* **16** (in press).

Harlow, H. F. (1958). The nature of love. *Am. J. Psychol.* **13**, 673-85.

Hasan, F. and Leonard, B. E. (1983). Changes in behaviour and neurotransmitter metabolism in the rat following acute and chronic sulpiride administration. In *Special aspects of psychopharmacology* (ed. M. Ackenheil and N. Matussek), pp. 67-82. Expansion Scientifique Française, Paris.

Jancsár, S. and Leonard, B. E. (1980). Effect of some antidepressant and other psychotropic drugs on the behaviour of olfactory bulbectomized rats in the 'open field' apparatus. *Ir. J. med. Sci.* **149**, 80.

— and — (1981). The effects of olfactory bulbectomy on the behaviour of rats in the 'open field'. *Ir. J. med. Sci.* **150**, 3.

— and — (1983*a*). Behavioural and neurochemical interactions between chronic reserpine and chronic antidepressants: a possible model for the detection of atypical antidepressants. *Biochem. Pharmac.* **32**, 1569-71.

— and — (1983*b*). The olfactory bulbectomized rat model as a model of depression. In *Frontiers in neuropsychiatric research* (ed. E. Usdin, M. Goldstein, A. J. Friedhoff, and A. Georgotas), pp. 357-72. Macmillan, New York.

— and — (1984). Changes in neurotransmitter metabolism following olfactory bulbectomy in the rat. *Prog. neuro-psychopharmac. Biol. Psychiat.* (in press).

Kaufman, C. I. (1974). Mother/infant relations in monkeys and humans. In

Ethology and psychiatry (ed. N. F. White), pp. 47–68. University of Toronto Press, Canada.

Leonard, B. E. and Tuite, (1981). Anatomical, physiological and behavioural aspects of olfactory bulbectomy in the rat. *Int. Rev. Neurobiol.* 22, 251–86.

Lloyd, K. G., Morselli, P. L., Depoortere, H., Founier, V., Zivkovic, B., Scatton, B., Broekkamp, C., Worms, P., and Bartholini, G. (1983). The potential use of GABA agonists in psychiatric disorders: evidence from studies with progabide in animal models and clinical trials. *Pharmacol. Biochem. & Behav.* 18, 957–66.

McKinney, W. J., Young, L. D., Suomi, S. T., and Davis, J. M. (1973). Chlorpromazine treatment in disturbed monkeys. *Arch. gen. Psychiat.* 29, 490–4.

O'Neill, K. A. and Valentino, D. (1982). Escapability and generalization: effect on behavioural despair. *Eur. J. Pharmac.* 78, 379–80.

Peroutka, S. J. and Snyder, S. H. (1980). Chronic antidepressant treatment lowers spiro-peridol labelled serotonin receptor binding. *Science* 210, 88–90.

Porsolt, R. D., Anton, G., Blavet, N., and Jalfre, M. (1978). Behavioural despair in rats: a new model sensitive to antidepressant treatments. *Eur. J. Pharmac.* 47, 379–85.

Randrup, A. and Braestrup, C. (1977). Uptake inhibition of biogenic amines by newer antidepressant drugs: relevance to the dopamine hypothesis of depression. *Psychopharmacology* 53, 309–14.

Roth, M. and Kerr, T. A. (1970). Diagnosis of reactive depressive illness. In *Modern trends in psychological medicine*, vol. 2 (ed. H. Price), pp. 65–199. Butterworth, London.

Seligman, M. E. P. (1975). *Helplessness*. Freeman, San Francisco.

Serra, G., Argiolas, V., Fadda, F., and Gessa, G. L. (1979). Hyposensitivity of dopamine 'auto receptors' induced by chronic administration of tricyclic antidepressants. *Pharmac. Res. Commun.* 12, 619–24.

Sheard, M. (1969). The effect of p-chlorophenylalanine on behaviour in rats: relation to brain serotonin and 5-hydroxyindole acetic acid. *Brain Res.* 15, 524–8.

Smith, C. B., Hollingsworth, P. J., García-Sevilla, J. A., and Zis, A. P. (1983). Platelet alpha$_2$ adrenoceptors are decreased in numbers after antidepressant therapy. *Prog. neuro-psychopharmac. Biol. Psychiat.* 7, 241–7.

Sulser, F., Vetulani, J., and Mobley, P. L. (1978). Mode of action of antidepressant drugs. *Biochem. Pharmac.* 27, 257–61.

Van Riezen, H., Schnieden, H., and Wren, A. F. (1977). Olfactory bulb ablation in the rat: behavioural changes and their reversal by antidepressant drugs. *Br. J. Pharmac.* 60, 521–8.

Vernges, M. and Karli, P. (1963). De'clenchement du comportement d'agression interspecifique. Rat Souris par ablation bilatérale des bulbes olfactifs. *C.r. Séarnc. Soc. Biol.* 157, 1061–3.

Vergnes, M. and Kempf, E. (1982). Effect of hypothalamic injections of 5,7-dihydroxytryptamine on elicitation of mouse killing in rats. *Behav. & Brain Res.* 5, 387–97.

Vetulani, J., Stawarz, R. J., Dingell, J. V., and Sulser, F. (1976). A possible common mechanism of action of antidepressant treatments. *N.S. Arch. Pharmac.* 293, 109–14.

Wallach, F. A. and Hedley, . (1979). The effects of several antihistamines in a modified behavioural despair test. *Fed. Proc. Fedn Am. Socs exp. Biol.* 38, 861.

5

Antidepressant drugs of the future

ROGER M. PINDER

INTRODUCTION

The pharmacotherapy of depression began more than two decades ago with the almost simultaneous discovery of the mood-lifting properties of the anti-tuberculosis drug iproniazid and the tricyclic antihistamine imipramine. Despite the spectacular initial success of iproniazid and its successors, which came to be known as the monoamine oxidase inhibitors, they were subsequently used only sparingly, following early reports of the potentially disastrous consequences of their interaction with certain foodstuffs containing tyramine (the so-called 'cheese effect') and by a realization that they lacked efficacy in the general population of depressed patients. They have been reserved for the treatment of atypical and neurotic types of depression, while imipramine and its successors, the tricyclic antidepressants, became the standard drugs for antidepressant therapy (Hollister 1981).

Reliance upon traditional antidepressants of the tricyclic type has lessened in recent years with substantial use of newer drugs termed second generation antidepressants. Development and introduction of the new drugs was prompted by a desire to eliminate some of the many troublesome side-effects of the tricyclics, particularly those of an anticholinergic and cardiovascular nature, and to reduce their pronounced toxicity upon overdosage (Blackwell 1981). The term second generation antidepressants includes new tricyclics like amoxapine, dothiepin, lofepramine, and the bridged tricyclic maprotiline, which largely retain tricyclic-like properties, as well as new drugs which are atypical in both structure and pharmacology, such as mianserin, nomifensin, trazodone, viloxazine, and zimeldine (Blackwell 1981; Hollister 1981).

The second generation drugs, however, have not provided the ideal solution to safe and effective antidepressant therapy. Like the traditional tricyclics they are slow to take effect and leave a substantial proportion of patients unaffected. Moreover, they are not entirely free from adverse effects. Of the new tricyclics only lofepramine may offer some advantage over the older drugs in terms of less anticholinergic and cardiovascular effects. Amoxapine, dothiepin, and maprotiline do not, and are at least as toxic in overdosage as traditional tricyclics (Crome 1982; Litovitz and Troutman 1983). Amoxapine and maprotiline are both markedly epileptogenic and carry additional hazards in the form of extra-pyramidal reactions and skin rashes respectively (Blackwell 1981; Hollister 1981). The atypical antidepressants do indeed tend to lack anticholinergic properties, to induce minimal cardiotoxity and to be much safer in overdosage. However, viloxazine commonly causes nausea and vomiting with occasional migraine (Blackwell 1981), while trazodone has been associated with severe priapism (Scher, Kreiger, and Juergens 1983) and aggravation of ventricular arrhythmias (Janowsky, Curtis, Zisook, Kuhn, Kesovsky, and Le Winter 1983), nomifensin with various immunoallergic reactions including fever, hepatitis and haemolytic anaemia (Blackwell 1981; Lylloff, Jersild, Bacher, and Slot 1982), and mianserin with blood dyscrasias (Adams, Reid, Robinson, Vishu, and Livingston 1983). Zimeldine was recently withdrawn from all markets because of neurological and hypersensitivity reactions, particularly Guillain-Barré syndrome.

NEW ANTIDEPRESSANTS

Despite the adverse effects of the second generation atypical antidepressants, the therapeutic balance is still in their favour over both traditional and new tricyclics, if only from the viewpoint of safety in overdosage (Crome 1982). The search for new drugs continues, with the primary objectives being to introduce greater efficacy at an earlier stage of treatment while retaining the gains already made in reduced anticholinergic and cardiovascular effects and greater safety. Several new antidepressants are about to be introduced, none of which seems likely to satisfy fully these objectives, while many more candidates are in various stages of clinical development (see Table 5.1). A complete list is beyond the scope of this review; the selection is a personal one and restricted to those substances which are in clinical development or were recently introduced.

TABLE 5.1. *Status of antidepressant development 1983*

– 17 new substances introduced for the first time since 1975
– 4 substances in preintroduction phase
– 10 substances in clinical phase III
– 15 substances in clinical phase II
– 11 substances in clinical phase I
– 24 substances under clinical study, phase unknown

Tricyclics

Several new tricyclic drugs have been studied clinically, of which four have been recently introduced. Three of these – amitriptyline-*N*-oxide, dimexiptyline and quinupramine – have typical tricyclic-like properties and are of little interest. The fourth drug, amineptine, is tricyclic in structure but contains an atypical aminoacid side-chain (Table 5.2). Amineptine produces central stimulation in animals via its inhibitory effects upon dopamine (DA) reuptake and by facilitating release of DA and noradrenaline (NA). At daily dosages of 150–200 mg amineptine is equivalent in efficacy to standard tricyclics, has an activating effect with minimal anticholinergic properties, but may need combining with a sedative anxiolytic to overcome initial side-effects of anxiety and insomnia (Kamoun 1979). Recent substantial reports of amineptine-induced cholestatic hepatitis (Bel and Girard 1981) do not encourage wide introduction of the drug.

Two successor compounds to the established tricyclics clomipramine and maprotiline are in clinical phase II (Table 5.2). Cianopramine is a highly selective inhibitor of serotonin (5-HT) reuptake, being about six times more potent than clomipramine and ten times more potent than imipramine in human blood platelets and second only to citalopram (see Table 5.4) in potency in rat brain synaptosomes. Initial clinical studies suggest antidepressant effects at much lower dosages than clomipramine and a positive inotropic effect on the heart (Gasic, Korn, and Omer 1982). Oxaprotiline is a mixture of two enantiomeric forms, of which the S(+)-enantiomer possesses the potential therapeutic properties of NA reuptake inhibition and antidepressant-like pharmacology but also the possible side-effect properties of anticholinergic and sympathomimetic activity (Nickolson and Pinder 1984). In the first major efficacy trials, anti-

TABLE 5.2. *New tricyclic antidepressants*

Drug name	Structure	Remarks
Amineptine	NH.$(CH_2)_6$.CO_2H	Introduced in France 1978. Stimulant profile; inhibits DA reuptake and releases DA and NA.
Cianopramine	CN $(CH_2)_3$.NMe_2	In phase II. Analogue of clomipramine; potent and selective inhibitor of 5-HT reuptake.
Oxaprotiline	CH_2.CH.CH_2.NHMe OH	In phase II. Analogue of maprotiline; selective inhibitor of NA reuptake.

cholinergic side-effects were similar in overall frequency and severity with oxaprotiline and amitriptyline although different in pattern (Roffman, Gould, Brewer, Lav, Sachais, Dixon, Kalzmarek, and Le Sher 1983). Neither ciano-pramine nor oxaprotiline seem likely to offer any major advantages over the standard tricyclics from which they were derived.

Selective inhibitors of 5-HT reuptake

Several highly selective inhibitors of 5-HT reuptake are ready to take the place of zimeldine, the first non-tricyclic antidepressant of this type to be introduced and which was withdrawn in 1983 (Table 5.3A and 5.3B). Most of them are at least as potent as zimeldine in inhibiting 5-HT reuptake in rat brain preparations *in vitro* and all are more selective than the standard drug of this type clomi-pramine (Diggory, Stephens, Dickinson, Moser, and Wood 1980). However, only citalopram and the tricyclic cianopramine (see Table 5.2) are more potent than clomipramine *in vivo*. Etoperidone, a close structural and pharmacological relative of trazodone (Cioli, Corradino, Piccinelli, Rocchi, and Valeri 1984), and alaproclate, which preferentially blocks 5-HT reuptake in the hippocampus and may have applications in Alzheimer's disease as well as depression (Bergman, Brane, Gottfries, Jostell, Karlsson, and Svennerholm 1983), are only weak inhibitors of 5-HT reuptake. Effective antidepressant doses found in clinical trials reflect to some extent the order of potency as 5-HT reuptake inhibitors, running from 40–60 mg daily for citalopram through 150 mg for indalpine and

TABLE 5.3A. *New antidepressants: selective inhibitors of 5-HT reuptake (introduced)*

Drug name	Structure	Remarks
Etoperidone		Introduced in Italy 1977. Trazodone analogue, weak inhibitor. Daily dosage 100–600 mg.
Indalpine		Introduced in France 1982. Daily dosage about 150 mg.
Fluvoxamine		Introduced in Switzerland 1983, daily dosage 100–300 mg. The 4-chloro analogue (clovoxamine), presently in phase III, inhibits both 5-HT and NA reuptake.

TABLE 5.3B. *New antidepressants: selective inhibitors of 5-HT reuptake (not yet introduced)*

Drug name	Structure	Remarks
Fluoxetine		In phase III. Daily dosage 40–80 mg.
Femoxetine		In phase III. Daily dosage 400–600 mg.
Paroxetine		In phase III. Daily dosage 20–80 mg.
Citalopram		In phase III. Daily dosage 40–60 mg. The most potent non-tricyclic inhibitor of 5-HT reuptake.
Alaproclate		Successor to zimeldine, in phase III. Weak inhibitor, daily dosage 100–400 mg.

100–300 mg for fluvoxamine to up to 400 mg for alaproclate and more for etoperidone, but the antidepressant dosages of fluoxetine and paroxetine are lower than might be expected. The therapeutic profiles of the new inhibitors are similar to that of zimeldine; that is, equivalent efficacy to the traditional tricyclics but with minimal anticholinergic and cardiovascular effects and in general no sedative properties (Feighner 1983). Etoperidone, however, resembles trazodone in being sedative and having a wide dosage range. Whether the safety in overdosage of the new drugs will be similar to that of zimeldine, whose only serious complication was occasional convulsions, or to the longer established safety of mianserin and nomifensin can only be determined with widespread use (Crome 1982). All of them cause gastrointestinal distress to some degree and, with the exception of the sedative etoperidone, they all cause sleep disturbances, particularly insomnia. This similarity to zimeldine in side-effect profile may lie in their common pharmacological actions, but there is as yet little evidence to suggest that the hypersensitivity reactions of zimeldine are common to antidepressants of this type.

Mianserin analogues

The antidepressant activity of mianserin has stimulated interest in structural and pharmacological analogues (Table 5.4). The postulated mechanism of

TABLE 5.4. *New antidepressants: mianserin analogues*

Drug name	Structure	Remarks
Org 3770		α_2-Antagonist without NA reuptake inhibition. In phase II, daily dose 20–40 mg.
Org 8282		No effect on reuptake or release of NA. In phase III, daily dose 6–9 mg.
Aptazapine		α_2-Antagonist without NA reuptake inhibition. Less 5-HT antagonism than Org 8282, Org 3770 or mianserin. In phase I.
Idazoxan (RX 78 1094)		Mixed α_2-antagonist and partial agonist. In phase II.

antidepressant action of mianserin is facilitation of noradrenergic transmission involving release of NA mediated by blockade of presynaptic α_2-adrenergic autoreceptors, a property which resides stereoselectively in the S(+)-enantiomer of mianserin (Nickolson and Pinder 1984). Although mianserin has additional inhibitory effects on NA reuptake *in vitro*, its 6-aza analogue Org 3770 retains only the α_2-autoreceptor antagonism also in a stereoselective manner (Nickolson and Pinder 1984). However, as with the mianserin enantiomers, Org 3770 shows no stereoselectivity in antidepressant-like activity in pharmaco-EEG in healthy volunteers, and it is likely that the racemates of both chiral drugs represent the optimal antidepressant moiety. Preliminary clinical studies with Org 3770 suggest a mianserin-like profile of antidepressant plus anxiolytic activity, sedative side-effects and an effective daily dose of 20 to 40 mg.

Org 8282 is a mianserin analogue without enantiomeric forms, since it lacks chirality at the 14b-carbon atom. Org 8282 resembles mianserin in being a potent histamine and 5-HT antagonist but has little effect *in vitro* upon release or reuptake of NA. *In vivo* it blocks some effects of the α_2-agonist clonidine and shows antidepressant-like activity in behavioural models in animals and in pharmaco-EEG in humans. Preliminary open and controlled efficacy trials suggest an antidepressant daily dose of 6–9 mg. Aptazapine is another mianserin analogue with antagonistic activity at α_2-autoreceptors. It was less active *in vitro* than mianserin in blocking NA reuptake and markedly less active as a 5-HT antagonist (Liebman, Lovell, Braunwalder, Stone, Bernard, Barbaz, Welch, Kim, Wasley, and Robson 1983). No clinical results are yet available, but aptazapine may provide a clue to the relative contribution of 5-HT antagonism and α_2-adrenoceptor blockade to the antidepressant activity of mianserin. However, the similarity of the antihistaminergic and anticholinergic properties of aptazapine and mianserin suggest that the former is unlikely to have any clinical advantage in terms of side-effects particularly sedation.

The possible therapeutic application of more specific α_2-antagonists in depression is also being investigated. The classical antagonist yohimbine, although more selective than mianserin, is rather less potent, has a variety of other receptor interactions, and is too toxic for regular clinical use. Attention has focused on the design of new centrally active α_2-autoreceptor antagonists, of which the first to reach the clinic is idazoxan (Table 5.4). Idazoxan is structurally based on the potent but non-selective α-antagonist piperoxan; it is many times more potent and selective at presynaptic α_2-autoreceptors than yohimbine and appears to be without other receptor interactions (Doxey, Roach, and Smith 1983). Intravenous or oral idazoxan fully reversed the hypotensive and sedative effects of clonidine in healthy humans, but no measures were made of the autoreceptor-mediated influence of clonidine upon NA release (Clifford and Price 1984). The anticipated antidepressant dose is 20 mg daily, but the value of idazoxan in assessing the role of specific α_2-antagonists as antidepressants is marred by reports that it also acts as a partial α_2-agonist in the CNS (Goldstein, Knobloch, and Malick 1983). A second candidate α_2-antagonist, imiloxan, which is not yet in the clinical phase, contains an additional methylene group between the benzodioxan ring and the imidazole moiety (Dye, Page, and Whiting 1983).

Drugs acting on central dopaminergic mechanisms

The introduction of nomifensin as an activating type of antidepressant whose primary mechanism of action seemed to be inhibition of DA reuptake in the brain has led to development of at least three new antidepressants which facilitate dopaminergic transmission (Table 5.5). All three drugs resemble nomifensin to some extent in being non-sedative and causing minimal anticholinergic effects, but they do produce agitation and insomnia. Whether the similarity to nomifensin will extend to its lack of cardiotoxicity and its safety in overdosage remains to be seen.

The drug most closely related to nomifensin is diclofensin, which was designed to prevent oxidative metabolism of nomifensin at the positions now occupied by chlorine atoms. Indeed, the plasma elimination half-life of diclofensin is several times that of nomifensin. Diclofensin appears to be the most potent known inhibitor of DA reuptake *in vitro*, although it also inhibits reuptake of NA and 5-HT at similar concentrations and may act *in vivo* mainly on the

TABLE 5.5 *New antidepressants: drugs acting on central dopaminergic mechanisms*

Drug name	Structure	Remarks
Minaprine	(phenyl)-pyridazine ring with Me substituent, $-NH.CH_2.CH_2.N$(morpholine, O)	Introduced in France 1980. Activating antidepressant. Inhibits DA reuptake *in vivo* but not *in vitro*.
Bupropion	(phenyl, Cl-substituted)$-CO.CHMe.NH.CMe_3$	In registration phase. Weak effects on DA reuptake. Activating antidepressant, convulsions may be a problem.
Diclofensine	tetrahydroisoquinoline with MeO, N–Me, and dichlorophenyl (Cl, Cl) substituent	The most potent known inhibitor of DA reuptake. Also inhibits reuptake of NA and 5-HT. Activating antidepressant in phase II.

noradrenergic system. Originally investigated clinically as an anti-Parkinson drug, diclofensin is now studied as an antidepressant (Omer 1982). Daily doses are somewhat lower than those of nomifensin, and diclofensin is particularly effective in neurotic-reactive depression but less so in endogenous depression. Tremor and anticholinergic effects as well as agitation and insomnia are fairly common, but lack of efficacy was the major reason for withdrawal in clinical trials. Minaprine was originally developed as a disinhibiting drug to treat withdrawn neurotic and psychotic patients, but it is now being established as an antidepressant (Biziere, Kan, Souilhac, Muyard, and Roncucci 1982). Although virtually inactive in models for DA reuptake *in vitro*, minaprine probably is active *in vivo* since it facilitates dopaminergic transmission in a similar manner to nomifensin.

The propiophenone derivative bupropion differs from other antidepressants in having no marked influence upon monoamine reuptake after acute administration and in producing no sensitivity changes in any central receptor after chronic administration (Feighner 1983). Its weak dopaminergic effects mediated by a weak inhibition of DA reuptake are probably not clinically relevant, although the high therapeutic dosage of bupropion in depression (300–750 mg daily) suggests that even modest pharmacological effects may become important in man. Bupropion has no anticholinergic or antihistaminic effects and produces no adverse cardiovascular effects. Common side-effects include agitation, insomnia, dizziness, and nausea. The occurrence of convulsions during clinical trials with an incidence of 0.5 to 1 per cent suggests that its epileptogenic potential may be a problem in clinical practice. Advantages of bupropion may include a broader spectrum of effect in that it was effective in patients who had previously failed to respond to tricyclics and was effective in both unipolar and bipolar patients.

Benzodiazepine analogues

Benzodiazepines have been investigated in depression for the same reasons as the non-tricyclic antidepressants — less cardiotoxicity, lower incidence of serious adverse effects, lack of anticholinergic effects and greater safety in overdosage. However, antidepressant activity in animal models and in man is shown not by classical benzodiazepines but by those of the triazolo or pyrazolo types (Table 5.6). Drugs such as alprazolam, adinazolam, and zometapine show a mixture of anxiolytic and antidepressant properties. Incorporation of the triazole or pyrazole moiety leads to an altered metabolic path and to drugs with a more rapid absorption and elimination; all three drugs have short half-lives and must be given in divided doses.

Alprazolam is the most potent of the three benzodiazepine analogues as an antidepressant, showing efficacy superior to placebo and equivalent to imipramine in the major six-week trial in 906 moderately depressed out-patients (Dawson, Jue, and Brogden 1984). Divided daily doses of 1–4 mg, with the major part given at bedtime, produced a claimed faster onset of action than

TABLE 5.6. *New antidepressants: benzodiazepine analogues*

Drug name	Structure	Remarks
Alprazolam		Introduced in many countries (USA 1981) for treatment of anxiety and anxiety/depression. As antidepressant, requires long-term dependence studies. Anti-depressant dosage 2–4 mg daily.
Adinazolam		In phase II. Similar profile to alprazolam. Antidepressant dosage 20–90 mg daily.
Zometapine		In phase II. Antidepressant dosage 200–400 mg daily.

imipramine with typical benzodiazepine-like side-effects of drowsiness and lethargy, but optimal doses have still to be established in depression. Alprazolam is currently registered in many countries only for the treatment of anxiety or anxiety with depression. Broadening of the indication to depression awaits the results of long-term studies in depressed patients looking at dependence, habituation, and withdrawal, although no such effects were seen in short-term efficacy trials. Adinazolam is less potent than alprazolam in animal models of depression and in contrast also shows a modest level of inhibition of NA reuptake and potentiates noradrenergic transmission (Pento 1983). Preliminary efficacy studies indicate an effective daily dose of between 20 and 90 mg given on a divided schedule, with a rapid onset of action within seven days. Side-effects included sedation, euphoria, and some anticholinergic effects, but no dependence or

withdrawal. Zometapine is the least potent of the three benzodiazepine analogues, requiring daily doses of up to 600 mg, but is rapidly absorbed and
eliminated almost unchanged in the urine. Nausea is common during zometapine
treatment, with occasional vomiting, which effects may limit its usefulness
despite a general lack of other adverse effects (Thorpe 1980*a*).

Monoamine oxidase inhibitors

The availability of monoamine oxidase inhibitors (MAOI) that discriminate
between MAO type A and type B has offered the opportunity for establishing
selective MAOI as major antidepressants (Youdim 1983). Since the monoamines
believed to be involved in depression, NA and 5-HT, are metabolized predominantly by the A-form of MAO, studies of antidepressant activity have tended to
focus on reversible selective inhibitors of MAO-A free of the cheese effect.
However, MAO activity is not the rate-limiting step in monoamine metabolic
pathways and considerable (> 80 per cent) inhibition is required before changes
in brain monoamine concentrations are evident. Irreversible inhibition of either
form of MAO over a prolonged period will, given a sufficient dose of the
inhibitor, inhibit both forms — *in vivo* selectivity is less marked than *in vitro*
selectivity. Both types of inhibitor may therefore have antidepressant potential.
However, of the compounds listed in Table 5.7, only pirlindole has established
efficacy in placebo-controlled trials; the rest have either not been studied in
depressed patients or the results so far are equivocal. Pirlindole is a tetracyclic
inhibitor of MAO-A, structurally related to the harmala alkaloids and with
additional inhibiting effects on NA reuptake. Placebo-controlled trials in endogenous depression have established an effective daily dose of 300 mg, with
a dose range in all types of depression of 75 to 300 mg. Pirlindole has been
given to cardiac patients without untoward effect. The most frequent side-
effects are extrapyramidal in nature — tremor and akathisia — with also hypo-
tension, hypersalivation, and insomnia (Thorpe 1980*b*). Toloxatone and
cimoxatone are members of a series of oxazolidinone derivatives developed as
reversible and selective inhibitors of MAO-A, although other members of the
same series are selective for MAO-B. Cimoxatone is more potent than toloxatone
and is equipotent with, though less selective than, the known antidepressant
MAO-A inhibitor clorgyline. No reports are avilable on the antidepressant
activity of these drugs; toloxatone appeared to be safe in healthy volunteers
after intravenous or oral administration, but was rapidly absorbed and eliminated with a half-life of less than two hours (Benedetti, Rovei, Dencke, Nagy,
and Johansson 1982). The benzamide derivative moclobemide is a short-acting
reversible MAO-A inhibitor which also has an extremely rapid elimination in
man with a plasma half-life of about 1 h. Open and controlled efficacy trials
have suggested antidepressant efficacy equivalent to amitriptyline at doses of
100 to 400 mg daily and a possible lack of interaction with tyramine (Raaflaub,
Haefelfinger, and Trautman 1984). However, no selective MAO-A inhibitor has
yet emerged that is entirely free of the cheese effect, perhaps because intestinal

TABLE 5.7. *New antidepressants: selective inhibitors of monoamine oxidase*

Drug name	Structure	Remarks
Pirlindole		Short-acting, reversible inhibitor of MAO-A. Introduced in USSR in 1980, phase III in western Europe. Daily dosage 75–300 mg.
Toloxatone ($R_1=R_2=H$, $R_3=Me$) Cimoxatone ($R_1=Me$, R_2=3-cyano-benzyloxy, $R_3=H$)		Short-acting, reversible inhibitors of MAO-A. Cimoxatone (phase I) is more potent and MAO-A selective than toloxatone (phase II).
Moclobemide		Short-acting, reversible inhibitor of MAO-A. In phase II. Daily dosage 100–400 mg.
Selegiline		Also known as L-deprenyl. Irreversible suicide inhibitor of MAO-B. Introduced in many countries as adjunct to L-DOPA in Parkinsonism. In phase II in depression. No cheese effect.
MDL 72145		Irreversible suicide inhibitor of MAO-B. Not metabolized to amphetamine derivatives. In phase I. No cheese effect.

MAO responsible for tyramine oxidation is of the A-type. Two irreversible, so-called 'suicide', inhibitors of MAO-B are being investigated as antidepressants, both of which lack the cheese effect (Table 5.7). Unlike the short-acting reversible MAO–A inhibitors these drugs produce long-lasting MAO inhibition after single doses. Selegiline, which is the R(−)-enantiomer of *N*-propynylmethamphetamine and is also known as L-deprenyl, is used principally as an adjunct to L-DOPA therapy in Parkinson's disease but has also antidepressant-like properties in animals. Clinical trials in depression have given equivocal results (Nickolson and Pinder 1984). Selegiline certainly potentiated the antidepressant effects of 5-hydroxytryptophan and seemed to be effective alone in open trials, but was indistinguishable from placebo in a double-blind trial in 31 patients with primary depressive disorders. The most recent placebo-controlled trial showed significantly better efficacy for selegiline 15 mg daily over six weeks (Mendlewicz and Youdim 1983). Selegiline resembled the classical non-selective MAO in producing a better response in patients lacking endogenous features, and response was associated with a greater than 90 per cent inhibition of total platelet MAO. Selegiline inhibits reuptake of NA and 5-HT to some extent and is metabolized in man to methamphetamine and amphetamine, which complicates interpretation of its antidepressant activity in terms solely of MAO-B inhibition (Nickolson and Pinder 1984). The irreversible MAO-B inhibitor MDL 72145, a derivative of 3-fluoroallylamine, is not metabolized to amphetamine derivatives and lacks sympathomimetic activity or effects upon monoamine-reuptake. Following single doses of 4 to 10 mg to healthy volunteers, MDL 72145 produced greater than 90 per cent inhibition of MAO-B in the absence of cardiovascular and central effects or interaction with tyramine (Alken, Palfreyman, Brown, Davies, Lewis, and Schechter 1984). No information is available on the antidepressant effects of MDL 72145.

It is still unclear whether any of the selective MAOI will offer a therapeutic advantage over the non-selective drugs in terms of efficacy in all types of depression. The MAO-A inhibitor pirlindole seems to be effective in endogenous depression but the MAO-B inhibitors less so. Selective inhibitors lacking the cheese effect may offer the opportunity of safe combination therapy with other antidepressants including both NA and 5-HT reuptake inhibitors (Marley and Wozniak 1983). Furthermore, since amitryptyline appears to diminish greatly the pressor response to tyramine in patients treated with classical MAOI (Pare, Hallstrom, Kline, and Cooper 1982) there may be a general case for revising the use of combined treatment with MAOI as one way of achieving a broader spectrum of antidepressant effects.

NEW PHARMACOLOGICAL APPROACHES TO THE TREATMENT OF DEPRESSION

The effects of antidepressants on central monoamine availability are immediate whereas clinical improvement may take some weeks, while several highly effective reuptake inhibitors immediately raise central levels of monoamines but are not known to be antidepressant (Sugrue 1983). Although the concept of altered receptor sensitivity in depression has been introduced to explain such discrepancies, acute effects on monoamine availability still provide a useful basis for the detection and selection of potential antidepressants. The search for new drugs includes both single·substances and combinations which might have mutual additive effects on a single neurotransmitter and thereby potentiate transmission. Studies of receptor sensitivity have also suggested potential new ways to treat depression.

Transmitter potentiation

Appreciation of the NA-releasing properties of mianserin has led not only to the development of more potent and specific α_2-antagonists but to a revival of interest in alternative ways of increasing synaptic availability of NA (Table 5.8). Release of NA is controlled presynaptically by a negative feedback mechanism triggered by the activation of α_2-autoreceptors and by a positive feedback mechanism operating at lower synaptic NA concentrations which is triggered by activation of β_2-adrenoceptors (Langer 1980). Combination of a β_2-agonist like salbutamol with an α_2-antagonist like mianserin could lead to more marked effects upon NA release. The availability of more potent and specific α_2-antagonists and the introduction into β_2-agonists of presynaptic selectivity could lead to further potentiation. It also seems quite feasible to design into the same molecule the attributes of α_2-antagonism and β_2-agonism, given the present advanced state of knowledge regarding structure-activity relationships for the two receptors. While the negative feedback mechanism controlling NA release operates by restriction of calcium availability, the positive feedback mechanism appears to be mediated through an increase of cyclic AMP(cAMP) levels in noradrenergic nerve endings. cAMP is also coupled to the postsynaptic noradrenergic receptor, and the increased cAMP produced during release and postsynaptic stimulation is degraded by the enzyme cAMP phosphodiesterase. Centrally active phosphodiesterase inhibitors, exemplified by rolipram, enhance the release of NA via presynaptic mechanisms and potentiate its postsynaptic action by preventing degradation of cAMP coupled to the postsynaptic receptor. As might be expected, phosphodiesterase inhibitors produce rapid desensitization of β-adrenoceptors in rat brain, while rolipram appears to have antidepressant effects in man (Wachtel 1983). Release of 5-HT is also not controlled entirely by 5-HT autoreceptors but is additionally under the influence of α_2-adrenoceptors located presynaptically on the serotonergic neurons, activation of which by α_2-agonists inhibits 5-HT release (Maura and Raiteri 1984). 5-HT autoreceptors are not blocked by most 5-HT antagonists such as mianserin and are believed to be 5-HT$_1$ in nature, but mianserin does stimulate release of

TABLE 5.8. *Some possibilities for transmitter potentiation*

Transmitter	Presynaptic effect	Postsynaptic effect	Examples
NA	Phosphodiesterase inhibition	Phosphodiesterase inhibition	Rolipram
NA	α_2-antagonism β_2-agonism	— —	Mianserin Salbutamol
5-HT	5-HT$_1$-antagonism α_2-antagonism	— —	Methiothepin Mianserin

5-HT in rat brain by blocking α_2-adrenoceptors located on 5-HT neurons. Methiothepin and quipazine are the only examples of 5-HT autoreceptor antagonists, but are not specific and have additional postsynaptic effects. Potent and specific 5-HT_1 antagonists selective for presynaptic receptors combined with α_2-antagonists could lead to enhanced serotonergic transmission and possibly to enhanced antidepressant activity (Table 5.8). In recent studies (Maura and Raiteri 1984) methiothepin produced cortical 5-HT autoreceptor supersensitivity following chronic administration to rats.

Receptor sensitivity

Chronic antidepressant treatment in animals produces a variety of adaptive changes in the sensitivity of central monoaminergic receptors, and there is a growing awareness that such changes have more to do with the mechanism of action of antidepressants than do acute effects upon reuptake, storage, synthesis, and release (Sugrue 1983). The pattern of changes in functional response and density of central receptors after chronic administration of antidepressants is shown in Table 5.9, which is a gross oversimplification since there appears to be no common mechanism of antidepressant action and several individual drugs fall outside the general trend. Mianserin, for example, produces α_2-supersensitivity and does not alter β-adrenoceptor binding upon chronic administration, while bupropion appears not to influence receptor sensitivity. Differences in receptor sensitivity have also been observed between depressive patients and normals, and such differences may normalize during treatment. The differences are far from consistent, particularly for adrenoceptors, where postsynaptic α_2-function certainly declines but changes in presynaptic α_2-function and density are less clear; α_2-agonist binding is increased in depression but α_2-antagonist binding is no different from normals (Table 5.9).

Studies of receptor sensitivity have suggested ways in which antidepressant treatment might be utilized to induce adaptive changes and thereby perhaps bring about a faster onset of action. It has been suggested that rapid downregulation of 5-HT_2 receptor binding, as occurs in rat brain during combined administration of tricyclic antidepressants and α_2-antagonists, could provide a faster onset of clinical antidepressant action (Crews, Scott, and Shorstein 1983). However, a faster onset of action is not associated with either mianserin or amoxapine, both of which decrease 5-HT_2 receptor binding after single doses in rats (Helmeste and Tang 1983). Furthermore, mianserin might have been expected to be the ideal drug for this purpose, combining α_2-antagonism and downregulation of 5-HT_2 receptors in the same molecule. The hypothesis may be better tested by giving combined treatment of a tricyclic or mianserin with a potent and specific α_2-antagonist like idazoxan. Increased sensitivity of central 5-HT receptors is induced by chronic administration of most antidepressants and can be enhanced rapidly by addition of lithium. Depressed patients who had failed to respond to full doses of tricyclics or mianserin showed significant improvement within 48 h of lithium being added to their treatment (De

TABLE 5.9. *Receptor sensitivity and antidepressants*

(a) *Changes in rat brain receptors during chronic antidepressant treatment*

	5-HT	α_1	α_2	β
Functional response	+	+	–	–
Receptor density	–	0	0	–

(b) *Differences in depressed patients compared with normals*

	5HT	α_1	α_2	β
Functional response	–	±	–	±
Receptor density	?	?	+,0	+

(+) = increased, (–) = decreased, (0) = no change, (?) = no information.

Montigny, Cournoyer, Morissette, Langlois, and Caillé 1983; Heninger, Charney, and Sternberg 1983). Although lithium is now accepted as having acute anti-depressant effects as well as prophylactic action, there is no evidence that it can alone produce a more rapid improvement than tricyclics or mianserin.

β-Adrenoceptor density in rat brain can be rapidly decreased by antidepressant administration together with α_2-antagonists or β-agonists (U'Prichard and Enna 1979; Scott and Crews 1983). No clinical studies have been reported on the effects of such combined treatment in depression, although the α_2-antagonist mianserin alone neither induces faster or any downregulation in β-adrenoceptors nor more rapid therapeutic effects. However, the more potent and specific α_2-antagonist imiloxan downregulates rat cortical β-adrenoceptor density more rapidly than tricyclic antidepressants (Dye *et al.* 1983). The β-agonist salbutamol may have antidepressant activity and certainly reduces functional β-adrenoceptor sensitivity in depressed patients (Lerer, Epstein, and Belmaker 1981). Central α_1-adrenoceptors might be expected to become supersensitive after administration of α_1-antagonists like prazosin, but although most anti-depressants are modest α_1-antagonists and do produce α_1-supersensitivity after chronic treatment, there is no evidence that prazosin-like drugs are effective in depression. As far as α_2-adrenoceptors are concerned, tricyclic antidepressants produce subsensitivity after chronic administration while mianserin causes supersensitivity (Sugrue 1983). Clonidine, which rapidly downregulates α_2-adrenoceptors in human platelets (Brodde, Anlauf, Graben and Bock 1982), appears to be without antidepressant properties. It will be interesting to see whether potent and specific α_2-antagonists like idazoxan and imiloxan will be antidepressant since they rapidly downregulate β-adrenoceptors and are likely to upregulate rapidly presynaptic α_2-adrenoceptors.

CONCLUSION

The pharmacotherapy of depression is still dominated by drugs which in acute doses raise central synaptic levels of monoamines. Although studies of receptor adaptation during chronic antidepressant treatment have provided a better analogy to the therapeutic actions of the drugs, antidepressants of the near future will remain firmly based upon traditional concepts of monoamine availability. A better understanding of the biological basis for depression in humans might help us to design better antidepressants, but clinical research is also to a large extent devoted to monoamines. The introduction of new drugs possessing a specificity of pharmacological action may help to delineate better the mechanisms involved. Nevertheless, several possibilities for improved therapy with already available drugs do exist, based upon pharmacological considerations, and some seem worthy of a clinical trial.

The search for a common mechanism of antidepressant action has also tended to focus upon monoamines. Such a search may seem futile when we are not sure that depression is a homogeneous entity by either diagnostic or biochemical criteria. However, the common mechanism may not lie with monoamines at all but rather with factors such as cerebral permeability, circadian rhythms, and availability of neuropeptide cotransmitters, all of which have recently been implicated as being influenced by antidepressant treatment. In the longer-term, we should not be too surprised if new antidepressant therapies are developed which seem to bear little relation to the uptake blockers and receptor modifiers of today.

REFERENCES

Adams, P. C., Reid, M. M., Robinson, A., Vishu, M. C., and Livingston, M. (1983). Blood dyscrasias and mianserin. *Post-grad. med. J.* **59**, 31-3.

Alken, R. G., Palfreyman, M. E., Brown, M. J., Davies, D. S., Lewis, P. I., and Schechter, P. J. (1984). Selective inhibition of MAO type B in normal volunteers by MDL 72145. *Br. J. clin. Pharmac.* **17**, 615-16.

Bel, A. and Girard, D. (1981). Hepatite, cholestase et amineptine. *Sem. Hôp. Paris* **57**, 1992-6.

Benedetti, M. S., Rovei, V., Dencke, S. I., Nagy, A., and Johansson, L. (1982). Pharmacokinetics of toloxatone in man following intravenous and oral administration. *Arzneimittel-Forschung* **32**, 276-9.

Bergman, I., Brane, G., Gottfries, C. G., Jostell, K. G., Karlsson, I., and Svennerholm, L. (1983). Alaproclate. A pharmacokinetic and biochemical study in patients with dementia of the Alzheimer type. *Psychopharmacology* **80**, 279-83.

Biziere, K., Kan, J. P., Souilhac, I., Muyard, J. P., and Roncucci, R. (1982). Pharmacological evaluation of minaprine dihydrochloride, a new psychotropic drug. *Arzneimittel-Forschung* **32**, 824-31.

Blackwell, B. (1981). Adverse effects of antidepressant drugs. Part 1: Monoamine oxidase inhibitors and tricyclics; Part 2: Second generation antidepressants and rational decision making in antidepressant therapy. *Drugs* 21, 201–19, 273–82.

Brodde, O. E., Anlauf, M., Graben, N., and Bock, K. D. (1982). *In vitro* and *in vivo* down regulation of human platelet α_2-adrenoceptors by clonidine. *Eur. J. Pharmac.* 23, 403–9.

Cioli, V., Corradino, C., Piccinelli, D., Rocchi, M. G., and Valeri, P. (1984). A comparative pharmacological study of trazodone, etoperidone and 1-(m-chlorophenyl)piperazine. *Pharmac. Res. Comm.* 16, 85–101.

Clifford, J. M. and Price, M. (1984). The reversal of some clonidine-induced effects by single oral doses of idazoxan, an α_2-adrenoceptor antagonist. *Br. J. clin. Pharmac.* 17, 602 p.

Crews, F. T., Scott, J. A., and Shorstein, N. H. (1983). Rapid downregulation of serotonin$_2$ receptor binding during combined administration of tricyclic antidepressant drugs and α_2-antagonists. *Neuropharmacology* 22, 1203–9.

Crome, P. (1982). Antidepressant overdosage. *Drugs* 23, 431–61.

Dawson, G. W., Jue, S. G., and Brogden, R. N. (1984). Alprazolam. A review of its pharmacodynamic properties and efficacy in the treatment of anxiety and depression. *Drugs* 27, 132–47.

De Montigny, C., Cournoyer, G., Morissette, R., Langlois, R., and Caillé, G. (1983). Lithium carbonate addition in tricyclic antidepressant-resistant unipolar depression. *Arch. gen. Psychiat.* 40, 1327–34.

Diggory, G. L., Stephens, R. J. Dickison, S. E., Moser, P., and Wood, M. D. (1980). Behavioural and neurochemical properties of Wy 25093 in rodents. *Archs. int. Pharmacodyn. Ther.* 248, 86–104.

Doxey, J. C., Roach, A. G., and Smith, C. F. C. (1983). Studies on RX 781094. A selective, potent and specific antagonist of α_2-adrenoceptors. *Br. J. Pharmac.* 78, 489–505.

Dye, A., Page, C. M. and Whiting, R. L. (1983). The time course of rat cerebro-cortical β-adrenoceptor down-regulation following RS–21361 and desmethyl-imipramine treatment. *Br. J. Pharmac.* 80, 665P.

Feighner, J. P. (1983). The new generation of antidepressants. *J. clin. Psychiat.* 44 (5, sect. 2), 49–55.

Gasic, S., Korn, A., and Omer, L. M. O. (1982). Cardiocirculatory effects of Ro 11–2465, a selective 5-HT uptake inhibitor, in healthy volunteers. *Eur. J. clin. Pharmac.* 21, 357–61.

Goldstein, J. M., Knobloch, L. C., and Malick, J. B. (1983). Electro-physiological demonstration of both α_2-agonist and antagonist properties of RX 781094. *Eur. J. Pharmac.* 91, 101–5.

Helmeste, D. M. and Tang, S. W. (1983). Unusual effects of antidepressants and neuroleptics on S$_2$-serotoninergic receptors. *Life Sci.* 33, 2527–33.

Heninger, G. R., Charney, D. S., and Sternberg, D. E. (1983). Lithium carbonate augmentation of antidepressant treatment. *Arch. gen. Psychiat.* 40, 1335–42.

Hollister, L. E. (1981). Current antidepressant drugs. Their clinical use. *Drugs* 22, 129–52.

Janowsky, D., Curtis, G., Zisook, S., Kuhn, K., Kesovsky, K., and Le Winter, M. (1983). Trazodone-aggravated ventricular arrhythmias. *J. clin. Psychopharmac.* 3, 372–6.

Kamoun, A. (1979). L'amineptine: synthèse des travaux cliniques. *L'Encéphale* 5, 721–35.

Langer, S. Z. (1980). Presynaptic regulation of the release of catecholamines. *Pharmac. Rev.* 32, 337–62.

Lerer, B., Epstein, R. P., and Belmaker, R. H. (1981). Subsensitivity of human β-adrenergic adenylate cyclase after salbutamol treatment of depression. *Psychopharmacology* **75**, 169–72.

Liebman, J. M., Lovell, R. A., Braunwalder, A., Stone, G., Bernard, P., Barbaz, B., Welch, J., Kim, H. S., Wasley, J. W. F., and Robson, R. D. (1983). CGS 7525 A. A new centrally active α₂-adrenoceptor antagonist. *Life Sci.* **32**, 355–63.

Litovitz, T. L. and Troutman, W. G. (1983). Amoxapine overdose. Seizures and fatalities. *J. Am. med. Assoc.* **250**, 1069–71.

Lylloff, K., Jersild, C., Bacher, T., and Slot,). (1982). Massive intravascular haemolysis during treatment with nomifensin. *Lancet* **2**, 41.

Marley, E. and Wozniak, K. M. (1983). Clinical and experimental aspects of interactions between amine oxidase inhibitors and amine reuptake inhibitors. *Psychol. Med.* **13**, 735–49.

Maura, G. and Raiteri, M. (1984). Functional evidence that chronic drugs induce adaptive changes of central autoreceptors regulating serotonin release. *Eur. J. Pharmac.* **97**, 309–13.

Mendlewicz, J. and Youdim, M. S. H. (1983). L-Deprenil, a selective monoamine oxidase type B inhibitor in the treatment of depression: A double-blind evaluation. *Br. J. Psychiat.* **142**, 508–11.

Nickolson, V. J. and Pinder, R. M. (1984). Antidepressant drugs: chiral stereo-isomers. In *Handbook of stereoisomers: Drugs in Psychopharmacology* (ed. D. F. Smith), pp. 215–40. CRC Press, Boca Raton.

Omer, L. M. O. (1982). Pilot trials with diclofensin, a new psychoactive drug, in depressed patients. *Int. J. clin. Pharmac., Ther. & Tox.* **20**, 320–6.

Pare, C. M. B., Hallstrom, C., Kline, N., and Cooper, T. B. (1982). Will ami-triptyline prevent the cheese reaction of monoamine oxidase inhibitors? *Lancet* **2** 183–6.

Pento, J. T. (1983). Adinazolam. *Drugs of the Future* **8**, 87–91.

Raaflaub, J., Haefelfinger, P., and Trautman, K. H. (1984). Single-dose pharma-cokinetics of the MAO-inhibitor moclobemide in man. *Arzneimittel-Forschung* **34**, 80–2.

Roffman, M., Gould, E., Brewer, S., Lau, H., Sachais, B., Dixon, N., Kaczmarek, L., and Le Sher, A. (1983). Comparative anticholinergic activity of oxa-protiline and amitriptyline. *Drug Dev. Res.* **3**, 561–6.

Scher, M., Krieger, J. N., and Juergens, S. (1983). Trazodone and priapism. *Am. J. Psychiat.* **140**, 1362–3.

Scott, J. S. and Crews, F. T. (1983). Rapid decrease in rat brain β-adrenergic receptor binding during combined antidepressant and α₂-antagonist treatment. *J. Pharmac. exp. Ther.* **224**, 640–6.

Sugrue, M. F. (1983). Chronic antidepressant therapy and associated changes in central monoaminergic functioning. *Pharmac. & Ther.* **21**, 1–33.

Thorpe, P. J. (1980a). Zometapine. *Drugs of the Future* **5**, 514–15.

—— (1980b). Pirlindole. *Drugs of the Future* **5**, 39–41 (see also 7, 61 and 8, 68).

U'Prichard, D. C. and Enna, S. J. (1979). *In vitro* modulation of CNS β-receptor number by antidepressants and β-agonists. *Eur. J. Pharmac.* **59**, 297–301.

Wachtel, H. (1983). Potential antidepressant activity of rolipram and other selective cyclic adenosine 3′,5′-monophosphate phosphodiesterase inhibitors. *Neuropharmacology* **22**, 267–72.

Youdim, M. B. H. (1983). Implications of MAO-A and MAO-B inhibition for antidepressant therapy. *Mod. Prob. Pharmacopsychiat.* **19**, 63–74.

PART 2
Anxiolytics

6

Anxiolytics in society

ANTHONY W. CLARE

INTRODUCTION

The term 'anxiolytic' has all the seductive charm of the jargon word that appears to be translucently clear but in fact is as semantically obscure as it is etymologically ugly. At first glance it would seem perfectly comprehensible – anxiolytic, meaning to lyse or dissolve anxiety. But what is anxiety? At the end of a lengthy and scholarly analysis of the Latin and Greek origins of the term, its French, German, Italian, and Spanish equivalents, psychodynamic formulations and phenomenological constructions, and having apologized for his failure to search the literature of Russia, Scandinavia, Japan, Holland, and many other countries, Sir Aubrey Lewis concluded that while 'many voices proclaim that anxiety is the alpha and omega of psychopathology' there are even more voices insisting 'that anxiety means what they choose it to mean' (Lewis 1967). For my purposes, I borrow heavily on Lewis's own definition of anxiety as an emotional state with the subjectively experienced quality of fear or a closely related emotion, which is unpleasant, is directed towards the future, in which there is either no recognizable threat or the threat is, by reasonable standards, out of proportion to the emotion it seemingly evokes, there are subjective bodily discomforts during the period of the anxiety and there are manifest bodily disturbances. Anxiety may be normal, mild or severe, episodic or persistent, due to physical disease, may accompany other features of mental disorder, or be alone and may, for the duration of the attack, affect perception and memory or may leave them intact.

ANXIETY IN SOCIETY

But anxiety, like poverty, has always been with us. Most of us are familiar with current community and general practice findings which suggest that minor affective disorders, characterized by anxiety and depression, are common and may account for up to 14 per cent of general practice consultations (Shepherd *et al.* 1981). However, anxiety as a presenting complaint was not exactly unknown to the predecessors of today's GP.

Recently, the manuscript notebooks of Richard Napier, a clergyman and astrological physician who treated over two thousand mentally-disturbed patients between 1597 and 1634 have been explored (MacDonald 1981) and a vivid picture of the symptoms and complaints presented by patients of that time has been provided. As MacDonald reminds us, seventeenth-century people were as convinced as we are that social and psychological distress disturbed the minds and corroded the health of its victims. Doctors, astrologers, preachers, and philosophers drew up almost identical lists of commonplace misfortune allegedly imperilling the mental health of ordinary people. Over 800 of the troubled people Napier treated had suffered some terrifying or distressing experience. The most common stresses were family conflicts, lovers' quarrels, disputes with neighbours, bereavement, fear of poverty, and desperate need. Table 6.1 shows the symptoms singled out for special attention either because preliminary counts showed that they were very numerous or because contemporary literature made it plain that they were important signs of mental disorder. Examination of the meaning of such terms as 'Troubled in mind', 'Light-headed' and 'Fearful' confirms that symptoms we commonly associate with anxiety were included. Many of the examples of melancholy fear that Robert Burton provides in *The Anatomy of Melancholy* (Burton 1621) are common anxieties that troubled psychologically healthy men and women as well (Table 6.2). The fears complained of by Napier's patients, fears about devils, death, illness, accident, disgrace, robbery, and witches, were fears experienced by almost everybody at least occasionally. Exaggeration of fears and dangers was a common symptom of mental ill-health according to Baxter's *A Christian Directory*, published in 1673 (Table 6.3). Like Burton, Baxter was a clergyman with medical training but whereas Burton drew upon all the relevant medical texts of his time and earlier, Baxter drew almost completely on his own experience as the only person with some medical knowledge in a rural district where he had

TABLE 6.1. *Symptoms presented by patients to Richard Napier (1559–1634)*

Symptom	Consultations	Per cent
Troubled in mind	794	32.0
Melancholy	493	19.9
Mopishness	377	15.2
Light-headed	372	15.0
All sensory symptoms	330	13.3
Took grief	328	13.2
Fearful	305	12.3
All religious symptoms	293	11.8
Moodiness	194	7.8
Simply sad	182	7.3

Michael MacDonald, *Mystical Bedlam* (1981).

TABLE 6.2. *Symptoms of melancholy according to Burton*

By type of disorder	Symptoms in the body	Symptoms in the mind
Common	Ill Digestion Wind Dry Brains Palpitations Heaviness of Heart	Fear Without Cause Restless Thoughts Vain Imaginings
Hypochondriacal Melancholy	Rumbling in Guts Shortness of Wind Cold Sweat Belly Ache	Anxiety Troublesome

TABLE 6.3. *Symptoms of melancholy according to Baxter*

Common symptoms	Occasional symptoms
Exaggeration of fears and dangers	Ruminations
Gloomy mood and frequent weeping	Circularity and confusion of thought
Self-reproach regarding cheerfulness	Inaction; tendency to keep to bed
Self-accusations	Obsessive scruples, rituals, prohibitions
Despair regarding future salvation	Accusatory hallucinations
Identification with others' miseries	Coprolalic and blasphemous urges
Belief in the uniqueness of own case	Intense guilt over blasphemies
Rejection of comforting attention	Delusions of demonic possession
Conscience is punitive	Hallucinations, visual
Loss of religious beliefs and habits	Suicidal tendencies
Peevishness and resentment	Paranoid ideation
Avoidance of company	Mutism
Inability to control own thoughts	Loss of insight
	Relapses of intransigence

something of a reputation as someone able to help depressed persons and in consequence received patients from all over the country. Murphy (1982), comparing Burton's and Baxter's clinical descriptions, draws attention to the fact that the earlier description has a markedly somatic emphasis and virtual absence of mention of exaggerated guilt feelings whereas the symptoms described by Baxter involve several aspects of self-accusation familiar to the twentieth-century clinician. But both descriptions confirm the popularity of anxiety and fearfulness as symptoms of psychological distress.

The eighteenth and nineteenth centuries saw no diminution in interest in the prevalence and psychopathology of anxiety. By the end of the nineteenth century, the new psychoanalytical movement had taken anxiety neurosis as one of the core syndromes of the 'psychoneuroses' and, by the early part of the century, the foundations were being laid for what was to prove an unstable concept, namely 'psychosomatic disease', in which anxiety was identified as a significant causal factor in a variety of physical diseases, including peptic ulceration, hypertension, asthma, colitis and rheumatoid arthritis.

ANXIOLYTICS IN SOCIETY

Naper and his seventeenth-century contemporaries, employed an Arabic concoction of rhubarb, senna, and myrobalans to treat the troubled mind, which it appeared to do by purging the patients' bowels! Trade expansion in the seventeenth century introduced a wealth of organic medicines into English practice, while tobacco was endorsed by Burton for its tranquillizing and healing effects. In truth, however, the only pharmaceuticals which consistently provided patients with mental relief were the opiates which were freely administered as opium grains, unguents, and laudanum and were recommended as soporifics and analgesics. According to MacDonald, opiates are mentioned in only 8.2 per cent of Napier's consultations with melancholy patients, but they feature in 16.1 per cent of his sessions with madmen and lunatics, 21.6 per cent of his consultations with distracted people and in 18.4 per cent of his consultations with so-called light-headed patients. MacDonald adds that 'A similar pattern of prescription may be found in the practice books of other seventeenth-century physicians'.

Berridge's review of nineteenth-century opium use reveals the extent to which opiate use at that time had become endemic. Up to 1868, opiates were available over-the-counter without any form of restriction.

Acceptance of the drug went so far as to encourage enterprising farmers, doctors and market gardeners to experiment with the cultivation of a British variety . . . It was accepted that opiate use on a regular and sustained basis was endemic among a large proportion of the labouring population. Indeed the concept of addiction had little social meaning in a situation where many people were undoubtedly dependent but unconscious of the fact until supplies were for one reason or another curtailed, while others took the drug for a host of minor ailments — toothache, bruises, earache, sleeplessness — for which medical aid was unobtainable.

Berridge (1977)

Edwards, commenting on such a situation, pointedly observes that 'what counts as a problem' is as much 'a process of evolution as the evolution of use patterns and related morbidities and mortalities' (Edwards 1981). Today, there is much concern expressed regarding an apparent epidemic of tranquillizers over-use, abuse, and dependence, and of alcohol consumption and misuse. Taking alcohol first, the scale of ethyl-alcohol consumption in Britain can be seen to be enormous if compared to, for instance, that of medically legitimated drugs and medicines (Taylor 1981). The most frequently prescribed group of psychotropics, namely the benzodiazepine tranquillizers, accounted for some 30 million scripts filled in 1979. The cost to the NHS was a little over £30 million. In the same year, the British drank 40 million proof gallons of spirits, 1500 million gallons of beer and 100 million gallons of wine. This is equivalent to over 17 pints of absolute (pure) alcohol for every individual aged over 15 in the country. The cost to the public was almost £9000 million.

Between 1950 and 1976, the annual per capita consumption of alcohol rose from 5.2 litres to 9.7 litres per head. Such a trend has been accompanied by equally dramatic increases in alcohol-related conditions and problems. Between 1950 and 1977 the numbers of offences for drunkenness rose from 47 717 (14 per 1000) to 108 871 (27.9 per 1000). Cirrhosis deaths per million rose from 23 to 37 between 1950 and 1975, drinking and driving prosecutions over the ten years 1966-76 from just over 10 000 cases to approximately 60 000, while the number of premature deaths associated with alcohol use is somewhere in the order of between 5000 and 10 000 per annum (Taylor 1981). In March 1982 values, the total social and health costs of alcoholism to Britain have been estimated as lying somewhere between £698 million and £1064 million (Maynard and Kennan 1981) but, as an editorial in the *British Journal of Addiction* recently pointed out, 'the costs in suffering which lie behind these figures defy any easy reckoning' (Editorial 1982).

While the Government is concerned that alcohol misuse may be costing in excess of £1000 million, it is not that concerned, for the very good reason that the estimated figures for consumer expenditure on beer in 1981 are £6361 million, and on wine and spirits for the same year £4983 million. The net tax accruing from that £11 344 million is in the region of £4000 million. Add to the benefits 70 000 jobs provided by the brewing, distilling and alcohol sales business, and the £1000 million earned in exports, and you may begin to see why the well-founded medical and social arguments in favour of curbing the growth of alcohol consumption do not cut quite as much ice with our political masters as one might have anticipated.

The status of alcohol as an anxiolytic is not conclusively established although the idea that individuals drink to relieve anxiety is commonly held. Research into the hypothesis that alcohol reduces tension has actually produced contradictory findings with evidence that alcohol can either reduce tension (Hodgson *et al.* 1979) or increase it (Stockwell *et al.* 1982). However, as has recently been pointed out, one problem is that tension has been taken to mean almost any unpleasant mood state (Smail *et al.* 1984). Phobic alcoholics report that alcohol helps them cope in feared situations (Smail *et al.* 1984) but there is also evidence that phobic symptoms not only precede heavy drinking but may facilitate the development of alcoholism (Stockwell *et al.* 1984). There is some support for the view that some alcoholics manifest a high level of anxiety and it has been suggested that those who drink particularly for the psychotropic effects exercised by alcohol are especially prone to develop dependence, and encounter other alcohol-related problems (Edwards, Hensman, Chandler, and Peto 1972). However, as these workers pointed out, using alcohol 'to relax', 'to feel good', for its tranquillizing, antidepressant, or disinhibiting effects may well be determined in part by individual and group expectation, and the notion of 'personal' motivation needs to be anatomized.

As Paul Williams has pointed out, the last two decades have seen large increases in the number of psychotropic drugs that are prescribed and dispensed each year (Williams 1981). The scale of the increases are well known and are merely summarized here. In England and Wales, between 1965 and 1970, there was a 19 per cent increase in the prescribing of psychotropic drugs (Parish 1971). Prescribing of non-barbiturate hypnotics increased by 145 per cent, tranquillizers by 59 per cent and antidepressant prescribing by 83 per cent. The prescribing of barbiturate hypnotics fell by 24 per cent and stimulants and appetite suppressants by 36 per cent. Williams (1981) examined the position for the period 1970-5 and found that, taken as a whole, psychotropic drug prescribing had increased by 8 per cent over the study years, a slower rate of increase than in the previous five years and less than the increase, 15 per cent, in the prescribing of non-psychotropic drugs over the same period. There was a 45 per cent decrease in the prescription of barbiturate hypnotics and a 47 per cent increase in the prescription of non-barbiturate hypnotics. The trends for tranquillizer and antidepressant prescribing were very similar to each other with increases of 28 and 32 per cent respectively. In view of the remarkable fall in barbiturate, appetite suppressant, and stimulant prescribing, as well as the more publicized rise in non-barbiturate psychotropic drug prescribing, there may well be substance in Fry's claim that 'drug therapy has changed remarkably in content but less remarkably in volume', and that in respect of the total volume of prescriptions for psychotropic drugs in the NHS over the past 30 years 'there has been no great change' (Fry 1982). More recent figures, suggest a levelling-out and even a perceptible fall in the number of prescriptions filled for benzo-diazepines while the downward trend for barbiturate prescribing continues (Fig. 4.1).

At the present time, it is estimated that about 10 per cent of adults in the UK consume a psychotropic drug during any one year and that about 15 per cent of all prescriptions written by GPs are for psychotropic substances. Similar figures have been obtained from surveys in the United States. The US National Survey of Psychotherapeutic Drug Use reported that about 14 per cent of women and 7.5 per cent of men had used a medically prescribed antianxiety agent one or more times during the year prior to the interview (Mellinger and Balter 1981). It is important to put these usage figures into a context of social psychotropic use. Approximately 75 per cent of the adult population drink alcohol regularly while 40 per cent are regular smokers.

The use of tranquillizers has been criticized on at least three grounds (Williams and Clare 1979). First, such prescribing is criticized on clinical grounds. General

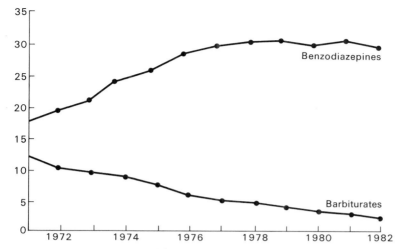

Fig. 6.1. Number of prescriptions (millions) in Great Britain 1971–82. (DHSS 1984).

practitioners, who are the main prescribers, are criticized for prescribing unnecessarily (Dunlop 1970; Trethowan 1975), and for using antidepressants and tranquillizers interchangeably (Weissman 1981). Attention has recently been drawn to the manner in which patients become long-term users of tranquillizers (Mellinger and Balter 1981) and in another study 20 per cent of patients prescribed a psychotropic for the first time for three months were still taking the drug six months later (Williams, Murray, and Clare 1982). Second, such prescribing is criticized on moral grounds; in the view of one critic, if 'man takes tranquillizers in order to withdraw from universal difficulties which man is born to cope with, this undermines social character' (Parry, Balter, Mellinger, Sisin, and Mannheimer 1973). Others regard psychotropic drug prescribing as a form of social exploitation (Stoessel 1973; Waldron 1977). Third, psychotropic drug use is criticized on financial grounds, attention being drawn to the cost of these drugs, with the implication that the money spent on tranquillizers and related drugs could and would be better spent elsewhere (Tyrer 1978).

Taking these criticisms in reverse order, financial criticisms seem weak. Williams (1981), in a thoughtful analysis, showed that the total tranquillizer bill for the period 1972-7 was £68.17 million. In 1977, just one of those years, the British spent over £6500 million on beer, wine, and spirits. Mellinger and his colleagues have wondered whether patients with psychological distress turn to alcohol when denied psychotropics (Mellinger, Balter, Mannheimer, Sisin, and Parry 1978), a query which led *The Lancet* to wonder about the wisdom of exhortations concerning the reduction of such prescribing given the fact that 'the problems of alcohol abuse are far greater than the mild degree of dependence that may result from absuing the alternatives' (Editorial 1978). Not all of us are quite so certain that we are concerned with a 'mild degree of dependence' but from the financial perspective at least it is difficult to contest William's view that psychotropic drugs account for a very small proportion of total health expenditure. It is equally difficult to see how the many treatments suggested to replace psychotropic drugs could be provided as cheaply.

The moral objections are more difficult to meet, being based, in part at any rate, on the view that the anxieties and stresses for which many people seek pharmacological relief are more appropriately faced with stoicism and overcome by drawing on personal coping skills and resources and non-medical supports.

The clinical objections would appear the most substantial. One of the reasons for the popularity of the modern non-barbiturate tranquillizers was the fact that they appeared to be non-addictive and they seemed extremely safe. In contrast with antidepressants, for example, it is quite difficult for patients to kill themselves by taking large doses of benzodiazepine tranquillizers. However, there is growing evidence that benzodiazepine tranquillizers are capable of inducing dependence, and can do so in normal dosages. While it is difficult to document such a phenomenon save in somewhat atypical groups, for example patients who have been taking such drugs for many years and who are well motivated to stop, the evidence from epidemiological surveys indicating quite substantial numbers of patients taking such drugs in normal and often quite low doses for lengthy periods of time does add support to the argument that the proportion of patients who are dependent may actually be quite high.

Does it matter that patients are regularly consuming such drugs if there is no evidence of escalation or serious sequelae? At the moment we cannot be sure of the actual and the long-term consequences of such use. Much interest is currently focused on the possible impact of such long-term use on levels of psychomotor performance and efficiency, and a number of researchers have examined the possible role of tranquillizers in road traffic accidents. While it is widely recognized that alcohol is an important factor in such accidents, the role of other psychotropic substances is much less clear. Yet such drugs could be related to road accidents as a result of their effects on driving skills, interaction with other substances, such as alcohol, or their effect on psychiatric ill-health (Clare 1983).

SUMMARY

The case records of seventeenth-century predecessors of today's general practitioners suggest a picture of anxiety and anxiolytic use which in these more pharmaceutically and phenomenologically sophisticated days are remarkably familiar. In seeking to understand and, perhaps, control the use of anxiolytic drugs it is important to see such a use in historical perspective. There is understandable concern regarding the benzodiazepine epidemic although the available evidence does suggest that the liberal provision of another apparent anxiolytic, with its associated consequences, should perhaps provoke even more concern.

However, tranquillizers lie more within the profession's power, but if the profession is to influence public attitudes towards drugs it does need to put their use into perspective. It may well be that simple guidelines concerning the use of tranquillizers in acute crises, their dangers when used chronically, the relationship between duration of use and the development of dependence, and appropriate clinical indications in addition to the consideration of practical alternatives to drugs in the management of anxiety, will prove to be more helpful in reducing inappropriate prescribing and indiscriminate use than fussing about their cost, moralizing over their effects, or demanding their prohibition.

REFERENCES

Baxter, R. A. (1673). A Christian directory. In *Collected works* (ed. W. Orme), vol. 3 (1830). Duncan, London.

Berridge, V. (1977). Opium and the historical perspective. *Lancet* i, 808–10.

Burton, R. (1621). *The anatomy of melancholy.*

Clare, A. W. (1983). Benzodiazepines, alcohol or nicotine? In *Benzodiazepines divided* (ed. M. R. Trimble), Chap. 1, pp. 1–15. John Wiley, Chichester.

Dunlop, D. (1970). The use and abuse of psychotropic drugs. *Proc. R. Soc. Med.* **63**, 1279–82.

Editorial (1978). Stress, distress and drug treatment. *Lancet* ii, 1347–8.

— (1982). Cirrhosis as a growth investment opportunity. *Br. J. Addict.* **77**, 113–22.

Edwards, G. (1981). The background. In *Drug problems in Britain: a review of ten years* (ed. G. Edwards and C. Busch). Academic Press, London.

—, Hensman, C., Chandler, J., and Peto, J. (1972). Motivation for drinking among men. *Psychol. Med.* **2**, 3, 260–71.

Fry, J. (1982). Psychiatric illness in general practice. In *Psychiatry and general practice* (ed. A. W. Clare and M. Lader), pp. 43–7. Academic Press, London.

Hodgson, R., Stockwell, T., and Rankin, H. (1979). Can alcohol reduce tension? *Behav. Res. Therapy* **17**, 459–66.

Lewis, A. (1967). Problems presented by the ambiguous word 'anxiety' as used in psychopathology. *Israel Ann. Psychiat. & rel. discipl.* **5**, 2, 105–21.

MacDonald, M. (1981). *Mystical Bedlam: madness, anxiety and healing in seventeenth-century England.* Cambridge University Press.

Maynard, A. and Kennan, P. (1981). The economics of alcohol abuse. *Br. J. Addict.* **76**, 339–45.

Mellinger, G. D. and Balter, M. B. (1981). Prevalence and patterns of use of psychotherapeutic drugs; results from a 1979 national survey of American adults. In *Epidemiological impact of psychotropic drugs* (ed. G. Tognoni, C. Bellantuono, and M. Lader), pp. 117–35. Elsevier/North Holland, Amsterdam.

—, —, Manheimer, D. I., Cisin, I. H., and Parry, H. J. (1978). Psychic distress, life crisis and use of psychotherapeutic medications. National Drug Survey data. *Arch. gen. Psychiat.* **35**, 1045–52.

Murphy, H. B. M. (1982). *Comparative psychiatry.* Springer-Verlag, Berlin/Heidelburg.

Parish, P. A. (1971). The prescribing of psychotropic drugs in general practice. *Jnl R. Coll. gen. Pract.* **21** suppl 4, 1–77.

Parry, H. J. (1978). Psychic distress, life crisis and use of psychotherapeutic

medications. National Drug Survey data. *Arch. gen. Psychiat.* **35**, 1045–52.
—, Balter, M. B., Mellinger, G. D., Cisin, I. H., and Mannheimer, D. I. (1973). National patterns of psychotherapeutic drug use. *Arch. gen. Psychiat.* **28**, 769–83.
Shepherd, M., Cooper, B., Brown, A. C., Kalton, G., and Clare, A. (1981). *Psychiatric illness in general practice*, 2nd edn. Oxford University Press, Oxford.
Smail, P., Stockwell, F., Canter, S., and Hodgson, R. (1984). Alcohol dependence and phobic anxiety states. I: A prevalence study. *Br. J. Psych.* **144**, 53–7.
Stoessell, J. (1973). *Psychopharmaka: die verordnete Anpassung.* Piper, München.
Stockwell, T., Smail, P., Hodgson, R., and Canter, S. (1984). Alcohol dependence and phobic anxiety states. II: A retrospective study. *Br. J. Psych.* **144**, 58–63.
Taylor, D. (1981). *Alcohol: Reducing the harm.* Office of Health Economics, London.
Trethowan, W. H. (1975). Pills for personal problems. *Brit. med. J.* **3**, 749–51.
Tyrer, P. (1978). Drug treatment of psychiatric patients in general practice. *Brt. med. J.* **2**, 1008–10.
Waldron, I. (1977). Increased prescribing of Valium, Librium and other drugs. *Int. J. Hlth Serv.* **1**, 37–62.
Weissman, M. M. (1981). Depression and its treatment in an U.S. urban community. *Arch. gen. Psychiat.* **38**, 417–21.
Williams, P. (1981). Trends in the prescribing of psychotropic drugs. In *The misuse of psychotropic drugs* (ed. R. Murray, H. Ghodse, C. Harris, D. Williams, and P. Williams). Gaskell Publications, Royal College of Psychiatrists, London.
— and Clare, A. (1979). Management of psychological disorder in general practice. In *Psychosocial disorders in general practice* (ed. P. Williams and A. Clare), pp. 133–4. Academic Press, London.
—, Murray, J., and Clare, A. W. (1982). A longitudinal study of psychotropic drug recipients. *Psychol. Med.* **12**, 201–6.

7

Where in the central nervous system do benzodiazepines act?

SUSAN D. IVERSEN

DISTRIBUTION OF BENZODIAZEPINE RECEPTORS IN CNS

Benzodiazepine drugs are used as anxiolytics, sedative/hypnotics, muscle relaxants and anticonvulsants. These drugs have been in use for more than two decades but it is only within the last few years that fundamental discoveries about their neuropharmacological mode of action have been made. With this information we can begin to specify the CNS substrates sensitive to these drugs and define their sites of action.

It has long been known that BZ inhibit the release of the catecholamine and indoleamine transmitters NA and 5-HT in brain (Corrodi, Fuxe, Linkbrink, and Olson 1971). But attention to these mechanisms waned with the discovery in biochemical binding-assay experiments that BZ bind to specific receptors in brain. We now know that the BZ receptor is part of a receptor complex which includes a $GABA_A$ receptor (Bowery, Price, Hudson, Hill, Wilkin, and Turnbull 1984) and that there exists a functional synergy between the BZ and GABA receptor (Fig. 7.1), such that activation of the BZ receptor enhances GABA transmission (Richards and Mohler 1984). Using specific radioactive ligands for BZ receptors it is possible with autoradiographic techniques to visualize in brain sections the location of these receptor types. Benzodiazepine receptors in human and rat brain have been described (Young and Kuhar 1980). The areas with the highest density include: olfactory bulb, fronto-limbic cortex, anterior medial forebrain bundle, septum, hippocampus and amygdala, cerebellum, substantia gelatinosa trigemini, and in spinal cord the dorsal laminae of the dorsal horn.

Quantitative autoradiography in more than 200 brain regions revealed that exogenous GABA increased BZ binding at all sites (Unnerstall, Kuhar, Niehoff, and Palacios 1981). Yet no correlation was observed between the magnitude of this stimulation and the distribution of high-affinity GABA binding sites. These findings indeed suggest that all BZ receptors are GABA-linked but the GABA receptors involved constitute a subpopulation of receptors of that class, i.e. there are GABA receptors in brain not linked with the BZ receptor complex.

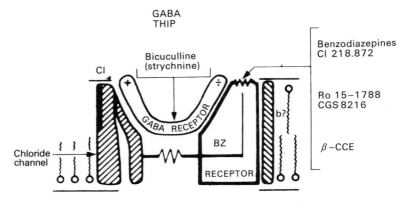

Fig. 7.1. A schematic representation of the GABA/benzodiazepine receptor chloride channel complex. Shown are drugs presumed to interact with the complex. (Reproduced from Braestrup, Nielsen, Honore, Jensen, and Petersen (1983).)

We do not yet know if BZ receptors are identical at different CNS sites. A number of novel BZ agonist, antagonist and mixed agonist/antagonist have been described recently which, unlike the classical BZ, have some but not all of their typical psychopharmacological properties. The evaluation of these new drugs is incomplete and the picture is confused but it is suggested that their properties imply the existence of multiple forms of the BZ receptor mediating the different effects of these drugs. Autoradiographic studies with different radioactive BZ ligands also suggest two forms of the BZ receptor with different CNS distributions (Lo, Niehoff, Kuhar, and Snyder 1983).

Electrophysiological experiments demonstrate that at widely different sites in CNS, BZ inhibit neuronal firing (Laurent, Margold, Humbel, and Haefely 1983) (Fig. 7.2). This is so at sites rich in specific neurotransmitter containing neurones such as dorsal raphe (5-HT), locus coeruleus (NA), substantia nigra, zona compacta (DA), and at chemically unspecified sites such as frontal cortex and hippocampus. The specificity of the response is demonstrated by the ability of the selective BZ antagonist, Ro 15-1788 to block the effects.

NEURAL BASIS OF THE ANXIOLYTIC EFFECT OF BZ

Animal models of anxiety

Anxiety or fear are readily conditioned in animals by the principle of classical conditioning. An aversive unconditioned stimulus elicits fear responses; if paired with a neutral stimulus, the latter conditioned stimulus will come reliably to elicit fear. This is the basis of the CONDITIONED EMOTIONAL RESPONSE test (Estes and Skinner 1941). Once the fear state exists it has a number of effects on

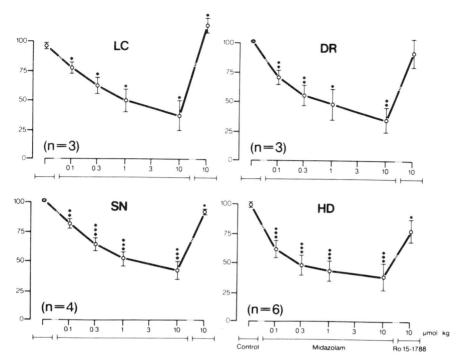

Fig. 7.2. Effect of midazolam in increasing i.v. doses on multiunit activity in the nucleus locus coeruleus (LC), dorsal raphe nucleus (DR), substantia nigra pars compacta (SN), and the dorsal hippocampus (HD) of unanesthetized 'encephale isole' rats. The injections were made at 7-min intervals. After the last dose of midazolam 10 μmoles/kg, Ro 15–1788, a specific benzodiazepine antagonist, was injected and completely reversed the effect of midazolam. The *ordinate* indicates multiunit activity in per cent of predrug control values: on the *abscissa* are the doses in μmoles/kg. (Reproduced from Haefely *et al.* (1983).)

behaviour; the production of species specific defensive reactions and the simultaneous inhibition of other motivated behaviours (Bolles and Faneslow 1980). For example, if a rat is trained to press a lever for food and then periodically a signal is presented followed by an electric shock to the animal, the signal will eventually reliably change behaviour and inhibit lever pressing without the shock being presented. Fear is conditioned to the neutral signal which predicts shock.

More commonly, the signal and the shock are presented simultaneously to the behaving animal (Geller and Seifter 1960). A rat presses a lever for food but simultaneously receives a shock as well as food; conflict is thought to exist between the urge to obtain food and the knowledge of the inevitable shock.

This procedure is termed PUNISHMENT. Although in theoretical terms is is supposed that the state of fear or anxiety elicits defensive behaviour as well as inhibiting other behaviour, we rarely measure these defensive reactions. Inhibition of rewarded lever-pressing or of unconditioned appetitive responses like exploration, eating, drinking, or social contact, which are simple to measure, are invariably used as an index of the emotional state. Benzodiazepine drugs and all known clinically effective anxiolytics attenuate responding suppressed on a CER or punishment paradigm.

SITES OF ANXIOLYTIC ACTIONS IN BRAIN

When we ask where in brain BZ act to relieve anxiety, a reconciliation of one body of facts can be made.

1. Biochemically, BZ inhibit the release of 5-HT (Jenner, Chadwick, Reynolds, and Marsden 1975; Saner and Pletscher 1979), an effect which does not show tolerance and correlates with the anxiolytic effect (Wise *et al.* 1972). Serotonergic drugs which result in reduced functional levels of 5-HT mimic the effect of BZ (Graeff 1981).
2. Electrophysiologically, BZ inhibit 5-HT neurones of the raphe (Laurent *et al.* 1983).
3. Anatomically, the 5-HT raphe system innervates limbic structures which on the basis of classical lesion studies are involved in emotional responsiveness, particularly to aversive stimuli, i.e. septo-hippocampal system and amygdala (Gray 1982).
4. Benzodiazepine receptors are found in high density in this limbic circuitry (Niehoff and Kuhar 1983) in close proximity to GABA-mimergic neurones with which they functionally interact (Gallager 1978; Haefely, Polc, Pieri, Schaffner, and Laurent 1983).

Let us turn to further experiments directly testing the hypothesis that an interaction of BZ with 5-HT neurones is involved in their anxiolytic action.

THE EFFECTS OF LESIONS TO THE 5-HT RAPHE NEURONES

The rostral raphe nuclei of the mesencephalon, including n. dorsalis, give rise to the 5-HT innervation of the limbic structures projecting in medial forebrain bundle. A selective lesion to this pathway (induced with the 5-HT toxin 5-hydroxytryptamine 5,7-DHT) at the level of the ventral tegmentum (i) releases response suppression acquired before the lesion; the magnitude of this release is as great as that seen with a BZ given systemically and after the lesion the BZ can induce no further release in lesioned rats (Tye, Everitt, and Iversen 1977), (ii) prevents the acquisition of response suppression on a punishment paradigm (Iversen 1983b). Thiebot, Hamon, and Soubrie (1984) report a similar release of response suppression on a CER paradigm after selective 5,7-DHT lesions to dorsal raphe nuclei.

THE EFFECTS OF APPLICATION OF BZ TO THE DORSAL RAPHE OR LIMBIC TERMINAL SITES

Thiebot and Sourbrie (1983) directly applied BZ to the dorsal raphe and reported release of response suppression on the CER task. At this site, iontophoretically applied GABA has been shown to inhibit the firing of 5-HT neurones and local infusions of GABA through chronically implanted cannulae released responding on a CER task, and thus mimicked the effect of BZ. Serotonin itself at the same site, which is likely, through activation of autoreceptors to lower functional activity in the 5-HT neurones of raphe, also released responding. Therefore, lowered 5-HT neuronal activity induced in the raphe by a variety of manipulations mimics the effect of systemically administered BZ.

BENZODIAZEPINE INTERACTIONS IN THE AMGYDALA

The ventral 5-HT pathway arising from raphe nuclei innervates a range of diencephalic and telencephalic limbic structures (Steinbusch and Nieuwewhuys 1983) which are also rich in BZ receptors, GABA, and implicated in emotional behaviour. Limbic structures include posterior hypothalamus, including mammillary bodies, septim, hippocampus, olfactory bulb, frontal cortex, and amygdala. This last site has been most intensively studied to date. The cortical and basolateral nuclei of the amygdala receive a uniform rich 5-HT innervation from the raphe nuclei and are rich in the GABA synthetic enzyme glutamic acid decarboxylase. Niehoff and Kuhar (1983) reported that BZ receptors are concentrated in the cortical and basolateral nuclei (Fig. 7.3), the site at which lesions in rats impair the response to fear-inducing novelty (Rolls and Rolls 1973; Aggleton, Petrides, and Iversen 1981). Local injection at this site of BZ are reported to release response suppression on a CER paradigm (Iversen 1983), Geller-Seifter punishment (Shibata, Kataoka, Gomita, and Veki 1982) Nagy, Zambo, and Desci 1979) and on the water-licking conflict test by Petersen, and Scheel-Kruger (1982), who have also shown that the GABA-agonist, muscimol, mimics the effect of midozalam in amygdala, and that this effect is reversed with bicuculline.

A substantial lesion literature exists, implicating the amygdala in the response to highly meaningful stimuli, particularly aversive events (Weiskrantz 1968). Amygdala lesions in monkeys impaired the CER response, whereas hippocampal lesions were without effect. In rats, Goddard (1964) reported that disruptive electrical stimulation of the amygdala impaired the acquisition of a CER response to shock without having an effect on food motivated learning. He demonstrated that the unconditioned fear response was not impaired but rather the con-

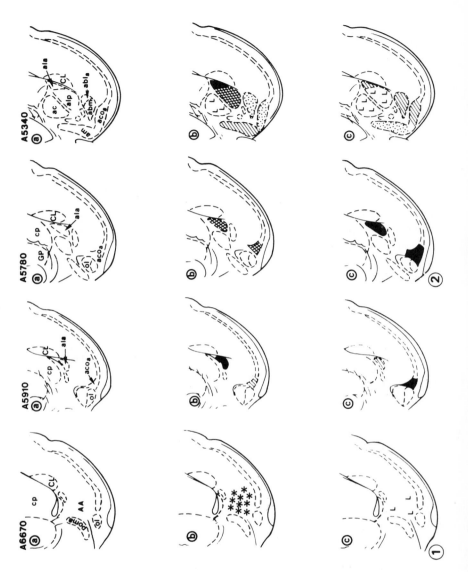

Fig. 7.3. A schematic representation of total BZ receptor density and type 1 receptor density in the rat amygdala at nine levels from anterior (1) to posterior (5) amygdala, as specified by the atlas of Konig and Klippel. The upper drawing (a) of each group depicts the amygdala nuclei according to Kretteck and Price (1978). The middle drawing (b) depicts total BZ density, black >95; cross hatch 75–95; diagnonal lines 50–75; dots 35–50; astericks 25–35 and L<25 (fentomoles/mg). The lower drawing (c) depicts type 1 BZ receptor density, black 70–100 per cent; cross hatch 10–70 per cent; dots 20–40 per cent and L<20 per cent. The anterior and posterior cortical nuclei (acoa; acop); the lateral (ala; alp) and the basolateral (abla; ablp) nuclei are very rich in BZ receptors. (Reproduced from Niehoff and Kuhar (1983).)

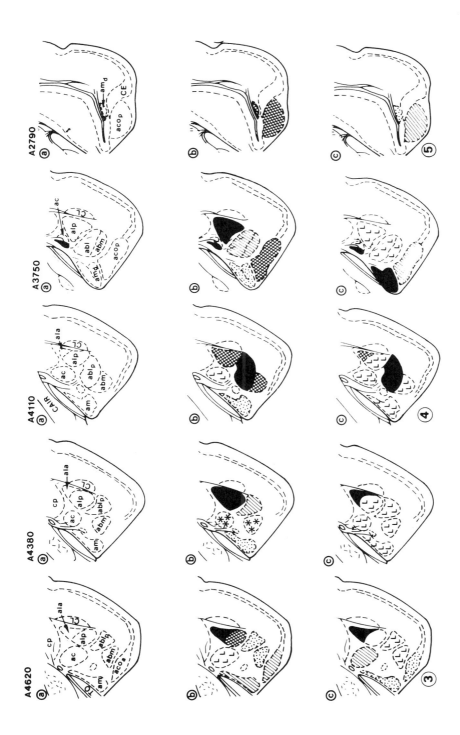

solidation of the relationship between the UCS and the CS. There is supporting evidence from lesion experiments in the monkey implicating the amygdala in memory consolidation processes (Mishkin and Aggleton 1983).

In summary, the limbic 5-HT pathways and the BZ/GABA complex are involved in the release of response suppression but the relationship between the BZ receptor complex and the indoleamine neurones remains obscure.

OTHER NEURAL SUBSTRATES INVOLVED IN ANXIETY

There is growing evidence that other neurochemically coded components of the limbic system may be sensitive to BZ drugs and contribute to their anxiolytic action.

(a) Dorsal noradrenaline pathway

The dorsal NA pathway originating in locus coeruleus (LC) and projecting to limbic system and cortex has been implicated in the processes of behavioural inhibition induced by unconditioned and conditioned aversive stimuli. Gray (1982) has used the lowered threshold of septal stimulation to drive hippo-campal theta-rhythm at 7.7 Hz as a correlate of the response to aversive stimuli and found that the ability of BZ to block this neurophysiological index of anxiety is dependent on the integrity of the dorsal NA input. 6-Hydroxy-dopamine lesions to the dorsal NA pathway or pharmacological manipulation to lower brain NA levels abolished the specific effect of BZ on 7.7 Hz theta rhythm. However, lesions to the dorsal NA bundle (or, indeed, hippocampus) do not release behavioural suppression induced with aversive stimuli in the dramatic way lesions to the ventral 5-HT pathway do. Since other experiments also implicate the LC in anxiety, it is possible that response suppression is not a relevant behavioural index of the aspect of anxiety dependent on hippocampal processing.

Redmond and his colleagues have focused attention on the LC in experiments with monkeys (Redmond and Huang 1979). Electrical stimulation of LC induced behavioural reactions of intense fear, whereas lesions to the LC rendered monkeys unperturbed when threatened by their handlers or by toy snakes placed in the cage. It is also reported that drugs which raise functional NA levels (yohimbine, piperoxan) are anxiogenic in monkeys. Drugs which lower NA function by postsynaptic receptor blockage (propranolol) or by blockade of $\alpha2$-adreno-autoreceptors on the LC neurones (clonidine) are anxiolytic in animals on CER tasks and in man. The efficacy of clonidine has been noted during the intense fear and panic associated with opiate withdrawal in addicts.

(b) Forebrain DA pathways

The dopamine (DA) neurones of the ventral tegmentum form three ascending projections to forebrain. The zona compacta of the substantia nigra forms the nigro-striatal pathway; the more medial A10 DA neurones gives rise to the meso-limbic DA innervation of nucleus accumbens, septum, amygdala, and olfactory tubercle, and a subpopulation of A10 neurones innervates limbic cortex, particularly frontal cortex.

5-Hydroxytryptamine neurones of the dorsal raphe innervate striatum via the dorsal 5-HT pathway; a medial 5-HT pathway innervates substantia nigra and a component of the ventral 5-HT pathway innervates the more medial ventral tegmental area. (Steinbusch and Nieuwenhuys, 1983). Few BZ receptors are found in striatum but the density is higher in substantia nigra. Intravenous BZ inhibit activity in SN neurones (Fig. 7.2) and thus the possibility must be considered that neurochemical interactions with the DA system contribute to the anxiolytic actions of BZ.

It is known that the 5-HT innervation of the nigro-striatal system serves an inhibitory role on motor output such that reduced 5-HT function results in enhancement of spontaneous motor behaviour and of motor responses to DA agonist and antagonist drugs (Gerson and Baldessarini 1980). Lowered 5-HT function in conflict situations, induced with drugs or lesions, results in a release of response suppression. Could this merely reflect general motor disinhibition without any fundamental change in the prevailing anxiety state? Thiebot et al. (1984) have raised this interpretation since they find that a 5,7-DHT lesion to the 5-HT input of the SN results in a release of responding on the CER paradigm. 5-Hydroxytryptamine depletion in SN is assumed to influence the functioning of DA neurones. If a release of behavioural inhibition is associated with a release of DA neurone activity from inhibitory 5-HT control it would be predicted:

(a) that the lesion in SN would release responding suppressed by punishment on conditioned anxiety but not equally low rates of responding maintained in non-aversive situations. This control experiment has not been performed.

(b) that enhanced DA function achieved by other lesion or drug manipulations would selectively release behavioural suppression. This is not the case with amphetamine which releases motor responding in general but is unable to release punished responding (Tye, Iversen, and Green 1979).

Although BZ receptors in SN may play some modulatory role in general motor function, it seems unlikely that the striatal DA system is the central mechanism for the behavioural inhibition associated with anxiety states and its release by BZ drugs.

It seems likely, however, that the frontal DA system through its links with the limbic circuitry (particularly the amygdala) is involved in the response to anxiety. Unavoidable mild foot-shock results in conditioned immobility in rats which can be reversed with BZ. It has also been shown that this form of stress enhances turnover of DA in frontal cortex (Rheinhard, Bannon, and Roth 1982) but not in striatum; 5-HT levels are unaffected. This biochemical response of the DA neurones can be blocked with BZ. But it must be remembered that the NA system as well as the DA system responds to stress under these experimental conditions, reinforcing the impression that a wide range of neurotransmitter substrates are both involved in the responses to aversive stimuli and the ability of BZ to modulate that response.

BENZODIAZEPINES AS ANTICONVULSANTS, MUSCLE RELAXANTS, HYPNOTICS, AND APPETITE STIMULATORS

Benzodiazepines have a number of behavioural effects in addition to their anxiolytic action. There is every reason to believe that the BZ/GABA receptor complex is involved in these effects since gabamimetic manipulations modify the effect of BZ in tests of convulsive activity, motor function, and appetitive behaviour. However, it is not clear how the anatomical distribution of BZ receptors relate to these different functions.

Young and Kuhar (1980) speculate (Table 7.1) that limbic system and cortex are involved in the anticonvulsant as well as the anxiolytic effects. Basic neurophysiological features of cortex and hippocampus/amygdala have been related to the propensity of these forebrain areas to show epileptic discharge. A lack of inhibitory function has been correlated with abnormal electrical activity and the ability of the BZ to enhance GABA receptor function could

TABLE 7.1. *A tentative correlation between pharmacological effects of benzodiazepines and brain areas with elevated levels of receptors*

Brain areas with receptor	Related drug effect
Limbic system (amygdala and hippocampus and frontal cortex)	Anxiolytic
Cortex, hippocampus, and amygdala	Anticonvulsant
Ventromedial hypothalamus	Appetite stimulation
Cerebellum (molecular layer)	Ataxia
Reticular formation	Muscle relaxation
Spinal cord	?
Substantia nigra, pars lateralis	?
Nucleus subthalamicus	?
Nucleus entopeduncularis	?
Zona incerta	?
Retina (inner plexiform layer)	?
Superior colliculus and others	?

(Reproduced from Young and Kuhar (1980).)

well account for their anticonvulsant activity. The BZ find a very special niche in the treatment of epilepsy (Trimble 1983). Benzodiazepines have not been found useful in the treatment of generalized seizures. It is within the partial seizures with focal limbic system involvement that the 1,4 and 1,5 benzodiazepines have been used with some success. It is interesting that many of these epileptic types with complex symptomatology, including cognitive and affective disorders, have many features of psychotic illness. It is at this interface of psychiatry and epilepsy within the limbic system that BZ have found clinical favour. It should be noted that long-term treatment with BZ can result in severe withdrawal symptoms including disturbed perception, panic and convulsions (Lader 1983).

It is interesting that the very structures implicated in anxiety are also involved in certain forms of experimental epileptiform excitability, at least in animals. (the amygdala, for example, in the process of epileptic kindling (Goddard, McNaughton, Douglas, and Barnes 1978)). Furthermore, Nagy, Zambo, and Decsi (1979) reported anticonvulsant activity of BZ injected directly into the amygdala of rabbit. Certainly in these limbic areas of temporal lobe there appears to be functional and anatomical relationships between the anxiolytic and anticonvulsant properties of BZ. Indeed, Haefely *et al.* (1983) have proposed 'that anxiety and emotional tension are caused by an abnormal activity of neuronal circuits in the limbic system. This neutral abnormality could consist in an excessive responsiveness to normal inputs, and result from any humoral or metabolic factor able to shift the fine-tuned balance between excitatory and inhibitory synaptic activity. Such a state might be a mild form of epileptiform neuronal activity. This mild form of epileptiform activity could be the neural basis of behavioural inhibition and increased arousal, and may evolve in plain .paroxysmal activity and panic attack'.

When first administered to experimental animals BZ produce muscle relaxation, sedation and often ataxia. The cerebellum, brain stem, and spinal cord have a high density of BZ receptors which are GABA related and are the likely sites for these effects of the drugs. The hypnotic effects of BZ, which accounts for one of their major clinical uses, may not be due to a direct effect on the CNS substrates directly controlling sleep processes. Rather, it has been suggested the reduction in anxiety and psychosomatic features of tension (e.g. muscle tone) enhances the endogenous sleep-promoting mechanism.

CONCLUSION

It seems likely that BZ/GABA receptor complexes at different levels of the CNS axis mediate the anxiolytic, anticonvulsant, muscle relaxant and hypnotic effects of the minor tranquillizers.

Surprisingly little is known about the neural sites essential for these behavioural effects. The systems mediating anxiolytic function involve certain limbic structures with rich monoamine innervation. However, little progress has been made in defining the interaction of the BZ/GABA complex and the mono-amine neurons at these sites. Such information would be useful in devising novel pharmacological approaches to the control of anxiety.

REFERENCES

Aggleton, J. P., Petrides, M., and Iversen, S. D. (1981). Differential effects of amygdaloid lesions on conditioned taste aversion learning by rats. *Physiol. Behav.* 27, 397-400.

Bolles, R. C. and Fanselow, M. S. (1980). A perceptual-defensive-recuperative model of fear and pain. *Behav. & Brain Sci.* 3, 291-323.

Bowery, N. G., Price, G. W., Hudson, A. L., Hill, D. R., Wilkin, G. P., and Turnbull, M. J. (1984). GABA receptor multiplicity. *Neuropharmacology* 23, 219-31.

Braestrup, C., Nielsen, M., Honore, T., Jensen, L. H., and Petersen, E. N. (1983). Benzodiazepine receptor ligands with positive and negative efficacy. *Neuropharmacology* 22, 1451-7.

Corrodi, H., Fuxe, K., Lindbrink, P., and Olson, L. (1971). Minor tranquillizers stress and central catecholamine neurones. *Brain Res.* 29, 1-6.

Estes, W. K. and Skinner, B. G. (1941). Some quantitative properties of anxiety. *J. exp. Psychol.* 29, 390-400.

Gallager, D. W. (1978). Benzodiazepines: Potentiation of a GABA inhibitory response in the dorsal raphe nucleus. *Eur. J. Pharmac.* 49, 133-43.

Geller, I. and Seifter, J. (1960). The effects of meprobomate, barbiturates, d-amphetamine and promazine on experimentally induced conflict in the rat. *Psychopharmacologia* 1, 482-92.

Gerson, S. C. and Baldessarini, R. J. (1980). Motor effects of serotonin in the central nervous system. *Life Sci.* 27, 1435-51.

Goddard, G. V. (1964). Amygdaloid stimulation and learning in the rat. *J. comp. Physiol. Psychol.* 58, 23-30.

——, McNaughton, B. L., Douglas, R. M., and Barnes, C. A. (1978). Synaptic change in the limbic system: evidence from studies using electrical stimulation with and without seizure activity. In *Limbic mechanisms* (ed. K. E. Livingston and O. Hornykiewicz), pp. 355-68. Plenum Press, New York.

Graeff, F. G. (1981). Minor tranquillizers and brain defense systems. *Braz. J. med. biol. Res.* 14, 239-65.

Gray, J. A. (1982). The neuropsychology of anxiety: An enquiry into the functions of the septo-hippocampal system. *Behav. & Brain Sci.* 5, 469-534.

Haefely, W., Polc, P., Pieri, L., Schaffner, R., and Laurent, J. P. (1983). Neuropharmacology of benzodiazepines: synaptic mechanisms and neural basis of action. In *The benzodiazepines: from molecular biology to clinical practice* (ed. E. Costa), pp. 21-66. Raven Press, New York.

Iversen, S. D. (1983). Where in the brain do benzodiazepines act? In *Benzodiazepines divided* (ed. M. R. Trimble), pp. 167-83. John Wiley, Chichester.

Jenner, P., Chadwick, D., Reynolds, E. J., and Marsden, C. D. (1975). Altered 5HT metabolism with clonazepam, diazepam and diphenyl hydantonin. *J. Pharmac.* 27, 707-10.

Kretteck, J. E. and Price, J. L. (1978). A description of the amygdaloid complex in the rat and cat, with observations on intra-amygdaloid axonal connections. *J. comp. Neurol.* 178, 255-80.

Lader, M. (1983). Benzodiazepine withdrawal states. In *Benzodiazepines divided* (ed. M. R. Trimble), pp. 17–31. John Wiley, Chichester.

Laurent, J-P., Margold, M., Humbel, V., and Haefely, W. (1983). Reduction by two benzodiazepines and pentobarbitone of the multiunit activity in substantia nigra, hippocampus, nucleus locus coeruleus and dorsal raphe nucleus of 'encephale isole' rats. *Neuro pharmacology* 22, 501–12.

Lo, M. M. S., Niehoff, D. L., Kuhar, M. J., and Snyder, S. H. (1983). Differential localization of type 1 and type 11 benzodiazepine binding sites in substantia nigra. *Nature, Lond.* 306, 57–60.

Mishkin, M. and Aggleton, J. (1983). Multiple functional contributions of the amygdala in the monkey. In *The amygdaloid complex* (ed. M. Y. Ben-Ari). Elsevier, Amsterdam.

Nagy, J., Zambo, K., and Decsi, L. (1979). Anti-anxiety action of diazepam after intra amygdaloid application in the rats. *Neuropharmacology* 18, 573–6.

Niehoff, D. L. and Kuhar, M. J. (1983). Benzodiazepine receptors: Localization in rat amygdala. *J. Neurosci.* 3, 2091–7.

Petersen, E. N. and Scheel-Kruger, J. (1982). The Gabaergic anticonflict effect of intra amygdaloid benzodiazepines demonstrated by a new water lick conflict paradigm. In *Behavioural models and the analysis of drug action*, Proc. 27th OHOLO Conference (ed. M. Y. Spiegelstein and A. Levy), pp. 467–73. Elsevier, Amsterdam.

Redmond, D. E. and Huang, Y. H. (1979). New evidence for a locus coeruleus norepinerphrine connection with anxiety. *Life Sci.* 25, 2149–62.

Reinhard, J. F., Bannon, M. J., and Roth, R. H. (1982). Acceleration by stress of dopamine synthesis and metabolism in prefrontal cortex: antagonism by diazepam. *N.S. Arch. Pharmac.* 318, 374–7.

Richards, J. G. and Mohler, H. (1984). Benzodiazepine receptors. *Neuropharmacology* 23, 233–42.

Rolls, E. T. and Rolls, B. J. (1973). Altered food preferences after lesions in the basolateral region of the amygdala in the rat. *J. comp. Physiol. Psychol.* 83, 248–59.

Saner and Pletscher, A. (1979). Effects of diazepam on cerebral 5-hydroxytriptamine synthesis. *Eur. J. Pharmac.* 55, 315–18.

Shibata, K., Kataoka, Y., Gomita, Y., and Veki, S. (1982). Localization of the site of the anticonflict action of benzodiazepines in the amygdaloid nucleus of rats. *Brain Res.* 234, 442–6.

Steinbusch, H. W. M. and Nieuwenhuys, R. (1983). The raphe nuclei of the rat brainstem: a cytoarchitectonic and immunohistochemical study. In *Chemical Neuroanatomy* (ed. P. Emson), pp. 131–20. Raven Press, New York.

Thiebot, M-H. and Soubrie, P. (1983). Behavioural pharmacology of the benzodiazepines. In *The benzodiazepines: from molecular biology to clinical practice* (ed. E. Costa), pp. 67–92. Raven Press, New York.

—, Hamon, M., and Soubrie, P. (1984). Serotonergic neurons and anxiety – related behaviour in rats. In *Psychopharmacology of the limbic system* (ed. E. Zarifian and M. Trimble). John Wiley (in press).

Trimble, M. R. (1983). Benzodiazepines in epilepsy. In *Benzodiazepines divided* (ed. M. R. Trimble), pp. 277–88. John Wiley, Chichester.

Tye, N. C., Everitt, B. J., and Iversen, S. D. (1977). 5-hydroxytryptamine and punishment. *Nature, Lond.* 268, 741–3.

—, Iversen, S. D., and Green, A. R. (1979). The effects of benzodiazepines and serotonergic manipulations on punished responding. *Neuropharmacology* 18, 689-95.

Unnerstall, J. R., Kuhar, M. J., Niehoff, D. L., and Palacios, J. M. (1981). Benzodiazepine receptors are coupled to a subpopulation of -aminobutyric and (GABA) receptors: Evidence from a quantitative autoradiographic study. *J. Pharmac. exp. Ther.* 218, 797-804.

Weiskrantz, L. (1968) (ed.). *Emotion: analysis of behavioural change*, pp. 50-90. Harper & Row, New York.

Wise, C. D., Berger, B. D., and Stein, L. (1972). Benzodiazepines: Anxiety-reducing activity by reduction of serotonin turnover in the brain. *Science* 177, 180-3.

Young, W. S. and Kuhar, M. J. (1980). Radiohistochemical localization of benzodiazepine receptors in rat brain. *J. Pharmac. exp. Ther.* 212, 337-46.

8

Pharmacokinetic and pharmacodynamic relationships with benzodiazepines

A. RICHENS AND A. N. GRIFFITHS

INTRODUCTION

All of the marketed 1,4-benzodiazepine drugs have broadly the same pharmaco-logical profile, demonstrating anxiolytic, sedative hypnotic, anticonvulsant, and muscle relaxant activity, although the relative balance of these effects may differ to some extent between individual compounds. The 1,5-benzodiazepine, clobazam, displays a wider separation of anxiolytic effect from impairment of motor coordination and this is associated with a relative lack of muscle relaxant activity.

Pharmacokinetically, however, there are important differences between those benzodiazepine drugs currently marketed in the UK, and these differences determine their application.

PHARMACOKINETICS

There have been a number of extensive reviews of the benzodiazepine drugs (Breimer 1979; Whelpton 1979; Bellantuono, Reggi, Tognoni, and Garattini 1980; Breimer, Jochemsen, and Albert 1980; Richens 1983; Greenblatt, Divoll, Abernethy, Ochs, and Shader 1983), but our purpose here is to give only a brief summary of the features most relevant to their clinical use.

Their lipid solubility (which influences rate of absorption and distribution), the rate of metabolism and the presence or absence of active metabolites, and the duration of the plasma half-life of the active component are the features which are of immediate relevance. Lipid solubility (as measured by the octanol: water partition coefficient) determines the rate at which an individual com-pound will cross a lipid membrane such as the gut wall or the blood–brain barrier. A drug given orally exhibits a lag phase, during which the formulation is reaching the small bowel and disintegrating in the intestinal fluid. Once the drug is in solution, its absorption is rapid because most of the benzodiazepines have a high lipid solubility. Passage into the brain is also rapid but because the same physical property is responsible for both processes, the drug enters the brain from the blood as quickly as it enters the blood from the gut. The rate of absorption is therefore the prime determinant of the onset of action for orally administered benzodiazepines. The same is in general true of intramuscular and rectal administration, but when a drug is given intravenously, the rate at which it moves across the blood–brain barrier will determine the speed of onset of action. Some drugs, e.g. diazepam, are quicker in onset than others, e.g. lorazepam, because the former have a higher lipid solubility than the latter. This is illustrated in Fig. 8.1, in which the peak velocity of saccadic eye movements have been used as a marker of the benzodiazepine drugs' effects on the brain. Diazepam, in fact, has one of the highest lipid solubilities of any of the drugs in this class and therefore remains a treatment of first choice in status epilepticus.

Relative to its size, the brain receives a higher proportion of the cardiac output than any other organ, and benzodiazepine drugs rapidly reach high concentrations within it. However, redistribution to less perfused tissues occurs, particularly to skeletal muscle and fat. This redistribution accounts for the

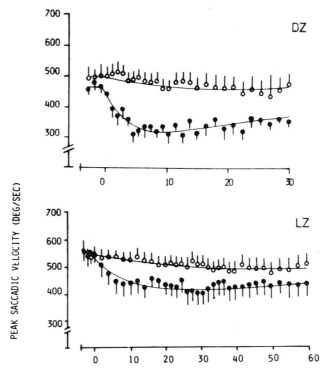

Fig. 8.1. Peak saccade velocity following intravenous injection of 2 mg of lorazepam (LZ) and 5 mg of diazepam (DZ). In both cases ● is the active treatment and ○ is placebo. Computer analysis indicated that the peak effect of diazepam occurred at 8.2 min and lorazepam 23.3 min. (Reproduced with permission from Tedeschi *et al.* 1983.)

first phase of the plasma concentration-time profile and is called the α-phase. The decline during this phase is log-linear and can be characterized by a rate constant (α) and a distribution half-life ($t_{\frac{1}{2}}\alpha$). For some drugs, e.g. midazolam, the α-phase is more prominant, and the significance of this is taken up later.

Once redistribution has occurred, the rate of decline in plasma concentration is determined by hepatic metabolism and renal elimination (the contribution of the latter is usually small for the parent compounds because they are poorly water-soluble; conjugation to more water-soluble metabolites as necessary before renal excretion can occur to any extent). This elimination phase is called the β-phase and can be characterized by a rate constant (β) and an elimination half-life ($t_{\frac{1}{2}\beta}$). As well as influencing the duration of action, the $t_{\frac{1}{2}\beta}$ will determine whether significant accumulation of a drug takes place when used nightly for hypnotic purposes. Nitrazepam ($t_{\frac{1}{2}\beta} = 18$–$31$ h) for example, will accumulate more than temazepam ($t_{\frac{1}{2}\beta} = 8$–16 h) and the accumulation of triazolam ($t_{\frac{1}{2}\beta} = 2$–5 h) will be negligible. The importance of this, and the relative contribution of the α- and β-phase in determing the duration of action of a hypnotic benzodiazepine drug are discussed below. A summary of the pharmacokinetic properties of the commonly-used drugs is given in Table 8.1.

The presence of active metabolites (Table 8.2) is important in determining duration of action because some of them have much longer plasma elimination half-lives than their parent compounds. For example, diazepam has a half-life of 20-40 h, whereas its major active metabolite has a half-life of 50–100 h and will accumulate with chronic dosing and account for much of diazepam's background pharmacological effect. Some compounds, e.g. clorazepate and prazepam, have such short plasma half-lives that they can be considered as little more than prodrugs for desmethyldiazepam, to which they are largely converted On the other hand, the duration of action of drugs without active metabolites, e.g. lorazepam, oxazepam, is determined by the rate of elimination of the parent drug only.

CLINICAL USE AND PLASMA LEVEL PROFILES

Benzodiazepines used chronically as anxiolytics and anticonvulsants require a constant non-sedative effect while for hypnotic use, drug action needs to be intermittent. Hypnotics are usually required to produce a fast onset of action, i.e. to induce sleep quickly. In this respect nitrazepam and flurazepam are satisfactory hypnotics, despite their long elimination half-lives, because they have a high lipid solubility and rapid rate of absorption. Oxazepam and lorazepam are more suitable for use as anxiolytics as their rate of absorption is too slow for hypnotic use, in spite of their having short elimination half-lives, a quality which is desirable for a drug used as an hypnotic. None the less, the elimination half-life is an important factor in determining duration of drug action. Figure 8.2 shows the effect of different elimination half-lives on accumulation after chronic administration. Clearly the compound with an 8 h half-life is preferable to the

TABLE 8.1. *Pharmacokinetic data for selected benzodiazepines*

	$t_{\frac{1}{2}\beta}$ (hours)	Volume of distribution (l/kg)	% bound to plasma proteins
Alprazolam	10-20	1-1.5	70-75
Chlordiazepoxide	6-28	0.26-0.58	94-97
Clobazam	16-50	0.8-1.8	87-92
Clorazepate	Very short	NA	82
Demoxepam	14-95	NA	NA
Diazepam	20-40	0.95-2	96.8-98.6
N-Desmethyldiazepam	50-100	0.93-1.27	97.6
N-Desalkylflurazepam	51-100	NA	NA
Flurazepam	Very short	NA	NA
Lorazepam	9-22	0.7-1	85
Lormetazepam	9-15	NA	NA
Medazepam	1-2	NA	98.7-99.5
Midazolam	1.3-3.1	0.8-1.8	NA
Nitrazepam	18-31	1.5-2.76	86-87
Oxazepam	4-13	0.6	87-90
Temazepam	8-16	1.3-1.6	96-98
Triazolam	2-5	NA	78-85

TABLE 8.2. *Clinically-important active metabolites of benzodiazepine drugs*

Alprazolam	None
Chlordiazepoxide	Desmethylchlordiazepoxide, demoxepam, desmethyldiazepam
Clobazam	Desmethylclobazam
Clorazepate	Diazepam
Diazepam	Desmethyldiazepam
Flurazepam	Desalkylflurazepam
Ketazolam	Desmethyldiazepam
Lorazepam	None
Lormetazepam	None
Medazepam	Desmethyldiazepam
Midazolam	None
Nitrazepam	None
Oxazepam	None
Temazepam	None
Triazolam	None

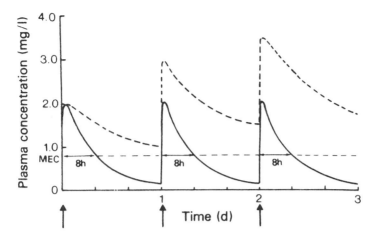

Fig. 8.2. Theoretical plasma concentration profile of two hypnotics with different elimination half-lives: solid line 6 h; dotted line 24 h during nightly administration. MEC refers to the minimal effective concentration; in hypnotic therapy the drug effect should last 8 h or less. D = 100 mg; $\triangle_t$ = 24 h; V_d = 50 l. (Taken from Breimer (1979) with permission.)

compound with a 24 h half-life as an hypnotic, whereas for an anxiolytic or anticonvulsant the reverse is true. The duration of action and likelihood of accumulation of a benzodiazepine is dependent on elimination half-life of both parent compound and any active metabolite present. However, this simplistic view may need modifying in the light of recent concepts concerning the relationship between the pharmacokinetic and pharmacodynamic effects of benzodiazepine drugs. Their pharmacokinetics are generally held to be best represented by a two-compartment model, although on occasion a single- or three-compartment model has been used. Figure 8.3 represents an idealized two compartment system after oral dosing. One must assume that drug effects last for the time the concentration is above the threshold for effect. Curry and Whelpton (1979) pointed out that initially there is a delay before onset of action and that the effect may wear off either during the α-phase (the distribution phase) or below the α/β inflection (i.e. during the β- or elimination phase). The relative importance of the two phases may thus determine the duration of action and the degree to which they influence the latter is a function of the compartment sizes and of volume of distribution. The profound effect on serum levels of a difference in the ratio between volume of distribution in two phases despite identical absorption rates (K_a), and is shown in Fig. 8.4. This figure clearly shows that the traditional classification of benzodiazepines purely on $t_{\frac{1}{2}\beta}$ is unreliable and potentially misleading. Amrein, Eckert, Haefely, and Leishman (1983) have suggested an alternative parameter 'residual fraction ($r_{12.1}$)' which is calculated from the plasma drug concentration 12 h following drug intake and the maximum plasma drug concentration. This parameter is

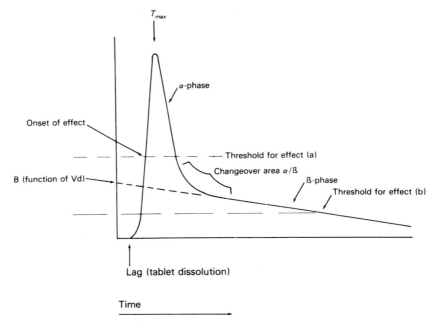

Fig. 8.3. Annotated model plasma concentration graph (semi-log plot) for a two compartment system and oral dosing. (Taken from Curry and Whelpton (1979) with permission.)

claimed to be a predictive guide of a benzodiazepine's therapeutic applications. Compounds with a small $r_{12.1}$ are suitable for hypnotic use, i.e. they are rapidly removed from the central compartment, while a large $r_{12.1}$ would suggest that the compound is best used as an anxiolytic; intermediate $r_{12.1}$ benzodiazepines are suggested to be hypnoanxiolytics (see Table 8.3). This new parameter is more helpful than elimination (β-phase) half-life but still has limitations in that it does not take accumulation of drug and tolerance to drug into account. These two factors are of major importance when benzodiazepines are used chronically.

Tolerance has the effect of gradually increasing the minimum effective concentration. The actual time course and the extent of tolerance to benzodiazepines in man has not been clearly investigated. Our studies of nitrazepam have led us to believe that tolerance to the sedative effects of nitrazepam has appeared within six days. The therapeutic implications of this are not clear, as nitrazepam has been reported to be effective as an hypnotic for up to 24 weeks (Oswald, French, Adam, and Gilham 1982).

SERUM LEVEL MONITORING

The routine measurement of plasma benzodiazepine drug concentrations cannot be justified at present because the therapeutic ranges for these compounds

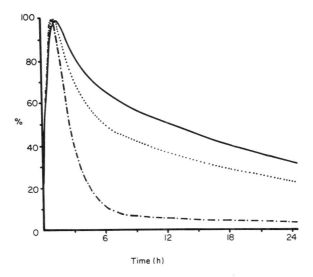

Time (h)

Fig. 8.4. Three theoretical plasma concentration profiles (percentage of maximum concentration against time) for which the following are the same:
1. absorption rate K_a = 2.0 (= invasion t_3 of 20 min);
2. diffusion rate α = 0.693 ($t\frac{1}{2}_\alpha$ = 1 h);
3. elimination rate β = 0.0395 (= $t\frac{1}{2}_\beta$ = 20 h).

The differences amongst the curves are due solely to the differences in the ratio between volumes of distribution in each individual curve, _____ A:B = 2:3; . . . . . . :B = 3:2; _ . _ . _ . A:B = 19:1. (Taken from Amrein *et al.* (1983) with permission.)

TABLE 8.3. *Residual fraction* ($r_{12.1}$) *and half-life* ($t\frac{1}{2}_\beta$) *of several benzodiazepines*

	$r_{12.1}$	$t\frac{1}{2}$ (hours)
Midazolam	$\leqslant 0.01$	2
Triazolam	0.16	2
Flunitrazepam	0.25	22
Oxazepam	0.40	8
Temazepam	0.42	8
Nitrazepam	0.70	25
Desmethyldiazepam	0.71	84

$r_{12.1}$ = quotient of plasma concentration of 12 h after drug intake to plasma C_{max}.
Modified from Amrein *et al.* (1983).

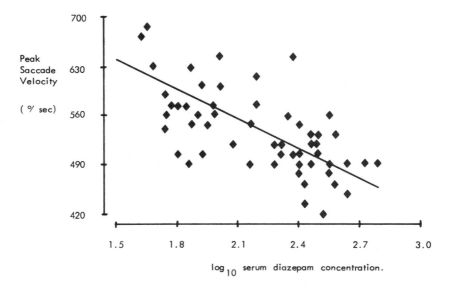

Fig. 8.5. Relationship between serum diazepam concentration and peak saccade velocity. The data are pooled from six subjects ignoring time; the observations were made over 6 h after intravenous administration of 5 mg of diazepam. The correlation coefficient (r) was −0.673, which was significant at $p < 0.001$.

have not been defined and because a poor relationship appears to exist between serum level and effects with chronic dosing, probably partly as a result of the development of tolerance. Furthermore, therapeutic ratios are relatively large and sedation is usually a satisfactory clinical indicator that the dose is excessive.

It has, on occasion, proved possible to relate plasma levels to effect in acute situations. Fink, Irwin, Weinfeld, Schwartz, and Conney (1976) demonstrated a linear correlation between the amount of EEG activity and serum diazepam concentration. Aschoff (1968) found a linear correlation between dosage of diazepam and the decrease of peak velocity of saccadic eye movements. Bittencourt, Wade, Smith, and Richens (1981) took this further and demonstrated a log-linear relationship between peak saccadic velocity and log concentration of temazepam, nitrazepam, and diazepam, and some recent unpublished data from our laboratory have confirmed this (Fig. 8.5). It would seem that inter-individual variation in benzodiazepine sensitivity may be the main reason why plasma level : effect relationships have so seldom been found even in an acute situation.

Also using eye movements, Griffiths, Tedeschi, Smith, and Richens (1983) investigated the effects of chronic administration of nitrazepam (long $t_{\frac{1}{2}}$) and temazepam (short $t_{\frac{1}{2}}$) on normal subjects, and showed that the residual performance impairment produced by nitrazepam on the first day of treatment had disappeared by day 6, despite much higher serum levels (Fig. 8.6). Temazepam,

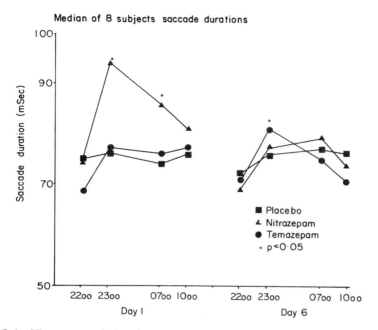

Fig. 8.6. Nitrazepam (10 mg), temazepam (20 mg) and placebo were given nightly for six days. Ok the first and sixth night saccade duration was measured at 22.00 (time of drug intake), 23.00, 07.00 and 10.00. Significant performance impairment (between drug and placebo) occurred with nitrazepam on day 1 at 23.00 and 07.00 with temazepam on day 6 at 23.00 ($p < 0.05$ in all cases). Eight subjects took part in the study.

on the other hand, produced no residual effects on day 1 but by day 6, with slightly higher serum levels, a significant performance impairment was seen. This would suggest that nitrazepam has produced tolerance to itself, possibly by desensitization of the benzodiazepine receptor, while temazepam had not. One explanation of this is that the receptors in the central nervous system are exposed for much longer periods to a high concentration of nitrazepam, but less so with temazepam. Desensitization to the effects of nitrazepam therefore predominates. Cross-tolerance between different benzodiazepine drugs also occurs. In a recent study from our laboratory (Fig. 8.7), six days pretreatment with nitrazepam reduced the effect of a single dose of diazepam on peak saccade velocity (Griffiths *et al.* 1984).

The reverse side of tolerance is withdrawal. Benzodiazepines do produce withdrawal symptoms, notably rebound insomnia and anxiety though this may in part be due to the removal of the pill taking ritual. The actual withdrawal effects may take some days to develop due to the long half-life of some of the metabolites, notably desmethyldiazepam. This gradual decrease of drug level may in some patients cushion the withdrawal. Short-acting benzodiazepines used

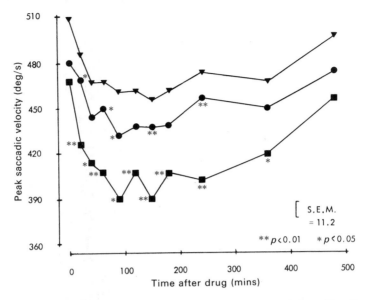

Fig. 8.7. Seven volunteers received three treatment regimes: (i) nitrazepam (10 mg) nightly for six nights (ii) placebo for six nights (iii) nitrazepam (10 mg) for one night. The treatments were given orally at 23.00 h and were followed by diazepam (10 mg) at 09.00 h on the day following the last dose of nitrazepam. Mean saccade velocity following diazepam ingestion is shown in Fig. 8.7.
▼ placebo + diazepam (10 mg)
● 6 nights nitrazepam (10 mg) + diazepam (10 mg)
■ 1 night nitrazepam (10 mg) + diazepam (10 mg)
The asterisks marked against the ■ symbols represent significant differences from ▼; those against ● represent differences from ■. There were no significant differences between placebo and six nights nitrazepam pretreatment at any time point.

in large doses can produce rebound anxiety the morning following night time administration for insomnia. Morgan and Oswald (1982) have reported this effect for triazolam. If this is substantiated, there may be important implications for the future use and development of very short-acting drugs like triazolam and midazolam.

REFERENCES

Amrein, R., Eckert, M., Haefely, W., and Leishman, B. (1983). Pharmacokinetic and clinical considerations in the choice of a hypnotic. *Brit. J. clin. Pharmac.* **16**, 5S–10S.

Aschoff, C. J. (1968). Verandenugen rascher blick bewegungen (Saccaden) beim menschen inter diazepam (Valium). *Arch. Psychiat. u. Nervenkr.* **211**, 325–32.

Bellantuono, C., Reggi, V., Tognoni, G., and Garattini, S. (1980). Benzo-diazepines: clinical pharmacology and therapeutic use. *Drugs* **19**, 195–219.
Bittencourt, P. R. M., Wade, P., Smith, A. T., and Richens, A. (1981). The relationship between peak saccadic eye movements and serum benzodiazepine concentrations. *Br. J. clin. Pharmac.* **12**, 523–34.
Breimer, D. D. (1979). Pharmacokinetics and metabolism of various benzo-diazepines used as hypnotics. *Br. J. clin. Pharmac.* **8**, 7S–13S.
Breimer, D. D., Jochemsen, R. von, and Albert, H. H. (1980). Pharmacokinetics of benzodiazepines — short acting vs. long acting. *Arzneimittel- Forschung/Drug Res.* **30**, 875–82.
Curry, S. H. and Whelpton, R. (1979). Pharmacokinetics of closely related benzodiazepines. *Br. J. clin. Pharmac.* **8**, 15S–21S.
Fink, M., Irwin, P., Weinfeld, R. E., Schwartz, M. A., and Conney, A. H. (1976). Blood levels and EEG effects of diazepam and bromazepam. *Clin. Pharmac. Ther.* **20**, 184–91.
Griffiths, A., Marshall, R., and Richens, A. (1984). Tolerance to a sedative effect of drazepam after 6 nights nitrazepam pretreatment in man. *Br. J. clin. Pharmac.* **18**, 305p.
—, Tedeschi, G., Smith, A. T., and Richens, A. (1983). The effects of repeated doses of temazepam and nitrazepam on human psychomotor performance. *Br. J. clin. Pharmac.* **15**, 615P–16P.
Greenblatt, D. J., Divoll, M., Abernethy, D. R., Ochs, H. R., and Shader, R. I. (1983). Clinical pharmacokinetics of the newer benzodiazepines. *Clin. Pharmacokinet.* **8**, 233–52.
Morgan, K. and Oswald, I. (1982). Anxiety caused by a short life hypnotic. *Br. med. J.* **284**, 942.
Oswald, I., French, C., Adam, K., and Gilham, J. (1982). Benzodiazepine hypnotics remain effective for 24 weeks. *Br. med. J.* **284**, 860–3.
Richens, A. (1983). Clinical pharmacokinetics of benzodiazepines. In *Benzodiazepines divided* (ed. M. R. Trimble), pp. 187–205. John Wiley, Chichester.
Tedeschi, G., Smith, A. T., Dhillon, S., and Richens, A. (1983). Rate of entrance of benzodiazepines into the brain determined by eye movement recording. *Br. J. clin. Pharmac.* **15**, 103–7.
Whelpton, R. (1979). Data compilation: benzodiazepine compounds. *Biopharmaceut. & Drug Disposition* **1**, 37–45.

9

Anxiety and its generation by pharmacological means

R. DOROW

Anxiety is a universal experience in humans which has various psychic and somatic expressions. Those who repeatedly experience severe anxiety states, including generalized anxiety and panic disorder, suffer a dramatic impairment in their daily life. The large number of patients with these symptoms is reflected by the plethora of anxiolytics prescribed. Recent surveys have shown that in one year 10-20 per cent of the adult population take benzodiazepines (Marks 1978; Tallman, Paul, Skolnick, and Gallager 1980). Besides benzodiazepines, a number of drugs such as meprobamate, barbiturates, antidepressants, propranolol, and alcohol are used for the treatment of anxiety states. Yet, the problem of anxiety is by no means solely a modern concern. An opposite approach was taken by Plato who in the *Nomoi* debated the usefulness of a theoretical substance, 'phobou pharmakon', which might *induce* anxiety. Although he certainly did not pursue medical interests when proposing the use of such a substance to test the bravery of soldiers, he raised some points which could be considered as a rationale for the pharmacological induction of anxiety: 'phobou pharmakon' should be easily controllable with respect to onset, duration, and intensity of action, and should lack after-effects. Besides its use as a test to identify a population at a high biological risk of anxiety, it could also be applied as a therapeutic tool in order to desensitize anxious citizens. Indeed, in the wake of the First World War, Wearn and Sturgis (1919) challenged soldiers suffering from 'irritable heart', a typical anxiety disorder of the period, with adrenaline infusions, in an attempt to validate a pharmacological model which could distinguish normal from anxiety-prone individuals. A similar idea led Bonn, Harrison, and Rees (1971) to use lactate-induced anxiety as part of their therapy.

Other exposures to anxiogenic paradigms, including isoproterenol infusion (Frohlich, Tarazi, and Dustan 1969) and inhalation of CO_2/O_2 (Griez and van den Hout 1983), were put forward as a possible treatment of anxiety states and phobias. In addition to the criteria envisaged by Plato, such a drug should offer some insight into the pathophysiology of anxiety and ultimately lead to the evaluation of new treatment paradigms, including novel agents that might prevent anxiety episodes. Guttmacher, Murphy, and Insel (1983) further proposed that the ideal pharmacological model of anxiety should meet the following criteria: It should mimic naturally occurring anxiety leading to the typical peripheral and central manifestations, should be replicable, and reflect the potential for a state response: successfully treated patients should not respond or should respond far less than those who have had no treatment.

The following is a short review of three different categories of drug-induced anxiety, i.e.

1. anxiety induced by drugs with a specific anxiomimetic profile;
2. anxiety induced as indirect secondary sequelae of other drug effects;
3. anxiety induced as withdrawal reaction from psychotropic agents.

ANXIETY INDUCED BY DRUGS WITH A SPECIFIC ANXIOMIMETIC PROFILE

Drugs acting at the benzodiazepine-/GABA-receptor chloride ionophore complex

Pentylenetetrazole, a convulsant agent formerly used in the treatment of depressive states (Meduna and Friedman 1939), was reported to induce anxiety in subconvulsive doses (Hildebrandt 1937; Rodin 1958). This compound is known to decrease functionally chloride conductance and thereby suppress the inhibitory effects of GABA. Besides pentylenetetrazole, a number of CNS-stimulant drugs which interact with the benzodiazepine-/GABA-receptor ionophore complex, such as bemegride, certain barbiturate derivatives, and picrotoxin, have been shown to induce anxiety in some cases. Moreover, drug discriminative paradigms designed to indicate 'anxiety' in animals have demonstrated the anxiogenic efficacy of some of these compounds (Lal and Emmett-Osglesby 1983).

The effective therapy of anxiety states with benzodiazepines and the discovery of specific benzodiazepine receptors and their functional interaction with the GABA-ionophore complex, have led to the assumption that the CNS has certain neuronal systems which mediate anxiety and anxiety-related behaviour. Braestrup, Nielsen, and Olsen (1980) isolated ethyl-β-carboline-3-carboxylate (β-CCE) from human urine and identified its affinity to benzodiazepine receptors. At that time it was thought that β-CCE was a possible candidate for the endogenous ligand to BZ-receptors, but it was later shown to be an isolation artefact. On the basis of this assumption, however, N-methyl-β-carboline-3-carboxamide (FG 7142), a metabolically more stable congener of β-CCE, was chosen for clinical pharmacological studies in healthy volunteers. Like β-CCE, FG 7142 lacks anticonvulsive or anticonflict effects, but antagonizes the pharmacological and electrophysiological effects of benzodiazepines (Petersen, Paschelke, Kehr, Nielsen, Braestrup 1982). Acute doses of FG 7142 stimulated locomotor activity without inducing convulsions in experimental animals. When the first human trials were started early in 1981, FG 7142 surprisingly induced severe anxiety attacks in two volunteers, which in one case could be antagonized by treatment with lormetazepam, a benzodiazepine hypnotic (Dorow 1982; Dorow, Horowski, Paschelke, Amin, and Braestrup 1983). The central and peripheral effects elicited by FG 7142 were those typically associated with anxiety, such as severe inner tension, restlessness, a feeling of impending doom, palpitations, increase in heart rate, elevation of blood pressure and stress-related hormones (see Table 9.1). Consequently, compounds like FG 7142, which induce biochemical, pharmacological, behavioural, and clinical effects opposite to those of benzodiazepines, are classified as 'inverse agonists' to the benzodiazepine receptor (Polc, Bonetti, Schaffner, Haefely 1982; Braestrup, Nielsen, Honore, Jensen, and Petersen 1983).

β-CCE and FG 7142 have since been shown to elicit responses in animals akin to anxiety in man (Ninan, Insel, Cohen, Cook, Skolnick, and Paul 1982; Stephens, Shearman, and Kehr 1984) and have been established as tools to induce pharmacological anxiety. In humans, oral application of FG 7142 is an unsuitable test model, due to the large variations in bioavailability and, consequently, the unpredictability of drug plasma levels (Dorow *et al.* 1983).

TABLE 9.1. *Effects of FG 7142-treatment associated with anxiety attacks*

I. CENTRAL EFFECTS
Restlessness
Hyperkinesis
Dizziness
Tremor
Inner tension
Excitation
Feeling of impending death

II. AUTONOMOUS AND CARDIOVASCULAR SYMPTOMS
Cold sweat
Nausea
Flushes of warmth
Redding of hands and face
Heavy breathing
Palpitations
Tightness in the chest
Paresthesias
Increase in blood pressure and pulse rate

III. EFFECT ON HORMONE SECRETION
Increase in serum — prolactin
— growth hormone
— cortisol

Furthermore, recent reports have offered evidence that chronic treatment with FG 7142 kindles epileptic seizures in rats (Little and Nutt 1984), suggesting a shift in the pharmacological effects towards stronger inverse agonistic influence on the chloride channel, i.e. reduction of chloride conduction. This chronic influence results in effects similar to those seen after acute administration of DMCM, a full inverse agonist at the benzodiazepine receptor (Braestrup, Schmiechen, Neef, Nielsen, and Petersen 1982; Petersen 1983). Moreover, an intravenous formulation in propyleneglycol could not reverse sedation in healthy subjects pretreated with 1 mg lormetazepam or induce anxiety as only 5 mg FG 7142 can be administered due to its unfavourable physiochemical properties (Dorow, Paschelke, and Horowski 1984). Recently it was shown that other β-carbolines may act as benzodiazepine receptor agonists, partial agonists, or antagonists in animals (Braestrup *et al.* 1983; Stephens, Kehr, Wachtel, Schmiechen 1985), a finding which was confirmed in healthy volunteers; e.g. a partial agonist with anticonvulsant and anxiolytic properties in animal tests was able to reverse sedative properties of lormetazepam (Dorow, Duka, unpublished data). The trial was conducted in part with the same volunteers and similar conditions as in the FG 7142 study. The findings corroborate that it is not β-carbolines in general, but inverse agonists like FG 7142 which cause the specific anxiomimetic effects.

Compounds which interact with the adrenergic system

It is well known that many adrenergic agents, such as adrenaline or isoprenaline, may induce anxiety responses in healthy volunteers and patients although individual responses may vary considerably (Wearn and Sturgis 1919; Cantril and Hunt 1932; Lindemann 1935). The indirect adrenergic drugs like cocaine, amphetamine, and its derivatives are known to induce psychotic reactions, but also anxiety and anxiety-related behaviour. The α_2-adrenergic autoreceptor antagonists piperoxane and yohimbine clearly display anxiomimetic activity in patients and normal volunteers (Holmberg and Gershon 1961; Ingram 1962; Garfield, Gershon, and Sletten 1967; Charney, Heninger, and Redmond 1983). Yohimbine is considered to be a reliable test substance and a more effective anxiogenic agent than adrenaline. Charney *et al.* (1983) showed that 30 mg yohimbine produced significant increases in subjective anxiety, autonomic symptoms, blood pressure, and plasma 3-methoxy-4-hydroxy-phenylethylene-glycol (MHPG) in healthy volunteers. They succeeded in demonstrating that both diazepam and clonidine antagonize the yohimbine-induced anxiety, whereas only clonidine, an α_2-receptor agonist, significantly attenuated autonomic symptoms, plasma MHPG levels, and blood pressure. Electrical or pharmacological activation of the locus coeruleus, the major norepinephrine-containing nucleus, leads to biochemical, behavioural, and physiological effects in monkeys, similar to the naturally occuring animal behaviour likened to anxiety in humans (Redmond and Huang 1979). Lesions of the locus coeruleus produce the opposite effects.

These findings corroborate the concept that noradrenergic hyperactivity, such as induced by yohimbine, may play an important role in the production of certain anxiety states in humans, and that clonidine exerts its antianxiety effects via a receptor-mediated decrease in noradrenergic activity.

A number of other anxiety-provoking situations, such as the discontinuation of opiates or antidepressive drugs and the withdrawal of clonidine, can be associated with anxiety states similar to those observed in patients suffering panic attacks, as they are likewise accompanied by increases in plasma MHPG. Some anxiety conditions may therefore be related to enhanced brain noradrenergic activity.

Further evidence that the adrenergic system might play a role in the generation of anxiety was offered by Frohlich, Dustan, and Page (1966). They reported that two patients who displayed palpitations, tachycardia, and severe anxiety on exertion, or on assuming an upright posture, could be successfully treated with propranolol. Moreover, β-adrenergic stimulation by isoproterenol in asymptomatic patients led to anxiety states and related symptoms which were then reversed by propanolol. The authors termed the underlying cause of the condition 'β-adrenergic hyperactivity'. A number of more recent reports suggest that propranolol may be useful in the treatment of certain anxiety states and the hyperventilation syndrome (Suzman 1968; Easton and Sherman 1976). Frohlich *et al.* proposed (1969) that the reaction to isoproterenol may constitute a test for the underlying disease and for the successful response to propranolol treatment, since only patients and not subjects react to the isoproterenol infusion.

The general conclusion from the above-mentioned reports that drugs affecting the central adrenergic system may attenuate or induce anxiety, implies that adrenergic pathways can play an important role in the generation of anxiety.

Lactate-induced anxiety

The infusion of sodium lactate leads to panic attacks which closely resemble spontaneous attacks in patients suffering from panic disorders, but rarely has an effect in normal controls (Pitts and McClure 1967; Bonn *et al.* 1971; Kelly, Mitchell-Heggs, and Sherman 1971). Lactate infusions are usually administered for 20 min, with symptoms peaking after 15 min and regressing immediately after discontinuation with few residual effects. These attacks are indeed a good model for investigating the biological manifestations that accompany the psychopathology, yet the site of action and mechanism of lactate effect remain unclear (Appleby, Klein, Sachar, and Levitt, 1981).

This test has, however, a drawback in that no adequate biological marker is available. Physiological measures implemented after an infusion of lactate are generally unable to distinguish controls from patients. Nevertheless, the test has been used to identify a subgroup of anxiety patients who are responsive to tricyclic antidepressants, but not to benzodiazepines (Rifkin, Klein, Dillon, and Levitt 1981). Treatment with imipramine can block real-life attacks and those induced experimentally with lactate (Appleby *et al.* 1981), whereas propanolol, a β-adrenergic blocker, cannot prevent panic attacks provoked by lactate (Gorman, Levy, Leibowitz, McGrath, Appleby, Dillon, Davies, and Klein 1983).

Other drugs

Caffeine

Caffeine is one of the widely used social stimulants and is generally believed to possess overall benevolent effects. However, it was shown that high levels of caffeine consumption (1.0–1.5 g/d) relate directly to high anxiety levels (Greden 1974) and that a reduction of caffeine by diet results in alleviation of symptoms which then reoccur after challenge with large amounts of the substance. Caffeine may also produce anxiety as part of a caffeine-withdrawal syndrome (White, Lincoln, Pearce, Reeb, and Varda 1980). Recently, Boulenger and Uhde (1982) could show that caffeine consumption positively correlated with trait-anxiety in patients with phobic disorders but not in controls. The mechanism of caffeine-induced anxiety still remains unclear. An increase in synthesis of catechol-amine release may mediate caffeine effects which, via a direct postsynaptic action, may in turn elevate cAMP levels through inhibition of phosphodiesterase activity (Rall 1980). It has also been reported that caffeine binds to benzo-diazepine receptors at high concentrations and reverses the effects of benzo-diazepines (Marangos, Paul, Goodwin, Syapin, and Skolnick 1979). Such high concentrations, however, cannot arise with normal caffeine consumption. At lower concentrations, caffeine binds to adenosine receptors in the brain. The biological significance of these observations is apparent from reports that the affinities of various caffeine analogues to these receptors parallel their be-havioural effects in animals.

Strychnine

Although strychnine, an alkaloid commonly used as a pesticide, has no proven therapeutic value, it has for centuries been employed as an ingredient in a number of drug preparations. Nowadays, the adulteration of street drugs with strychnine is a frequent source of poisoning. Strychnine poisoning induces severe convulsions which are accompanied by extreme anxiety and a fear of impending death. The convulsive activity results from the compound's suppres-sion of inhibitory impulses, i.e. by antagonizing glycine, a postsynaptic inhibitory transmitter (Kuno and Weakly 1972). The severe convulsive activity of strychnine prohibits its application as an anxiety-inducing agent, although diazepam is indeed an effective antidote.

Organophosphates

Exposure to organophosphates, a group of widely used insecticides, evokes a number of behavioural effects which most commonly include anxiety. Intoxica-tion leads to anxiety, giddiness, restlessness, and tension, insomnia, and excessive dreaming (Levin, Rodnitzky, and Mick 1976). The toxicological effects of these compounds relate to their potent inhibition of cholinesterase enzymes, which in turn leads to the accumulation of acetylcholine at peripheral and central sites. The severe adverse effects of organophosphate poisoning prohibits their use as a model to induce anxiety.

All the above known types of pharmacological influence on the CNS are presumably based on different underlying biochemical and physiological mechanisms and different topographical sites of the brain.

The relevant denominator here is that they all result in similar anxiety states and related symptoms.

ANXIETY INDUCED AS INDIRECT SECONDARY SEQUELAE OF OTHER DRUG EFFECTS

It is well known that a number of psychotropic agents, such as marijuana, amphetamine, psilocybin, and LSD, may induce psychotic reactions with hallucinations or delusions often associated with states of severe anxiety. 'Bad trips' are defined as drug-induced emotional conditions ranging from acute panic states or severe anxiety episodes to overt psychotic experiences. In his review, Abruzzi (1977) reported that frightening or psychotic drug experiences are frequent occurrences after abuse of these drugs. Abruzzi documented over 5000 cases of bad trips, of which far more were attributed to LSD than any other single drug, presumably due to the compound's strong hallucinogenic properties. By way of comparison, THC and THC-containing drugs, which are more widely available, produced far less bad trips.

Despite early attempts to implement such drugs in the treatment and diagnoses of certain psychiatric illnesses, their well-known psychic and untoward effects rule out their use in the treatment of anxiety. An indication that these drug effects are indirect is evidenced by the difficulty in finding a suitable drug treatment for this cause of anxiety.

ANXIETY INDUCED BY WITHDRAWAL REACTIONS FROM PSYCHOTROPIC AGENTS

Discontinuation of psychotropic drugs, especially those with CNS-depressant activity like alcohol, barbiturates, benzodiazepines, meprobamate, but also drugs like opiates and lithium, may lead to pronounced withdrawal reactions. These symptoms most commonly include sleep disturbances, irritability, dysphoria, and anxiety. In severe cases, delirium and seizures have been observed (Fraser, Wikler, Essig, and Isbell 1958; Schöpf 1983; Lader 1983). Dose, duration of treatment, and pharmacokinetic parameters, e.g. half-life, appear to influence occurrence, severity, and onset of withdrawal symptoms.

Animal experiments have shown that withdrawal reactions after chronic benzodiazepine treatment could be precipitated by the administration of Ro

15-1788, a specific benzodiazepine receptor antagonist (Cumin, Bonetti, Scherschlicht, and Haefely 1981; Lukas and Griffiths 1982; Emmett-Oglesby, Spencer, Lewis, Elmesallamy, and Lal 1983*a*, 1983*b*). The receptor antagonist alone had no overt pharmacological activity. Ro 15-1788 induced withdrawal reactions after a period as short as one week (Lukas and Griffiths 1982). In a recent study in humans it could be shown that even after a single, very high intravenous dose of benzodiazepines, some withdrawal reactions, including anxiety, could be precipitated by Ro 15-1788 24 h after benzodiazepine treatment. However, no withdrawl symptoms were observed when Ro 15-1788 was administered 15 min after benzodiazepine treatment (Dorow *et al.*, in preparation).

These findings indicate that benzodiazepines may produce functional changes in the GABA-benzodiazepine receptor complex by a rapid mechanism leading to anxiety in some healthy non-anxious subjects on withdrawal.

CONCLUSIONS

In the attempt to draw up meaningful rationales for the pharmacological induction of anxiety, it is convenient to consider five areas in which possible advantages can be derived: (1) Such a procedure may detect populations at a high risk of anxiety disorders. (2) An anxiogenic drug could be used to discern specific subgroups of anxiety-prone patients and, by dint of the patients' reactions to a specific anxiolytic compound, help find the appropriate treatment. (3) Challenging subjects with anxiogenic preparations could help assess the anxiolytic properties of new compounds and other treatment regimens. (4) The pharmacological induction of anxiety may also be used as a therapeutic means of desensitizing anxious patients. (5) Knowledge derived from e.g. biochemical and behavioural studies of anxiogenic compounds in animals, may offer an insight into the basic mechanisms and the pathophysiology of anxiety in humans. This in turn demands an adequate understanding of the compounds' specific mechanisms of action.

The last aspect broaches another area of discussion: anxiety is a state of subjective experience that can be described exclusively by humans. It can perhaps be modelled, but not reproduced in animals, which leads to the question as to whether animal experiments exist for anxiety and whether they could indeed provide insight into basic mechanisms and into the prevention and treatment of anxiety. In their review, Lal and Emmett-Osglesby (1983) discussed animal models of anxiety which either expose animals to aversive stimuli, resulting in overt behavioural changes, or which are based on introceptive stimuli. The former paradigms usually include punishment procedures as used, for example, in the Geller-Seifter conflict-test, the latter may consist of electrical stimulation of certain brain areas or pharmacological stimuli known to induce anxiety in humans, as applied in the drug discrimination test with pentylenetetrazole. The detection of anxiogenic substances in humans is a prerequisite for validating pharmacological models of anxiety in animals, which in turn can be implemented to discover anxiogenic compounds. Returning to the criteria which an anxiogenic drug should ideally fulfil, recourse may be had to the *Nomoi*, for Plato's proposals evidently still hold true: 'phobou pharmakon' should have a rapid onset of action, a linear dose-response relationship and thus be easily controllable without after-effects — an antidote should be available.

Table 9.2 offers a summary of certain models of pharmacologically induced anxiety in the light of the above mentioned criteria. Withdrawal reactions and indirect sequelae to drug effects, e.g. 'bad trips', cannot be regarded as an appropriate method of evoking anxiety in view of the unpredictability of response, the duration and severity of action and consequent poor controllability. A promising contribution to the understanding of the biological basis of anxiety came to light with the discovery of unexpected anxiogenic effects of inverse agonists to benzodiazepine receptors. As a large number of biochemical, behavioural, and electrophysiological animal tests have been used to characterize the effects of this kind of compound, more information is available on their mechanism of action at the cellular level than is for other anxiogenic drugs. FG 7142, however, is not a safe drug to use as a test model, due to its unfavourable bioavailability and hence its unpredictable onset of action. Once active, this compound elicits severe fits of anxiety, and as already observed in animals, chronic application may lead to convulsions.

Both yohimbine and lactate fulfil most of the criteria, yet very little is known about the mechanism of lactate's action and there are, to date, no biological markers for its effects. A drawback of the lactate model is that its efficacy is restricted to panic-attack patients although it indeed meets the rationale for identifying subgroups of anxious patients. Yohimbine seems to meet the 'criteria' of 'phobou pharmakon' best. It is active in patients with

TABLE 9.2. *Some models of pharmacologically-induced anxiety in humans*

Challenge	Blocker	Receptor	Possible site of action	Proposed clinical correlate
FG 7142	Lormetazepam Ro 15-1788(?)	Benzo-diazepine	Limbic(?) system	Generalized anxiety disorder
Yohimbine	Clonidine	α_2	Locus ceruleus	Anxiety and panic disorder
Na Lactate	Imipramine	?	?	Panic disorder

Adapted from Insel, Ninan, Aloi, Jimerson, Skolnick, and Paul (1984).

anxiety disorders and in normal subjects. Anxiety and related symptoms are induced dose-dependently, a biological marker is at hand and the symptoms are readily reversed by clonidine and diazepam.

In conclusion, the generation of anxiety by pharmacological means, applied with the necessary ethical considerations and caution, ought to be the object of further research. Such an approach could evidently lead to a greater insight into its pathophysiology and novel procedures for the treatment of anxiety.

ACKNOWLEDGEMENTS

I gratefully acknowledge the help of H. Haghgou, J. Horkulak, and E. Staab-Renner in the preparation of the manuscript.

REFERENCES

Abruzzi, W. (1977). Drug-induced psychosis. *Int. J. Addict.* **12**, 183–93.

Appleby, I. L., Klein, D. F., Sachar, E. J., and Levitt, M. (1981). Biochemical indices of lactate-induced panic: A preliminary report. In *Anxiety: new research and changing concepts* (ed. D. F. Klein and J. Rabkin). Raven Press, New York.

Bonn, J. A., Harrison, J., and Rees, W. L. (1971). Lactate-induced anxiety: Therapeutic application. *Br. J. Psychiat.* **119**, 468–71.

Boulenger, J.-P. and Uhde, T. W. (1982). Caffeine consumption and anxiety: Preliminary results of a survey comparing patients with anxiety disorders and normal controls. *Psychopharmac. Bull.* **18**, 53–7.

Braestrup, C., Nielsen, M., and Olsen, C. E. (1980). Urinary and brain β-carboline-3-carboxylates as potent inhibitors of brain benzodiazepine receptors. *Proc. natn. Acad. Sci. U.S.A.* **77**, 2288–292.

——, ——, Honore, T., Jensen, L. H., and Petersen, E. N. (1983). Benzodiazepine receptor ligands with positive and negative efficacy. *Neuropharmacology* **22**, 1451–7.

——, Schmiechen, R., Neef, G., Nielsen, M., and Petersen, E. N. (1982). Interaction of convulsive ligands with benzodiazepine receptors. *Science* **216**, 1241–3.

Cantril, H. and Hunt, W. A. (1932). Emotional effects produced by the injection of adrenalin. *Am. J. Psychol.* **44**, 300–7.

Charney, D. S., Heninger, G. R., and Redmond, D. E. Jr. (1983). Yohimbine induced anxiety and increased noradrenergic function in humans: effects of diazepam and clonidine. *Life Sci.* **33**, 19–29.

Cumin, R., Bonetti, E. P., Scherschlicht, R., and Haefely, W. E. (1981). Use of the specific benzodiazepine antagonist, Ro 15–1788, in studies of physiological dependence on benzodiazepines. *Experientia* **38**, 833–4.

Dorow, R. (1982). β-carboline monomethylamide causes anxiety in man. 13th Collegium Internationale Neuro-Psychopharmacologicum Congress, Jerusalem, June 1982.

——, Paschelke, G., and Horowski, R. (1984). Clinical Pharmacology of FG 7142, an inverse agonist of benzodiazepine receptors. *Clin. Neuropharmacology* **7**, Suppl. 1, 676–7, Raven Press, New York.

——, Horowski, R., Paschelke, G., Amin, M., and Braestrup, C. (1983). Severe anxiety induced by FG 7142, a β-carboline ligand for benzodiazepine receptors. *Lancet* 8341, 98–9.

Easton, J. D. and Sherman, D. G. (1976). Somatic anxiety attacks and propanolol. *Arch. Neurol.* 33, 689–91.

Emmet-Oglesby, M., Spencer, D. G., Elmesallamy, F., and Lal, H. (1983*a*). The pentylenetetrazol model of anxiety detects withdrawal from diazepam in rats. *Life Sci.* 33, 161–8.

—, —, Lewis, M., Elmesallamy, F., and Lal, H. (1983*b*). Anxiogenic aspects of diazepam withdrawal can be detected in animals. *Eur. J. Pharmac.* 92, 127–30.

Fraser, H. F. Wikler, A., Essig, C. F., and Isbell, H. (1958). Degree of physical dependence induced by secobarbital or phenobarbital. *J. Am. med. Assoc.* 166, 126–9.

Frohlich, E. D., Dunstan, H. P., and Page, I. H. (1966). Hyperdynamic beta-adrenergic circulatory state. *Arch. int. Med.* 117, 614–19.

—, Tarazi, R. C., and Dustan, H. P. (1969). Hyperdynamic β-adrenergic state: Increased β-receptor responsiveness. *Arch. int. Med.* 123, 1–7.

Garfield, S. L., Gershon, S., Sletten, I., Sundland, D. M., and Ballou, S. (1967). Chemically induced anxiety. *Int. J. Neuropsychiat.* 3, 426–33.

Gorman, J. M., Levy, G. F., Leibowitz, M. R., McGrath, P., Appleby, I. L., Dillon, D. J., Davies, S. D., and Klein, D. F. (1983). Effect of acute β-adrenergic blockade on lactate-induced panic. *Arch. gen. Psychiat.* 40, 1079–82.

Greden, J. F. (1974). Anxiety and caffeinism: a diagnostic dilemma. *Am. J. Psychiat.* 131, 1089–92.

Griez, E. and van den Hout, M. A. (1983). Treatment of phobophobia by exposure to CO_2-induced anxiety symptoms. *J. nerv. ment. Dis.* 171 (8), 506–8.

Guttmacher, L. B., Murphy, D. L., and Insel, T. R. (1983). Pharmacologic models of anxiety. *Comp. Psychiat.* 24, 312–26.

Hildebrandt, F. (1937). Pentamethylenetetrazol (cardioxol). *Handbk exp. Pharmac.* 5, 151–8.

Holmberg, G. and Gershon, S. (1961). Autonomic and psychic effects of yohimbine hydrochloride. *Psychopharmacologia* 2, 93–106.

Ingram, C. G. (1962). Some pharmacologic actions of yohimbine and chlorpromazine in man. *Clin. Pharmac. Ther.* 3, 345–52.

Insel, T. R., Ninan, P. T., Aloi, J., Jimerson, D., Skolnick, P., and Paul, S. M. (1984). A benzodiazepine receptor mediated model of anxiety: Studies in non-human primates and clinical implications. *Arch. gen. Psychiat.* 41, 741–50.

Kelly, D., Mitchell-Heggs, N., and Sherman, D. (1971). Anxiety and the effects of sodium lactate assessed clinically and physiologically. *Br. J. Psychiat.* 119, 129–41.

Kuno, M. and Weakly, J. N. (1972). Quantal components of the inhibitory synaptic potential in spinal motoneurones of the cat. *J. Physiol.* 224, 287–303.

Lader, M. (1983). Dependence on benzodiazepines. *J. clin. Psychiat.* 44, 121–7.

Lal, H. and Emmett-Oglesby, M. W. (1983). Behavioral analogues of anxiety, animal models. *Neuropharmacology* 22, 1423–41.

Levin, H. S., Rodnitzky, R. L., and Mick, D. L. (1976). Anxiety associated with exposure to organophosphate compounds. *Arch. gen. Psychiat.* 33, 225–8.

Lindemann, E. (1935). The psychopathological effect of drugs affecting the vegetative system. *Am. J. Psychiat.* 91, 983–1008.

Little, H. J. and Nutt, D. J. (1984). Benzodiazepine contragonists cause kindling. *Br. J. Pharmac.* **81**, 28P.

Lukas, S. E. and Griffiths, R. R. (1982). Precipitated withdrawal by a benzodiazepine receptor antagonist (Ro 15–1788) after 7 days of diazepam. *Science* **217**, 1161–3.

Marangos, P., Paul, A., Goodwin, F., Syapin, P., and Skolnick, P. (1979). Purinergic inhibition of diazepam binding to rat brain. *Life Sci.* **24**, 851–8.

Marks, J. (1978). *The benzodiazepines. Use, overuse, misuse, abuse.* MTP Press, Lancaster, Penn., USA.

Meduna, L. J. and Friedman, E. (1939). The convulsive-irritative therapy of the psychoses. *J. Am. med. Assoc.* **112**, 6.

Ninan, P. T., Insel, T. M., Cohen, R. M., Cook, J. M., Skolnick, P., and Paul, S. M. (1982). Benzodiazepine receptor-mediated experimental 'anxiety' in primates. *Science* **218**, 1332–4.

Petersen, E. N., Paschelke, G., Kehr, W., Nielsen, M., and Braestrup, C. (1982). Does the reversal of the anticonflict effect of phenobarbital by β-CCE and FG 7142 indicate benzodiazepine receptor-mediated anxiogenic properties. *Eur. J. Pharmac.* **82**, 217–21.

Petersen, E. N. (1983). DMCM: A potent convulsive benzodiazepine receptor ligand. *Eur. J. Pharmac.* **94**, 117–24.

Pitts, F. N. and McClure, J. N. (1967). Lactate metabolism in anxiety neurosis. *New Engl. J. Med.* **277**, 1329.

Plato. *Nomoi* 1, 15, 548.

Polc, P., Bonetti, E. P., Schaffner, R., and Haefely, W. (1982). A three-state model of the benzodiazepine receptor explains the interactions between the benzodiazepine antagonist Ro 15–1788, benzodiazepine tranquilizers, β-carbolines, and phenobarbitone. *Naunyn-Schmiedeberg's Arch. Pharmac.* **321**, 260–4.

Rall, T. W. (1980). Central nervous system stimulants. The xanthines. In *The pharmacological basis of therapeutics* (ed. A. Goodman Gilman, L. S. Gilman, and A. Gilman), 6th edn, pp. 592–607. Macmillan, New York.

Redmond, D. E. Jr. and Huang, Y. H. (1979). New evidence for a locus coeruleus-norepinephrine connection with anxiety. *Life Sci.* **25**, 2149–62.

Rifkin, A., Klein, D. F., Dillon, D., and Levitt, M. (1981). Blockade by imipramine or desipramine of panic induced by sodium lactate. *Am. J. Psychiat.* **138**, 676–7.

Rodin, E. (1958). Metrazol tolerance in a 'normal' volunteer population. *EEG clin. Neurophysiol.* **10**, 433–46.

Schöpf, J. (1983). Withdrawal phenomena after long-term administration of benzodiazepines. A review of recent investigations. *Pharmacopsychiatry* **16**, 1–8.

Stephens, D. N., Shearman, G. T., and Kehr, W. (1984). Discriminative stimulus properties of β-carbolines characterized as agonist and inverse agonists at central benzodiazepine receptors. *Psychopharmacology* **83**, 233–9.

—, Kehr, W., Wachtel, H., and Schmiechen R. (1985). The anxiolytic activity of β-carboline derivatives in mice, and its separation from ataxic properties. *Pharmacopsychiat.* **18**, 167–70.

Suzman, M. M. (1968). An evaluation of the effects of propanolol on the symptoms and electrocardiographic changes in patients with anxiety and the hyperventilation syndrome. Read before the 49th Annual Session of the American College of Physicians in association with the Royal College of Physicians of London, Boston, 2 April 1968.

Tallman, J. F., Paul, S. M., Skolnick, P., and Gallager, D. W. (1980). Receptors for the age of anxiety: pharmacology of the benzodiazepines. *Science* **207**, 274–81.

Wearn, J. T. and Sturgis, C. C. (1919). Studies on epinepherine: Effects of the injection of epinepherine in soldiers with 'irritable heart'. *Arch. int. Med.* **24**, 247–68.

White, B. C., Lincoln, C. A., Pearce, N. W., Reeb, R., and Varda, C. (1980). Anxiety and muscle tension as consequences of caffeine withdrawal. *Science* **209**, 1547–8.

10

Prospects in treating anxiety

PETER TRYER

In many ways the hopes and fears of psychopharmacology are exemplified in the history of anti-anxiety drugs. Each new anti-anxiety agent has been introduced as a major breakthrough, has received unqualified praise for a few years and then turned solidly towards a decline in a welter of recriminatory adverse effects. Perhaps it is related to anxiety being both an emotion and an essential drive; the emotion shouts out for attention and relief but the demands of the drive component are just as strong if far less strident. So any treatment for anxiety that removes the symptoms selectively and entirely will be far from ideal as it will almost certainly impair anxiety as a drive. There would be little problem if drive anxiety could be separated from symptom anxiety but this has to depend on the vagaries of clinical judgment. So, however we treat anxiety, it would be wrong to remove the symptom entirely even if at times it is painful.

The treatment of anxiety is therefore a two-edged sword, and a fine balance has be to struck. Perhaps even this is appropriate, as anxiety is predominantly concerned with choice and uncertainty.

It is useful to consider each of the important aspects of psychopharmacology with regard to anti-anxiety drugs. Each of them has made valuable and lasting contributions, but has also failed to detect important problems. For each discipline suggestions are made about overcoming these difficulties and the likely prospects for future developments. A full knowledge of past errors makes one unlikely to recapitulate them so it is valuable to take an historical perspective.

CLINICAL USE

The most striking feature of anti-anxiety drug treatment in the past two centuries has been fashion. At different times, opium, alcohol, chloral, barbiturates, propanediols, and benzodiazepines have been the most popular anti-anxiety drugs. Each time a new drug supplants the old it is hailed as having all the advantages of the old drugs and none of the adverse effects, and suggestions are made that the other drugs should be consigned to oblivion. The main adverse effects found are those of safety and drug dependence, dangers which are recognized surprisingly late in many cases.

The latest, and most pronounced, example of this 'boom-and-bust' pheno-menon is that of the benzodiazepines. At the time they were introduced in 1958 the drug treatment of anxiety was in disarray. Barbiturates had already been shown to be dangerous and addictive (Isbell, Altschul, Kornetsky, Eisen-man, Flanary, and Fraser 1950), meprobamate and the other propanediols were better but not particularly effective in reducing anxiety, and a new group of drugs was thought to be needed. When 'four hours after being given chlor-diazepoxide on New Year's Day 1958, one of twelve chronically anxious but therapeutically recalcitrant patients . . . telephoned that for the first time in many years he was totally free from symptoms' (Hordern 1968), the benzo-diazepine era began. Prescriptions for these drugs exceeded barbiturates within six years and by the 1970s they were the most commonly prescribed drugs in the world, with diazepam heading the list (Skegg, Doll, and Perry 1977). The demonstration that a significant proportion of patients on therapeutic doses of benzodiazepines develop pharmacological dependence (Petursson and Lader 1981; Tyrer, Rutherford, and Huggett 1981; Tyrer, Owen, and Dawling 1983; Ashton 1984) has led to a dramatic reversal in popularity and in the past four years there has been a significant drop in prescriptions for benzodiazepines throughout the western world.

The future must not reflect the past. There is now no more room for wonder drugs in anxiety. Even if a drug was found that was far superior to the benzo-diazepines and had no risks attached to its use, we would be in danger of approaching Aldous Huxley's *Brave New World*, in which the drug 'soma' was consumed by all and anxiety and strife no longer existed. It seems likely that anti-anxiety drugs will be used increasingly as adjuvants to other therapies and taken in flexible dosage for limited periods of time. The recent public reaction to the risks of dependence on benzodiazepines, which at times has assumed hysterical proportions, should not blind us to their merits. It would be a loss to psychiatry to have benzodiazepines no longer available and if they had been prescribed more rationally in the past much of the current concern would have been avoided.

Benzodiazepines, barbiturates, and propanediols are all sedative anti-anxiety agents which can cause drowsiness and other symptoms of central nervous depression in excessive, and sometimes in normal, dosage. Antipsychotic and tricyclic antidepressant drugs in low dosage also have anti-anxiety effects, primarily through their antihistaminic and anticholinergic properties and in this way act as sedatives. All such drugs will reduce anxiety both as a symptom and as a drive. This may be often unwanted in clinical practice and further refine-ments of this type of drug are unlikely to overcome this handicap.

An alternative means of overcoming anxiety is a stimulant drug that enhances self-confidence, removing the self-doubt and uncertainty that is such a feature of pathological anxiety. In the past amphetamines were valuable in treating anxiety in this way, but their euphoriant effects and high risk of dependence soon rendered them unacceptable. However, this is likely that the antiphobic and anti-panic effects of tricyclic antidepressants (Klein, 1964; McNair and Kahn 1981) and monoamine oxidase inhibitors (Tyrer, Candy, and Kelly 1973; Sheehan, Ballenger, and Jacobsen 1980) have the same pharmacodynamic action. This is independent of sedation as there is a time lag of between one and six weeks before onset of therapeutic effects and improvement is not related to their anticholinergic properties.

More attention could be paid to the possible anti-anxiety potential of drugs having an activating profile in early pharmacological studies. The monoamine oxidase inhibitors are highly effective anti-anxiety drugs and in anxiety and phobic disorders appear to be somewhat superior to tricyclic antidepressants (Tyrer and Shawcross 1984) but their potential adverse effects make it unlikely that they will be used widely. There is a place for similar agents, including monoamine oxidase inhibitors without the 'cheese effect', although unfortunately efficacy and potential toxicity seem to be intertwined (Sandler 1981). The main advantage of such drugs is that they can alleviate anxiety symptoms without affecting the drive component, and may even enhance this through their stimulant action.

Two other aspects of the treatment of clinical anxiety need refinement. The first is diagnosis, as without accurate diagnosis treatment will always be confused. After years in limbo, the classification of anxiety has now attracted new attention, most particularly in the United States where DSM-III now classifies the main anxiety disorders into Generalized Anxiety Disorder, Panic Disorder, Agoraphobia with Panic Attacks and Agoraphobia (alone) (American Psychiatric Association 1980). An important stimulus for reclassification has been the work of Klein and his colleagues (Klein 1964, 1980; Zitrin, Klein, and Woerner 1980) suggesting that drug response differs within anxious disorders and at the presence or absence of panic is an important predictor. This needs further enquiry and the DSM-III categories enable hypotheses to be tested.

The second aspect is combined drug and psychological therapy in anxiety. Anxiety disorders are an excellent example of the need for a combined approach, and as self-mastery of symptoms is the eventual aim it should be stimulated early in treatment. Unfortunately, studies involving combined drug and psychological treatments are remarkably few, and even long-established treatments such as relaxation training for anxiety have not been subjected to the rigorous clinical trials that would establish its efficacy without question. Studies of combined therapy are not easy to carry out as they have include at least three groups of patients – two with the treatment separate and one with them combined – but they will be essential for clinical progress.

PHARMACODYNAMIC ASPECTS

The effects of anxiety on the mind and body have been the subject of sound scientific enquiry since the time of Cannon. The science of psychophysiology owes a great deal to anxiety as many of its techniques have been stimulated through study of this mood (Lader 1975). Unfortunately, psychophysiology has not quite lived up to its initial expectations that it could be developed further into the objective measurement of anxiety and other mood states. The correlation between psychophysiological measures, both central and peripheral, and anxious mood are disappointingly low (Tyrer and Lader 1976), and the development of rating scales for anxiety have refined its assessment more than the most sophisticated of psychophysiological tests.

There has therefore been a shift away from laboratory tests and techniques such as the galvanic skin response and skin conductance, forearm blood flow, and auditory-evoked potentials towards more direct assessments of function. Anxiety only becomes a major clinical problem when it is of sufficient intensity to cause disintegration of normal function. Similarly, a drug treatment may be excellent at relieving the symptoms of anxiety but lead to marked impairment of functioning through its adverse effects. The development of ingenious quantitative tests of performance in real life by psychologists such as Hindmarch (e.g. Hindmarch and Gudgeon 1980) is likely to be extended in the future. One can envisage tests of function in specified activities becoming mandatory in the assessment of new anti-anxiety agents (and other drugs) as regulatory bodies become more sensitive to these aspects of drug function.

There is also a need to develop laboratory equivalents of pathological anxiety. Volunteer studies are always limited by the inability to generalize from drug effects in a normal person (whether or not they are under stress at the time of testing) to clinical anxiety in patients. There must be better laboratory correlates of clinical anxiety but we have yet to find them.

PHARMACOKINETICS

Pharmacokinetics probably has expanded faster than any other discipline within pharmacology in the past ten years. Before then there was very little interest in the metabolism of drugs, their relative concentrations in body fluids or in their speed of elimination. All has now changed and close study of the pharmacokinetics of a compound is essential if it is to receive approval for clinical use. There is much greater awareness of pharmacokinetics among doctors as a whole, and, whereas discussion of the half-life of a compound may have been greeted with blank faces a few years ago, now it is immediately recognized and understood.

Despite this, pharmacokinetics remains a secondary discipline within pharmacology and, in my view is at present overrated. Its expansion has led to a unnecessary proliferation of anti-anxiety drugs, which are really replicas of existing compounds. The minor variations in pharmacokinetics which separate them do not have any clinical significance (*Drugs and Therapeutics Bulletin* 1978; Greenblatt and Shader 1978). Pharmacokinetics as a separate discipline is in danger of overreaching itself. It must always be remembered that the pharmacokinetics of a drug explains rather than predicts, and that the pharmacodynamic effects of a drug will always be more important than its pharmacokinetic aspects. Ten years ago, Dollery was the first to point out these dangers in a prescient editorial and it is even more true today (Dollery 1973). Pharmacokinetics plays the same role in pharmacology as the Civil Service in a government. It organizes, refines and executes decisions and advances rather than initiates them. In the future it will probably be of lesser importance in psychopharmacology than it is today.

ANIMAL PHARMACOLOGY

There is a range of well-established tests for screening anxiety and other psychotropic drugs (Spencer 1976) and these have served psychopharmacology well in the past. These tests, such as the inhibition of condition avoidance responses to aversive stimuli, will continue to be used as essential routine experiments in the evaluation of potential anti-anxiety drugs. However, there are several other branches of animal pharmacology that are more fundamental in stimulating progress. A study of behaviour under optimal conditions after drug therapy in different animals (ethopsychopharmacology) and combined study of behaviour, neuropsychology, and pharmacology (neuropsychopharmacology), are likely to expand rapidly and have already led to exciting new theories about the mechanism of anxiety, its relationship with depression and the differences between normal and pathological anxiety (Seligman and Maier 1967; Gray 1982). These theories are helping to bridge the gap between animal and human psychopharmacology, and are doing so with the aid of complex cybernetic and behavioural arguments that can in no way be dismissed as reductionist.

NEUROCHEMISTRY

Neuropharmacology deals with the most fundamental aspects of drug treatment, and at its heart are the changes that take place at receptors and consequently in organ systems when drugs are administered. Thirty years ago all the neuropharmacology of psychotropic drugs could be written on the back of the proverbial postage stamp and most of it would have been speculation. Now we have almost a surfeit of receptors and mechanisms of drug action and the implications and nature of their interactions are proven more difficult to unravel than when they are studied alone. The discovery of benzodiazepine receptors in the central nervous system (Möhler and Okada 1977; Squires and Braestrup 1977) is likely to prove a landmark in understanding the nature of anxiety and the internal mechansims that are concerned with its generation and control.

We now know that the benzodiazepine receptors are closely lined to GABA-receptors in the central nervous system and that they often function as a single unit together with a chloride channel (Olsen 1980). Benzodiazepines facilitate GABA-transmission but this is a non-specific property possessed by both alcohol and barbiturates. Benzodiazepine receptors are found in reasonable concentrations in the limbic system (Möhler and Okada 1977) but are also found in greater concentrations in parts of the cerebellum, spinal cord and cortex (Braestrup and Squires 1977; Möhler and Okada 1977). It therefore appears unlikely that there is a simple relationship between benzodiazepine receptors and the anti-anxiety effects of either drugs or endogenous factors alleviating anxiety. The demonstration of a benzodiazepine receptor implies that there is an endogenous ligand that normally binds with the benzodiazepine receptor and has either an anxiogenic or anxiolytic effect. Determined efforts have been made to find the elusive ligand but it is still unknown. After so much searching without success it is likely that the ligand either does not exist as a single substance or is present for only a very short time in its active form. Already there is evidence for at least two types of benzodiazepine receptor (Klepner *et al.* 1979) and only one may be concerned with anxiety. It seems likely that further major advances are close at hand and these will undoubtedly be relevant to the drug treatment of anxiety.

SUMMARY

The past gains, present handicaps and likely future developments in treating anxiety are summarized for each of the main pharmacological disciplines (Table 10.1). Like anxiety itself, each discipline is uncertain and insecure about its own role but, with the possible exception of pharmacokinetics, is likely to grow in stature as it makes advances.

PREDICTION

It is entertaining, if not always informative, to attempt prediction of the future. If asked to guess what major advances in anti-anxiety treatment are likely in the remaining fifteen years of this century I would predict the following scenario.

Over the next five years the total number of prescriptions for anti-anxiety drugs will fall gradually and there will be no obvious replacements for the benzodiazepines. Sedative antidepressants such as trimipramine, amitriptyline, and mianserin will tend to be used increasingly for the relief of anxiety on the grounds that they are less likely to lead to long-term problems such as dependence and also protect the drive component of anxiety. The endogenous ligand for benzodiazepine receptors will be discovered by 1990; it will prove to be relevant to depression as well as anxiety and help to explain their clinical interrelationship. Synthesis of compounds derived from the endogenous ligand will introduce new anti-anxiety drugs but these, like the benzodiazepines, will be shown to produce pharmacological dependence and therefore only used occasionally.

In the last decade of the century a major new psychological treatment for anxiety will be discovered, which in retrospect will be seen to be a rediscovery of existing knowledge. This will replace much of anti-anxiety drug therapy but

TABLE 10.1. *Past, present, and future of anti-anxiety drugs*

Discipline	Past gains	Present handicaps	Future prospects
Clinical use	Steady development of safer and more effective drugs.	All the most effective drugs carry risk of dependence.	More sparing use, more emphasis on stimulant drugs.
Pharmacodynamics	Excellent record of drug effects on many organ systems.	Great difficulty in predicting drug effects and relating them to anxiety.	Closer links between drug effects and receptor changes.
Pharmacokinetics	Greater understanding of fate of drugs in body, particularly their metabolites.	Proliferation of un-necessary compounds differing only in pharmaco-kinetics.	Lesser importance given to subject.
Animal pharmacology	Good record of screening potential drugs.	Difficulty in interpreting across species to man.	Greater role of neuropsychology.
Neurochemistry	Demonstration of benzo-diazepine receptor and role of GABA in the central nervous system.	Inability to relate drug effects to receptor changes.	Identification of natural substances concerned with normal control of anxiety.

will also be used in combination with drugs given intermittently for short periods. By the end of the millenium very few patients will be taking anti-anxiety drugs regularly and most of these will be dependent patients who were first prescribed their drugs in the 1970s. Legislation will be passed which will place most anti-anxiety drugs in the same category as established addictive agents such as the opiates and amphetamines.

REFERENCES

American Psychiatric Association (1980). *Diagnostic and statistical manual of mental disorders*, 3rd edn. American Psychiatric Association, Washington.

Ashton, H. (1984). Benzodiazepine dependence: an unfinished story. *Br. med. J.* **288**, 1135–40.

Braestrup, C. and Squires, R. F. (1977). Specific benzodiazepine receptors in rat brain characterized by high-affinity [3-H]-diazepam binding. *Proc. natn Acad. Sci., U.S.A.* **74**, 3805–9.

Dollery, C. T. (1973). Pharmacokinetics – Master or servant? *Eur. J. clin. Pharmac.* **6**, 1–2.

Drug and Therapeutics Bulletin (1978). Therapeutic differences between benzodiazepines. **16**, 46–8.

Gray, J. A. (1982). *The neuropsychology of anxiety: an enquiry into the functions of the septo-hippocampal system.* Clarendon Press, Oxford.

Greenblatt, D. J. and Shader, R. I. (1978). Prazepam and lorazepam, two new benzodiazepines. *New Engl. J. Med.* **299**, 1342–4.

Hindmarch, I. and Gudgeon, A. C. (1980). The effects of clobazam and lorazepam on aspects of psychomoter performance and car handling ability. *Br. J. clin. Pharmac.* **10**, 145–50.

Hordern, A. (1968). Psychopharmacology: some historical considerations. In *Psychopharmacology: dimensions and perspectives* (ed. C. R. B. Joyce), p. 121. Tavistock Publications, London.

Isbell, H., Altschul, S., Kornetsky, C. H., Eisenman, A. J., Flanary, H. G., and Fraser, H. F. (1950). Chronic barbiturate intoxication. *Arch. Neurol. Psychiat.* **64**, 1–16.

Klein, D. F. (1964). Delineation of two drug-responsive anxiety syndromes. *Psychopharmacologia* **5**, 397–408.

—— (1980). Anxiety reconceptualized. *Comp. Psychiat.* **21**, 411–27.

Klepner, C. A., Lippa, A. S., Benson, D. I., Sano, M. C., and Beer, B. (1979). Resolution of two biochemically and pharmacologically distinct benzodiazepine receptors. *Pharmac. Biochem. & Behav.* **11**, 457–62.

Lader, M. (1975). *The psychophysiology of mental illness.* Routledge & Kegan Paul, London.

McNair, D. M. and Kahn, R. J. (1981). Imipramine compared with a benzodiazepine for agoraphobia. In *Anxiety: New research and changing concepts* (ed. D. F. Klein and J. G. Rabkin), pp. 69–80. Raven Press, New York.

Möhler, H. and Okada, T. (1977). Benzodiazepine receptor: demonstration in the central nervous system. *Science* **198**, 849–51.

Olsen, R. W. (1981). GABA-benzodiazepine-barbiturate receptor interactions. *J. Neurochem.* **37**, 1–13.

Petursson, H. and Lader, M. H. (1981). Withdrawal from long-term benzodiazepine treatment. *Br. med. J.* **283**, 643–5.

Sandler, M. (1981). Monoamine oxidase inhibitor efficacy in depression and the 'cheese effect'. *Psychol. Med.* **11**, 455-8.

Seligman, M. E. P. and Maier, S. F. (1967). Failure to escape traumatic shock. *J. exp. Psychol.* **74**, 1-9.

Sheehan, D. V., Ballenger, J., and Jacobsen, G. (1980). Treatment of endogenous anxiety with phobic, hysterical and hypochondriacal symptoms. *Arch. gen. Psychiat.* **37**, 51-9.

Skegg, D. C. G., Doll, R., and Perry, J. (1977). Use of medicines in general practice. *Br. med. J.* i, 1561-3.

Spencer, P. S. J. (1976). Animal models for screening new agents. *Br. J. clin. Pharmac.* **3**, suppl., 5-12.

Squires, R. F. and Braestrup, C. (1977). Benzodiazepine receptors in rat brain. *Nature, Lond.* **266**, 732-4.

Tyrer, P. J. and Lader, M. H. (1976). Central and peripheral correlates of anxiety. *J. nerv. ment. Dis.* **162**, 99-104.

— and Shawcross, C. (1984). Monoamine oxidase inhibitors in anxiety disorders. *J. clin. Psychopharmac.* (in press).

—, Candy, J., and Kelly, D. (1973). A study of the clinical effects of phenelzine and placebo in the treatment of phobic anxiety. *Psychopharmacologia* **32**, 237-54.

—, Owen, R., and Dawling, S. (1983). Gradual withdrawal of diazepam after long-term therapy. *Lancet* i, 1402-6.

—, Rutherford, D., and Huggett, T. (1981). Benzodiazepine withdrawal symptoms and propranolol. *Lancet* i, 520-2.

Zitrin, C. M., Klein, D. F., and Woerner, M. G. (1980). Treatment of agoraphobia with group exposure in vivo and imipramine. *Arch. gen. Psychiat.* **37**, 63-72.

PART 3
Psychopharmacology and cognition

11

Psychopharmacology of cognition

SUSAN D. IVERSEN

Cognition is defined as the 'action of knowing, perceiving, conceiving as opposed to emotion and volition', the highest level of neural integration in the brain. The study of cognitive function in patients who have sustained damage to the nervous system confirms the view that the hippocampus and neocortex are the key brain structures involved in cognitive mechanisms.

Focal damage to various sectors of the cortex in animals and in man impairs, in a highly selective manner, different aspects of cognitive processing; the coding of visual, auditory or tactile sensory stimuli, their perception, recognition, naming and memory. Precisely wired thalamo–cortical projections and intracortical connections ensure the processing of specific classes of stimuli in modality-specific sensory and association cortex.

The visual system has been studied in particular detail and it is well established that damage to the visual sensory cortex, while reducing the capacity for detailed vision or acuity, does not impair the ability to discriminate between objects. Striate and pre-striate visual cortex project to the visual association cortex in the posterior part of ventral temporal lobe. Lesions to this area in monkeys and in man impair the ability to distinguish visual forms and common objects (Iversen 1983). Similar studies have been performed in the auditory, tactile and olfactory cortex confirming the specialization of posterior cortex for perception. The organization is further extended in man, where the perception of verbal and non-verbal material involves different hemispheres.

Further convergence of highly processed information occurs in frontal cortex. Lesion studies indicate that the highest levels of cortical integration occur in this region. The ability to store and retrieve information depends on the integrity of structures in the limbic system and thalamus, notably the amygdala–hippocampal circuit and medial thalamus.

Recently, much attention has become focused on the psychopharmacology of cognition. Why? Three developments have converged to create this interest. First, the gradual unravelling of the anatomy of the neurotransmitter pathways of the mammalian brain and the discovery that a very large number of chemical transmitters exist in the cortex in highly organized relationships to the intrinsically layered cortical columns. Second, more attention has been given to the psychological evaluation of the diffuse disorders of cognition seen in dementia, particularly senile dementia of the Alzheimer's type (AD), which is characterized by memory loss, especially of recent events, learning disability, spatial and temporal disorientation, impaired speech, and loss of sensory and motor control. The range of impairments, their order of onset, and the rate of deterioration varies considerably between patients. Third, it has been established for some years that plaques and neurofibrillary tangles exist as neuropathological markers of AD and that the severity of the dementia correlates with their numbers in cortex and hippocampus.

In the late 1970s it was reported that marked loss of acetylcholinesterase and choline acetyltransferase could be measured in the cortex of patients dying with AD, and that the loss of cholinergic markers also correlated with the severity of dementia (Perry, Tomlinson, Blessed, Bergmann, Gibson, and Perry 1978) (for reveiw see Perry and Perry 1980, and Rossor, Emson, Mountjoy, Roth, and Iversen 1982). In subpopulations of patients dying with AD, losses of cortical noradrenaline, serotonin, and somatostatin have also been reported (Rossor 1982). Since these transmitter candidates are known to be widely distributed in cortex and since the global nature of the cognitive loss in AD implicates widespread cortical dysfunction, there is growing interest in the possibility that AD may represent a degenerative disease of certain neurotransmitter pathways. Many of the successful psychoactive drugs which have been developed for treating psychiatric and neurological conditions are known to act by modifying neurotransmitter function, raising hopes for a drug to restore in AD functional levels of neurotransmitters in cortex. In this symposium a number of these issues are dealt with in more detail. However, in view of the very considerable interest generated by these findings, it seems timely to raise some questions which are unresolved and should not be ignored.

1. *Is there a relationship between the neuropathological markers and the loss of ACh in AD?*

In post-mortem tissue there is no doubt that both the neuropathological markers and the cholinergic loss correlate with the dementia score (Perry *et al.* 1978; Rossor *et al.* 1982). If both reflect degenerative processes, do they proceed in parallel or is one secondary to the other? In aged animals of some species plaques and neurofibrillary tangles are observed and provide an experimental model for determining the biochemical mechanisms involved in the creation of these neuropathological features.

2. *Are the cell bodies of cortical projections as well as the cortical terminals degenerated in AD?*

The discovery of an ACh deficiency in AD has led to a rapid expansion in our knowledge of the anatomical organization of the cholinergic neurones in brain. In 1967 Shute and Lewis provided the first mapping of cholinergic neurones in brain using ACh-esterase as a marker. This may give a misleading picture, since the enzyme involved in the degradation of ACh is now known to exist also in non-cholinergic neurones and at synapses where ACh is not released (Rossier 1977). The development of sensitive assay and immuno-histochemical methods for evaluating levels and distribution of the specific enzyme involved in the synthesis of ACh, choline acetyltransferase, combined with the use of radioactive tracing agents, has now made it possible to define more precisely the cholinergic projections in mammalian brain (Fibiger 1982). The cholinergic neurones innervating cortex lie in the basal forebrain inter-mingled in substantia innominata (nucleus basalis of Meynert) with many non-cholinergic neurone groups. It should be noted that this anatomical fact creates a number of problems in experimental studies of the cholinergic system. A selective toxin for ACh neurones is not yet available and with non-specific mechanical or toxin lesions of this area it is difficult to confine damage to the cholinergic neurones. Equally, it is difficult to label selectively those neurones or distinguish them from surrounding tissue when they have been labelled.

However, despite these difficulties a consensus of fact is emerging about the cholinergic forebrain projections.

1. About 30 per cent of cortical ACh resides in neurones that are intrinsic to the cortex.
2. Within substantia innominata, the cholinergic neurones are concentrated in the nucleus basalis and extend to the diagonal band; these neurones innervate the cortical mantle topographically. Cholinergic neurones in the septal nuclei innervate hippocampus. Using specific choline acetyl-transferase immunohistochemistry, these projections have been defined in rat (Mesulam, Mufson, Wainer, and Levy 1983*b*) and monkey (Mesulam, Mufson, Levey, and Wainer 1983*a*).
3. In AD a substantial loss of cholinergic activity is observed in cortex and hippocampus (Perry and Perry 1980; Rossor *et al.* 1982).

But questions remain. Is the residual cholinergic activity in cortex due to undamaged terminals of the cholinergic neurones projecting from nucleus basalis to cortex or to the remaining intrinsic neurones? The ChAT activity in the intrinsic neurones is low and at the limits of resolution for the existing immunohistochemical techniques, making it difficult to answer the question. It is clear, however, that a substantial proportion of the cortical ChAT loss must be ascribed to degeneration of the ascending terminal projection. Whitehouse, Price, Struble, Clark, Coyle, and deLong (1982) have reported that in AD the degeneration proceeds to the cell body level in basal forebrain where a significant loss of the large ACh-containing neurones is observed. Perry, Candy, Perny, Irving, Blessed, Fairbairn, and Tomlinson (1982), however, found that the exten-sive loss of ChAT activity in the cortex of AD patients was not matched by an equally extensive loss of neurones from the nucleus of basalis of Meynert. Sofroniew, Pearson and Eckenstein, Cuello, and Powell (1983) have also claimed that in experimental degeneration of nucleus basalis in monkeys, induced by cortical lesions, and in AD (Pearson, Sofroniew, Cuello, Powell, Eckenstein,

Esiri, and Wilcock 1983), the cholinergic cell bodies in nucleus basalis are shrunken but not lost.

It is important to resolve these anatomical issues since they have important implications for the pharmacological treatment of AD, where the emphasis at present focuses on cholinergic replacement therapy. The potential response to direct or indirect agonist therapy is likely to vary with the degree and nature of the degeneration of the neurochemical pathways. Such information is also important for the development of animal models of AD. Animal models of mental illness play a key role in the search for novel drugs and attempts are being made to evaluate the effects of cholinergic lesions in animals. However, there remains the problem of modelling the essential symptoms of the human condition with an acute treatment in the animal model. Dopamine lesions in rats and monkeys do not result in Parkinsonian-like symptoms. Will acute cholinergic lesions induce the symptoms seen in AD? It may indeed by impossible to replicate in animal models the slow degenerative diseases of CNS. Perhaps combinations of partial ACh cell body and terminal lesions, induced sequentially or combinations of partial lesions to the various monoamine systems implicated in AD would provide interesting alternatives to the global, acute ACh lesions to nucleus basalis. But does a model need to reflect directly the disease state? In some instances, for example the use of dopamine agonists in Parkinson's disease or dopamine antagonists in schizophrenia, models inducing under or overactivity of the forebrain dopamine pathways with lesions or drugs have proved highly satisfactory for drug testing, despite the fact that the behavioural assay used does not resemble the clinical condition. In this sense any measure of cholinergic cortical function should be useful for detecting potential cholinergic agonists.

3. *Is a cholinergic loss in cortex unique to AD?*

Recently Dubois, Ruberg, Javoy-Agid, Ploska, and Agid (1983) have reported that in certain advanced forms of Parkinson's disease, dementia is seen, which is clinically difficult to distinguish from AD. It is known that in such patients the the degeneration of the dopamine system is more widespread and complete than in less severely affected patients. However, it now appears that in such patients the degeneration extends to other monoamine systems, and in particular a correlation between the loss of cholinergic markers in cortex and the severity of the dementia was found. Cholinomimetic agents may also find a clinical use in such Parkinsonian patients.

THE CONCEPT OF THE ISODENDRITIC CORE

It is becoming clear that a number of neuropsychiatric conditions which result in gross disturbances of cognition are associated with degeneration of the mono-aminergic innervation of neocortex and allo-cortex. The monoamine neurones in brain form a dense core (Rossor 1981) extending from brainstem to basal forebrain. These neurones collateralize, have extensive axon and terminal aborization in cortex, and physiologically appear to serve tonic modulatory (rather than phasic) roles in higher levels of integration. Further support for this functional interpretation of the monoamine core is provided by recent experiments on grafting of such neurones. Foetal monoamine neurones survive grafting to adult CNS, particularly to sites deprived of their monoamine innervation. Such grafts of dopamine (Dunnett, Bjorklund, Stenevi, and Iversen 1981) or cholinergic (Dunnett, Low, Iversen, Stenevi, and Bjorklund 1982) neurones, despite the fact that they are cut off from their normal *in situ* anatomical connections, survive, are metabolically active, form synapses, and manufacture transmitter which is released and which can be shown to afford functional compensation in the damaged adult brain.

In Parkinson's disease, Huntington's Chorea, and AD, a progressive degeneration of the so-called isodendritic core neurones occurs (Rossor 1982). If these systems release monoamines to regulate levels of neural integration rather than provide synaptic transmission of specific signals, their replacement with diffuse acting agonists should be functionally useful. L-DOPA treatment of Parkinson's disease provides a striking example of this approach and encourages the search for an equivalent therapy in AD. Further encouragement is afforded by findings of Crachman (1977) who found that the deterioration of cognitive performance (particularly short-term memory) induced by the cholinergic antagonist scopolamine in normal volunteers could be reversed by the AChE inhibitor, physostigmine, but not by the stimulant drug d-amphetamine.

The clinical evaluation of potential cerebroactive drugs in dementia is hampered by a failure to use the specific cognitive test batteries of the kind reported in the Drachman study. Too much weight is currently given to global geriatric rating scales, which include some general assessment of memory but are heavily weighted to the emotional and social responses of the patient. When more quantitative assessment of cognitive function is made a number of the widely used drugs appear to lack efficacy, and there is little evidence of any significant effects on cognition (McDonald 1982). In conclusion, the use of neurone replacement, centrally acting agonist drugs, or some combination of these two, holds promise for the treatment of degenerative diseases of the isodendritic core.

REFERENCES

Drachman, D. A. (1977). Memory and cognitive function in Man: Does the cholinergic system have a specific role? *Neurology* 27, 783–90.

Dubois, B., Ruberg, M., Javoy-Agid, F., Ploska, A., and Agid, Y. (1983). A subcortico-cortical cholinergic system is affected in Parkinson's disease. *Brain Res.* 288, 213–18.

Dunnett, S. B., Bjorklund, A., Stenevi, U., and Iversen, S. D. (1981). Behavioural recovery following transplantation of substantia nigra in rats subjected to 6-OHDA lesions of the nigro-striatal pathway. I. Unilateral lesions. *Brain Res.* 215, 147–61.

—, Low, W. C., Iversen, D. S., Stenevi, U., and Bjorklund, A. (1982). Septal transplants restore maze learning in rats with fornix-fimbria lesions. *Brain Res.* **251**, 335–48.

Fibiger, H. C. (1982). The organization and some projections of cholinergic neurons of the mammalian forebrain. *Brain Res. Rev.* **4**, 327–88.

Iversen, S. D. (1983). Brain lesions and memory in animals: a reappraisal. In *The physiological basis of memory* (ed. J. A. Deutsch), pp. 139–98. Academic Press, New York and London.

Mesulam, M-M., Mufson, E. J., Levey, A. I., and Wainer, B. H. (1983*a*). Cholinergic innervation of cortex by the basal forebrain: Cytochemistry and cortical connections of the septal area, diagonal band nuclei, nucleus basalis (substantia innominata) and hypothalamus in the Rhesus monkey. *J. comp. neurol.* **214**, 170–97.

—, —, Wainer, B. H., and Levey, A. I. (1983*b*). Central cholinergic pathways in the rat: an overview based on an alternative nomenclature (Ch.1–Ch.6). *Neuroscience* **10**, 1185–201.

McDonald, R. J. (1982). Drug treatment of senile dementia. In *Psychopharmacology of old age*, British Association for Psychopharmacology Monograph No. 3 (ed. D. Wheatley), pp. 113–38. Oxford University Press.

Pearson, R. C. A., Sofroniew, M. V., Cuello, A. C., Powell, T. P. S., Eckenstein, F., Esiri, M. M., and Wilcock, G. K. (1983). Persistence of cholinergic neurons in the basal nucleus in a brain with senile dementia of the Alzheimer's type demonstrated by immunohistochemical staining for choline acetyltransferase. *Brain Res.* **289**, 375–9.

Perry, E. K. and Perry, R. H. (1980). The cholinergic system in Alzheimer's disease. In *Biochemistry of dementia* (ed. P. J. Roberts), pp. 135–83. Wiley, Chichester, New York and Toronto.

—, Tomlinson, B. E., Blessed, G., Bergmann, K., Gibson, P. H., and Perry, R. H. (1978). Correlation of cholinergic abnormalities with senile plaque and mental test scores in senile dementia. *Brt. med. J.* **2**, 1457–9.

Perry, R. H., Candy, J. M., Perry, E. K., Irving, D., Blessed, G., Fairbairn, A. F., and Tomlinson, B. E. (1982). Extensive loss of choline acetyltransferase activity is not reflected by neuronal loss in the nucleus of Meynert in Alzheimer's disease. *Neurosci. Lett.* **33**, 311–15.

Rossier, J. (1977). Choline acetyltransferase: A review with special reference to its cellular and subcellular localization. *Int. Rev. Neurobiol.* **20**, 284–337.

Rossor, M. N. (1981). Parkinson's disease and Alzheimer's disease as disorders of the isodendritic core. *Brit. med. J.* **283**, 1–7.

— (1982). Neurotransmitters and CNS disease. *Lancet* 1200–4.

—, Emson, P. C., Mountjoy, C. Q., Roth, M., and Iversen, L. L. (1982). Neurotransmitters of the cerebral cortex in senile dementia of Alzheimer's type. *Exp. Brain Res.*, suppl. 5, 153–7.

Shute, C. C. D. and Lewis, P. R. (1967). The ascending cholinergic reticular systems: Neocortical, olfactory and subcortical projections. *Brain* **90**, 487–50.

Sofroniew, M. V., Pearson, R. C. A., Eckenstein, F., Cuello, A. C., and Powell, T. P. S. (1983). Retrograde changes in cholinergic neurons in the basal forebrain of the rat following cortical damage. *Brain Res.* **289**, 370–4.

Whitehouse, P. J., Price, D. L., Struble, R. G., Clark, A. W., Coyle, J. T., and deLong, M. R. (1982). Alzheimer's disease and senile dementia: Loss of neurons in the basal forebrain. *Science* **215**, 1237–9.

12

Alzheimer's disease and Parkinson's disease: pathological and biochemical changes associated with dementia

J. A. EDWARDSON, C. A. BLOXHAM, J. M. CANDY, A. E. OAKLEY,
R. H. PERRY, AND E. K. PERRY

INTRODUCTION

Both Alzheimer's and Parkinson's diseases are disorders of unknown aetiology involving degenerative changes in the brain. Cognitive impairment, whilst differing in prevalence and severity, is also common to both disorders. In Alzheimer's disease, dementia of insidious onset and progressive deterioration is invariable and is characterized by the following mental disabilities: profound memory loss; impairment of abstract thinking and judgement; aphasia, apraxia, and agnosia. In contrast, a less severe form of dementia occurs in a variable proportion of patients with Parkinson's disease and frequently includes disturbances in visuospatial skills whereas symptoms of aphasia, apraxia and agnosia are said to be absent (Mayeux 1982).

It is generally accepted that 'higher' mental functions in man are associated with the relatively great development of the neocortex. However, such complex activities depend not only on the integrity of the cerebral cortex but also on the integrity of connections between the cortex and various subcortical nuclei. Functional intellectual abnormalities in degenerative diseases of the brain may therefore reflect primary abnormalities at either level. Thus, Albert, Feldman, and Willis (1974), in attempting to relate mental changes in dementia to the involvement of particular brain areas, introduced the concept of distinct 'cortical' and 'subcortical' dementias and assigned Alzheimer's disease to the former and Parkinson's disease to the latter categories. Recent neuropathological and neurochemical observations on autopsy brain material have, however, challenged this notion. Several subcortical nuclei, in addition to the cerebral cortex, are now known to be involved in Alzheimer's disease whilst, in Parkinson's disease, neurochemical abnormalities of the cortex relating to the degree of dementia have recently been reported. It is probable that common neuroanatomical pathways are involved in the cognitive changes in Alzheimer's and Parkinson's disease but that the site of primary and secondary abnormalities differ. Thus, in

Alzheimer's disease present evidence suggests that primary lesions in the cortex may lead to secondary changes in subcortical nuclei, and, vice versa, in Parkinson's disease cortical abnormalities may be the result of primary subcortical degeneration.

NEUROPATHOLOGICAL CHANGES IN SUBCORTICAL NUCLEI

A comparison of the various regions known to be pathologically involved in Alzheimer's and Parkinson's disease (Table 12.1) suggests that there are in fact more areas of involvement common to the two disorders than areas specifically affected in one or other disorder. Thus, anatomically in both diseases, there are neuropathological abnormalities in at least three different subcortical nuclei — locus coeruleus, nucleus of Meynert, and dorsal raphe nucleus — all of which project to the cerebral cortex. As judged by evidence to date, neuronal loss in these nuclei is more extensive in Parkinson's compared with Alzheimer's disease (or at least the senile form of the latter). This observation in itself suggests that neuron numbers in these areas are not correlated closely with the severity of dementia, since dementia is generally of greater severity in Alzheimer's disease. In the locus coeruleus, for example, neuron loss in Alzheimer's disease is not closely associated with either the clinical or pathological features of the dementia (Tomlinson, Irving, and Blessed 1981). Furthermore, in the nucleus basalis of Meynert, neuronal loss is greater in non-demented cases of Parkinson's disease (Candy, Perry, Perry, Irving, Blessed, Fairbairn, and Tomlinson 1983; Whitehouse, Hedreen, White, and Price 1983) than in elderly (70–90 years) demented cases of Alzheimer's disease (Perry, Candy, Perry, Irving, Blessed, Fairbairn, and Tomlinson 1982). These observations support the concept that cognitive impairment is not necessarily a function of neuronal loss — at least in Alzheimer's disease. This conclusion does not exclude the possibility that there are important functional changes in these neuronal systems which are not initially manifest structurally. Indeed, abnormalities in cortical neurochemistry relating to the projections from these nuclei appear, at least in the instance of the cholinergic system, to correlate more closely with cognitive impairment in both diseases than do morphological changes in the subcortical nuclei.

One subcortical nucleus which clearly distinguishes Parkinson's from Alzheimer's disease is the substantia nigra. Extensive loss of neurons from this area, not seen in Alzheimer's disease, is considered to be the core abnormality related to the movement disorder of Parkinson's disease. A consistent correlation is reported between the severity of Parkinsonism and the presence of intellectual impairment, suggesting that basal ganglia dysfunction may, at least in part, be associated with Parkinsonian dementia. If this is so, then the normality — at least structurally — of the basal ganglia in Alzheimer's disease would indicate a major difference between the two diseases with respect to the cause and presumably also type of dementia. On the other hand, the relation between

TABLE 12.1. *Neuropathological abnormalities in Alzheimer's and Parkinson's disease*

Brain area	Alzheimer's disease	Parkinson's disease
Cerebral cortex	Senile plaques and neurofibrillary tangles throughout; Hirano bodies and granulovacuolar degeneration in archicortical structures; Neuronal loss probable in some areas; Reduction in dendritic arbour.	Conflicting reports, but probable that Alzheimer-type changes only occur in a minority of cases in excess of normal age-related changes; Lewy bodies rarely present.
Substantia nigra	Neuron population probably normal but not quantitatively assessed.	Degeneration usually severe, Lewy body formation.
A–10	Neuron population not quantitatively assessed; occasional tangles.	
Locus coeruleus	Degeneration in more advanced cases, tangles occasionally seen.	Degeneration usually severe; Lewy body formation.
Meynert nucleus	Neuronal loss depends on age of patient-only moderate in elderly cases; moderate tangle formation.	Degeneration usually severe – more marked in demented cases; Lewy body formation.
Raphe nuclei	Numerous tangles in dorsal raphe; neuronal loss if it occurs, not extensive.	Degeneration and Lewy bodies in dorsal raphe.
Dorsal motor vagus nucleus	Normal.	Degeneration.
Sympathetic ganglia	No tangles.	Degeneration and Lewy bodies.
Hypothalamus	Occasional tangles.	Degeneration and Lewy bodies in posterolateral portion.
Spinal column		Some reports of degeneration.

dementia and the severity of Parkinsonism may reflect the progressive involvement, as the disease advances, not only of the nigro-striatal pathway but also of other pathways, such as cortical projections from the other subcortical nuclei.

NEUROPATHOLOGICAL CHANGES IN THE CEREBRAL CORTEX

Whether or not the neuropathological involvement of the cortex distinguishes Alzheimer-type and Parkinsonian dementia is currently a controversial issue. Several reports have suggested that in those Parkinsonian cases with symptoms of dementia there is an increased prevalence of Alzheimer-type senile plaques and neurofibrillary tangles in the cortex. However, a recent survey indicates that such an association is not invariable and that in only a minor proportion of cognitively impaired Parkinson patients is the cortex affected by the classical neuropathological features of Alzheimer's disease (Perry, Tomlinson, Candy, Blessed, Foster, Bloxham, and Perry 1983; Tomlinson *et al.* unpublished observations). It thus seems likely that the more severe dementia of Alzheimer's compared with Parkinson's disease relates closely to cortical abnormalities and, indeed, a correlation between the clinical severity of dementia and extent of senile plaque formation was reported many years ago (Blessed, Tomlinson, and Roth 1968). In Alzheimer's disease there are, in addition to plaques and tangles, other morphological abnormalities in the cortex (Table 12.1). These include neuronal loss and reductions in dendritic aborizations — two aspects which have not yet been investigated in the cortex of demented patients with Lewy-body Parkinson's disease.

NEUROCHEMICAL CHANGES IN THE CEREBRAL CORTEX

Neurochemical analyses of post-mortem brain tissue in Alzheimer's and Parkinson's disease have mainly concentrated on, respectively, the cerebral cortex and basal ganglia or projecting nuclei. Thus, many transmitter and peptide systems have now been investigated in the cortex of Alzheimer-type patients, whereas in Parkinson's disease many transmitter abnormalities (dopaminergic, noradrenergic, serotonergic, cholinergic, and GABAergic) have been reported in nigral–striatal regions, although these have not been related to cognitive impairment. A direct comparison between neurochemical abnormalities in the two diseases is thus limited and in the present analysis is confined to the cortex.

Cortical neurochemical analyses in the two diseases are summarized in Table 12.2. As might be predicted from the common sites of neuropathological abnormalities (noradrenergic, serotonergic, and cholinergic nuclei) there are, in both Parkinson's and Alzheimer's disease, cortical neurochemical abnormalities relating to these transmitter systems (Ruberg, Ploska, Javoy-Agid, and Agid

TABLE 12.2. *Cortical neurochemistry in Alzheimer's and Parkinson's disease*

	Transmitter system	Alzheimer's disease	Parkinson's disease
Cholinergic:	Choline acetyltransferase	↓	↓●
	Acetylcholinesterase	↓	↓●
	Muscarinic receptor binding	→	↑
Noradrenergic:	Noradrenaline	↓	↓
	MHPG	↓	
	Dopamine B hydroxylase	↓	
	α_1 ⎫	→	
	α_2 ⎬ receptor binding	→	
	β ⎭	→	
Serotonergic:	Serotonin	↓	↓
	5-HIAA	↓	↓
	Receptor binding	↓	→
Dopaminergic:	Dopamine	→	↓
	HVA	→	↓
	Monoamine oxidase	↑	
	Spiroperidol binding	→	↑
γ-Aminobutyric acid:	Glutamate decarboxylase	↓○	↓○
	γ-Aminobutyric acid	→	↓
	Receptor binding (GABA, muscimol, or diazepam)	→	
Glutamic acid:	Glutamic acid level	→	
	Glutamate release	→	
Somatostatin:	Neuropeptide immunoreactivity	↓	↓●
	Receptor binding		↓●
Opioid peptides:	Enkephalin immunoreactivity	→	→
	Receptor binding (enkephalin)	→	↑
Neurotensin:	Neuropeptide immunoreactivity	↓	↓●
Other neuro-peptides:	Substance P Cholecystokinin Vasoactive intestinal peptide TRH	→	

● Abnormalities confined to/more extensive in demented subjects.
○ Probably non-specific, related to mode of death.

1982; Scatton, Javoy-Agid, Rouquier, and Agid 1983; Cross, Crow, Johnson, Joseph, Perry, Blessed, and Tomlinson 1983; Perry *et al.* 1983). Of particular interest are recent findings that cholinergic deficits are more prevalent in demented Parkinsonian cases whereas these losses are invariable in Alzheimer-type dementia. This evidence, together with pharmacological evidence that antagonism of the cholinergic system selectively affects cognitive function, suggests that a major component of cognitive impairment may, in both disorders, relate to cholinergic dysfunction.

Amongst various other transmitter systems, reductions in dopaminergic activities, whilst invariable in Parkinson's disease, are not consistently reported in Alzheimer's disease, although in the former these have not yet been related to cognitive impairment. γ-Aminobutyric acid is not consistently reduced in Alzheimer's disease (Perry, Attack, Perry, Hardy, Dodd, Edwardson, Blessed, Tomlinson, and Fairbairn 1984) although there is one report of a cortical reduction in this transmitter in Parkinson's disease (Teräväinen and Calne 1983). Reductions in somatostatin (Davies, Katzman, and Terry 1980; Rossor, Mountjoy, Roth, and Iversen 1980) and possibly also neurotensin (Candy, Perry, Perry, Biggins, Thompson, and Irving 1983) are found in Alzheimer's disease, and similar changes in Parkinson's disease appear to be confined to those cases with known cognitive impairment (Epelbaum, Ruberg, Moyse, Javoy-Agid, Dubois, and Agid 1983; Biggins, Perry, Candy, Perry, Bloxham, Johnson, and Edwardson 1983). Most other cortical neuropeptides are apparently normal in Alzheimer's disease and, where these have been analysed, also in Parkinson's disease. Thus, with respect to presynaptic transmitter function, dementia in both diseases is associated with marked reductions in cortical cholinergic and somatostatin activities and neither abnormality clearly distinguishes between the two types of dementia.

In contrast to measurements of presynaptic markers, receptor binding studies in the cerebral cortex may provide a possible basis for distinguishing the two disorders (Table 12.2). Thus, in Alzheimer's disease, the only consistent receptor abnormality so far reported is the loss of both S1 and S2 sub-types of serotonin receptor binding (Cross *et al.* 1983). In Parkinsonian cases, a range of cortical receptor abnormalities have been reported, including increases in muscarinic, dopaminergic and opioid receptor densities (Ruberg *et al.* 1982). Further analyses of these receptor changes in relation to mental function in Parkinson's disease should be worthwhile, although the question of whether some of these changes occur in response to drug treatment also needs to be investigated. Serotonin receptor density, in contrast to Alzheimer's disease, is reported to be normal in Parkinson's disease, and in a recent preliminary survey (Cross *et al.*, unpublished) was found to be similar in both mentally normal and cognitively impaired cases. The possibility thus arises that the more severe dementia of Alzheimer's disease may involve disturbances of serotonoceptive cortical neurons which, in turn, relate perhaps to the invariable appearance of cortical plaques and tangles in Alzheimer-type but not Parkinson-type dementia.

THE CHOLINERGIC SYSTEM AND DEMENTIA

In the absence of convincing evidence that any other transmitter involvement relates closely to cognitive impairment, it is worth considering the cholinergic involvement of Alzheimer's and Parkinson's disease in more detail (Table 12.3). Whilst reductions in cortical cholinergic activities are common to both forms of cognitive impairment and relate to some extent to the severity of dementia, there is no evidence that these abnormalities are more extensive in Alzheimer's disease, in which dementia is generally more severe (Fig. 12.1). Similarly, the loss of neurones from the nucleus of Meynert, being greater in Parkinson's disease, cannot account for the severe dementia of Alzheimer's disease, in which the neuronal population in this nucleus may be only slightly reduced in elderly cases, despite cortical abnormalities (Perry *et al.* 1982). There is thus no gross biochemical or structural aspect of the cholinergic system which distinguishes the more severe dementia of Alzheimer's disease, although microscopically, tangle-affected Meynert neurons are only found in Alzheimer's disease. However, since neurons with neurofibrillary tangles are prominent in many other brain areas, particularly in the cortex, where affected neurons are clearly non-cholinergic, it may be concluded that other neuronal systems are associated with Alzheimer-type dementia. It should be noted that, with respect to cholinergic cell bodies, those in the septum have not yet been subjected to quantitative comparison in Alzheimer's and Parkinson's disease.

TABLE 12.3. *Cholinergic system in dementia of Alzheimer's and Parkinson's disease*

A. CORTICAL NEUROCHEMISTRY

Choline acetyltransferase: reductions, particularly in temporal lobe, correlate with severity of dementia in both diseases.

Acetylcholinesterase: reductions in both disorders evident biochemically (selective loss of intermediate, 10S form in both instances) and histochemically.

Muscarinic receptor: increased binding activity reported in Parkinson's but not Alzheimer's disease.

B. MORPHOLOGICAL ASPECTS

Neuronal population in nucleus of Meynert: severely depleted in Parkinson's disease (particularly demented cases) but in only some (usually younger) cases of Alzheimer's disease; intraneuronal abnormalities include tangles in Alzheimer's disease and Lewy bodies in Parkinson's disease.

Cortical projections: senile plaques, much more prevalent in Alzheimer's disease, contain (at earlier stages) reactive cholinergic processes presumed to originate from nucleus of Meynert.

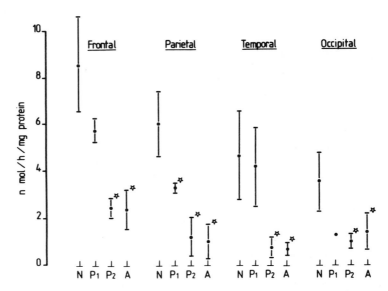

Fig. 12.1. Choline acetyltransferase activity in four neocortical areas from 8 control cases (N), 3 Parkinsonian cases without cognitive impairment (P1), 6 Parkinsonian cases with cognitive impairment/dementia (P2) and between 5–15 Alzheimer-type cases (A). Mean activity ± S.E. indicated; those significantly different ($p < 0.001$) from the control group marked with an asterisk.

The increased density of the muscarinic receptor in Parkinson's (Ruberg *et al.* 1982) but not Alzheimer's disease (Davies and Verth 1977; Perry, Perry, Blessed, and Tomlinson 1977) is of interest in view of a recent report that lesions of nucleus of Meynert result in increased cortical muscarinic binding. The absence of any such response in Alzheimer's disease might indicate a defect in cholinoceptive neuronal function and, in fact, the extent to which muscarinic receptors are actually functional has not yet been tested, since ligand binding assays do not *per se* provide this sort of information. It is possible that in Alzheimer's disease intrinsic cortical function is a primary abnormality and that this in turn results in a dying back of cholinergic and other projecting processes. So far, however, clear-cut neurochemical evidence of intrinsic cortical neuronal malfunction in Alzheimer's disease is lacking and may perhaps need to await the discovery of as yet unidentified neuronal types within the cortex.

The cholinergic involvement common to both Alzheimer's and Parkinson's disease is currently of considerable interest in view of evidence that in both diseases the cholinergic deficit may, at least to some extent, relate to the degree of cognitive impairment. In Parkinson's disease, however, many other cortical changes (dopaminergic, noradrenergic, and serotonergic, for example) also need to be examined in relation to the cognitive impairment. In Alzheimer's disease the evidence for a specific cholinergic involvement is more convincing since, amongst a range of transmitter and peptide activities in temporal cortex, the cholinergic deficit correlates most closely with, for example, mental impairment (Perry, Blessed, Tomlinson, Perry, Crow, Cross, Dockray, Dimaline, and Arregui 1981). However, it is unlikely that the cholinergic deficit accounts for more than a proportion of the clinical deficit, and it is possible that other as yet unidentified neuronal systems are involved in the severe dementia.

CORTICAL CHANGES: PRIMARY OR SECONDARY?

Anatomically, it is possible, although unproven, that subcortical abnormalities in Alzheimer's disease, such as loss of neurons from nucleus of Meynert, are a consequence of primary cortical changes. Thus, as far as is known, only nuclei projecting to the cortex are involved in Alzheimer's disease, and in general, pathological changes in these are less severe compared to the cortical involvement. In contrast, in Parkinson's disease there is extensive loss of neurons not only from nuclei projecting to cortex but also from nuclei such as the substantia nigra and dorsal vagus nucleus which project elsewhere, suggesting that subcortical neuronal loss is a primary feature of the disease.

In addition to neuronal loss, there are relatively specific microscopic abnormalities characteristic of the two diseases, and these may be relevant to this question of the primary site of the degenerative process. Thus, Lewy bodies in, for example, substantia nigra or locus coeruleus, are only rarely evident in cases of Alzheimer's disease and even then are not generally in excess of those seen in normal, age-matched controls. Conversely, recent evidence suggests that in idiopathic Parkinsonism with dementia, cortical tangles are uncommon (occurring perhaps in around 20 per cent of cases), and plaques are rarely present in numbers exceeding those seen in non-demented old people.

The precise chemical nature of Lewy bodies, plaques, and tangles remains an enigma, although there is now evidence that indirectly links all three. Both Lewy bodies and tangles are intracellular abnormalities consisting of — at least partly in the former — filaments of unknown origin. It has been suggested that neurofilament antigens are common to both lesions (Anderton, Breinburg, Downes, Green, Tomlinson, Ulrich, Wood, and Kahn 1982; Goldman, Yen, Chiv, and Peress 1983) although an earlier report suggested that the tangle constituent may not be a normal brain protein (Ihara, Abraham, and Selkoe 1982). However, this matter now appears to have been resolved in a more detailed study showing that neurofibrillary tangles in Alzheimer's disease are heterogeneous as regards their filamentous content, and contain both antigens cross-reacting with neurofilaments and antigens unique to paired helical filaments and not shared with normal neurofilaments (Rasool, Abraham, Anderton, Haugh, Kahn, and Selkoe 1984).

Neuronal perikarya do not appear to be primarily involved in the formation of senile plaques which, in addition to reactive glia, contain mainly dendritic and axonal processes and their terminals. Such an appearance suggests that the plaque is an area where neurotransmission would be impaired. The presence of cholinergic processes in plaques has been inferred from their histochemical reactivity for acetylcholinesterase (Perry, Candy, and Perry 1983), and a recent Golgi–Cox study has suggested that processes from many different neuronal types, including intrinsic cortical neurones, are present in the plaque area. Whether the neuronal processes are primarily derived from degenerated or tangle-affected neurones remains to be established; however, we have recently obtained evidence suggesting a relationship between neurofibrillary tangles and plaques. Following early reports that aluminium salts could induce neuro-fibrillary degeneration in the rabbit CNS (Klatzo, Wisniewski, and Streicher 1965; Terry and Peña 1965) it was reported the brain aluminium content of Alzheimer cases was significantly increased in areas rich in tangles (Crapper, Krishman, Dalton 1973). Subsequently, electronmicroscopy-X-ray-spectrometry has revealed evidence of intracellular accumulation of aluminium in tangle-bearing neurones associated with Alzheimer's disease and Guam Parkinsonism-dementia (Perl and Brody 1980; Perl 1983). In studies on the extracellular core material isolated from senile plaques of Alzheimer cases, we have recently observed a high content of aluminium (Figs 12.2 and 12.3). While the signifi-cance of this observation is being explored at the present time, it does suggest a link, albeit tenuous, between plaques and tangles, the latter in turn being

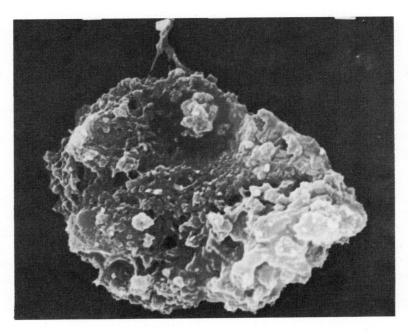

Fig. 12.2. Surface topography, as revealed by scanning electron microscopy, of a senile plaque core isolated from unfixed cerebral cortex (from an Alzheimer case) using enzyme digestion. Full details of the method are in preparation. Magnification ×3500.

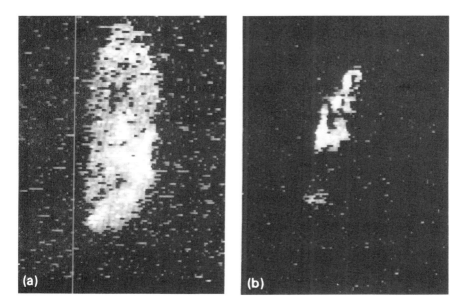

Fig. 12.3. X-ray analysis of a section of (3–4 μm) through the core of an isolated senile plaque embedded in epon. The distribution of sulphur (12.3(a)) reveals the whole cross-section of the core, while the distribution of aluminium (12.3(b)) shows a focalized concentration in the centre of the plaque core.

related to Lewy bodies by the presence of neurofilament antigens. It remains to be seen whether perikarya affected by Lewy bodies also demonstrate a raised content of aluminium. It is not known whether the increased aluminium associated with the major structural lesions of Alzheimer's disease has any role in the mechanisms of pathogenesis or whether it is a secondary response to cell damage.

CLINICAL IMPLICATIONS

With respect to defining clear-cut correlates of dementia in either Alzheimer's or Parkinson's disease, current evidence is obviously limited and present findings are only suggestive. An important issue which needs to be studied in far greater detail is the definition of the particular aspects of cognitive function which decline, especially at earlier stages in both disorders. Particular attention needs to be paid to determining if the dementia of Alzheimer's disease is quantitatively or qualitatively different from that of Parkinson's disease. In Parkinson's disease there may, for example, be similarities in the nature of the cognitive abnormality and deficiencies in the initiation of motor programmes (Bloxham, Mindel, and Frith 1984). Since the term 'cognitive function', clearly embraces a broad range of interacting mental activities, the involvement of specific neuronal pathways in particular functions such as memory or abstract thinking needs to be examined in individual groups with deficits predominantly in these areas. In this respect, comparison of patients with other more specific cognitive disorders, such as Korsakoff's psychosis, is likely to be of value.

As far as pharmacological treatment of either disorder is concerned there is not yet any clinically-useful approach in Alzheimer's disease, and in Parkinson's disease L-DOPA treatment, whilst to a certain extent rectifying the movement disorder, is not generally considered to influence cognitive ability. The cholinergic hypothesis of Alzheimer's disease has stimulated a large number of trials of putative cholinergic treatments and amongst these the only consistent improvements so far reported are found with physostigmine. It is possible that in this disorder more refined approaches to countering the defect in cholinergic neurotransmission will ultimately meet with greater success, especially at earlier stages of the disease. In Parkinson's disease, however, cholinomimetic therapy poses a major problem, since such agents exacerbate the movement disorder. Interestingly, two cases, examined in a recent series (Bloxham *et al.*, unpublished observations) with neuropathological evidence of Lewy-body Parkinsonism and extensive neurochemical cholinergic deficits presented clinically with clear-cut evidence of dementia but minimal movement disorder. The possibility arises with respect to movement dysfunction that in such cases the cholinergic deficit had partially compensated for the dopaminergic deficit and, in turn, this raises the question of whether cholinergic deficits in Parkinson's disease are in some way compensatory or secondary to a primary dopamine deficit. Rational treatment of dementia in Alzheimer's or Parkinson's diseases clearly depends on a greater understanding of the involvement of different neuronal systems. It may be anticipated that continued pathological and biochemical analysis of the brain in relation to the severity of mental impairment will lead more closely towards this objective.

SUMMARY

Structural and biochemical abnormalities of the brain are compared in Alzheimer's disease and Parkinson's disease which is also associated with dementia. Neuropathologically, the disorders are distinguished by the abundance of plaques and tangles in the neocortex in Alzheimer's disease but not Parkinson's disease, and the involvement of certain subcortical nuclei, other than those projecting to the cortex, in Parkinson's but not Alzheimer's disease. Neurochemically, the dementia in both diseases is related to cortical cholinergic defects and to loss of neurons from the nucleus of Meynert. These abnormalities are not greater in Alzheimer's disease, however, despite the more severe dementia. It is suggested that the cognitive impairment in Alzheimer's disease originates from a primary cortical abnormality with secondary changes in the ascending cholinergic system and other projections from subcortical nuclei. In Parkinson's disease, however, a primary degeneration of the subcortical cholinergic neurons may be responsible for the cortical cholinergic deficits and corresponding cognitive impairments. It is suggested that a tenous link may exist between the major structural features of both disorders since both Lewy bodies and tangles possess antigens for neurofilament proteins, whereas tangles and the extracellular core deposits of plaques show an abnormal concentration of aluminium.

REFERENCES

Albert, M. L., Feldman, R. G., and Willis, A. L. (1974). The 'subcortical dementia' of progressive supranuclear palsy. *J. Neurol. Neurosurg. Psychiat.* **37**, 121–30.

Anderton, B. H., Breinburg, D., Downes, M. J., Green, P. J., Tomlinson, B. E., Ulrich, J., Wood, J. N., and Kahn, J. (1982). Monoclonal antibodies show that neurofibrillary tangles and neurofilaments share antigenic determinants. *Nature, Lond.* **298**, 84–6.

Biggins, J. A., Perry, R. H., Candy, J. M., Perry, E. K., Bloxham, C. A., Johnson, M., and Edwardson, J. A. (1983). Neurotensin immunoreactivity and choline acetyltransferase activity in the cerebral cortex in Parkinson's disease. *Reg. Peptides* **7**, 277.

Blessed, G., Tomlinson, B. E., and Roth, M. (1968). The association between quantitative measures of dementia and of senile change in the cerebral grey matter of elderly subjects. *Br. J. Psychiat.* **114**, 797–801.

Bloxham, C. A., Mindel, T. A., and Frith, C. D. (1984). Initiation and prediction of movements in Parkinson's disease, *Brain* **107**, 371–84.

Candy, J. M., Perry, R. H., Perry, E. K., Biggins, J. A., Thompson, J., and Irving, D. (1983). Transmitter systems in Alzheimer's disease. In *Aging of the brain* (ed. W. H. Gispen and J. Traber), pp. 29–48. Elsevier, Amsterdam.

—, —, —, Irving, D., Blessed, G., Fairbairn, A. F., and Tomlinson, B. E. (1983). Pathological changes in the nucleus of Meynert in Alzheimer's and Parkinson's disease. *J. Neurol. Sci.* **59**, 277–89.

Crapper, D. R., Krishnan, S. S., and Dalton, A. J. (1973). Brain aluminium distribution in Alzheimer's disease and experimental neurofibrillary degeneration. *Science* **180**, 511–13.

Cross, A. J., Crow, T. J., Johnson, J. A., Joseph, M. H., Perry, E. K., Perry, R. H., Blessed, G., and Tomlinson, B. E. (1983). Monoamine metabolism in senile dementia of Alzheimer type. *J. Neurol. Sci.* **60**, 383–92.

Davies, P. and Verth, A. H. (1977). Regional distribution of muscarinic acetylcholine receptor in normal and Alzheimer's type dementia brains. *Brain Res.* **138**, 385–92.

—, Katzman, R., and Terry, R. D. (1980). Reduced somatostatin-like immunoreactivity in cerebral cortex from cases of Alzheimer's disease and Alzheimer's senile dementia. *Nature, Lond.* **288**, 279–80.

Epelbaum, J., Ruberg, M., Moyse, E., Javoy-Agid, F., Dubois, B., and Agid, Y. (1983). Somatostatin and dementia in Parkinson's disease. *Brain Res.* **278**, 376–9.

Goldman, J. E., Yen, S. H., Chiv, F. C., and Peress, N. S. (1983). Lewy bodies of Parkinson's disease contain neurofilament antigens. *Science* **221**, 1082–4.

Ihara, Y., Abraham, C., and Selkoe, D. J. (1982). Antibodies to paired helical filaments in Alzheimer's disease do not recognize normal human brain proteins. *Nature, Lond.* **304**, 327–9.

Klatzo, I., Wisniewski, H. M., and Streicher, E. (1965). Experimental production of neurofibrillary degeneration. I. Light microscopic observations. *J. Neuropath. exp. Neurol.* **24**, 187–99.

Mayeux, R. (1982). Depression and dementia in Parkinson's disease. In *Movement disorders* (ed. D. Marsden and S. Fahn), pp. 75–95. Butterworths Scientific Publications, London.

Perl, P. (1983). Trace element studies of neurofibrillary tangle bearing neurons — evidence of aluminium accumulation. In *Aging of the brain* (ed. W. H. Gispen and J. Traber), pp. 23–8. Elsevier, Amsterdam.

— and Brody, A. C. (1980). Alzheimer's disease: X-ray spectometric evidence of aluminium accumulation in neurofibrillary tangle-bearing neurons. *Science* **208**, 297–99.

Perry, R. H., Candy, J. M. and Perry, E. K. (1983). Some observations and speculations concerning the cholinergic system and neuropeptides in Alzheimer's disease. In *Banbury Report 15: Biological aspects of Alzheimer's disease* (ed. R. Katzman) pp. 3,51–61 Cold Spring Harbor Laboratory.

—, Perry, R. H., Blessed, G., and Tomlinson, B. E. (1977). Necropsy evidence of central cholinergic deficits in senile dementia. *Lancet* **1**, 189.

Perry, R. H., Candy, J. M., Perry, E. K., Irving, D., Blessed, G., Fairbairn, A., and Tomlinson, B. E. (1982). Extensive loss of choline acetyltransferase activity is not reflected by neuronal loss in the nucleus of Meynert in Alzheimer's disease. *Neurosci. Lett.* **33**, 311–15.

—, Tomlinson, B. E., Candy, J. M., Blessed, G., Foster, J. F., Bloxham, C. A., and Perry, E. K. (1983). Cortical cholinergic deficit in mentally impaired Parkinsonian patients. *Lancet* **2**, 789–90.

Perry, E. K., Attack, J. R., Perry, R. H., Hardy, J. A., Dodd, P. R., Edwardson, J. A., Blessed, G., Tomlinson, B. E., and Fairbairn, A. F. (1984). Intralaminar neurochemical distributions in human mid-temporal cortex — comparison between Alzheimer's disease and the normal. *J. Neurochem.* **42**, 1402–10.

—, Blessed, G., Tomlinson, B. E., Perry, R. H., Crow, T. J., Cross, A. J., Dockray, G. J., Dimaline, R., and Arregui, A. (1981). Neurochemical activities in the human temporal lobe related to aging and Alzheimer-type changes. *Neurobiol. Aging* **2**, 251–6.

Rasool, C. G., Abraham, C., Anderton, B. H., Haugh, M., Kahn, J., and Selkoe, D. J. (1984). Alzheimer's disease: immunoreactivity of neurofibrillary tangles with anti-neurofilament and anti-paired helical filament antibodies. *Brain Res.* **310**, 249–60.

Rossor, M. N., Mountjoy, C. Q., Roth, M., and Iversen, L. L. (1980). Reduced amounts of immunoreactive somatostatin in the temporal cortex in senile dementia of Alzheimer type. *Neurosci. Lett.* **20**, 373–7.

Ruberg, M., Ploska, A., Javoy-Agid, F., and Agid, Y. (1982). Muscarinic binding and choline acetyltransferase activity in Parkinsonian subjects with reference to dementia. *Brain Res.* **232**, 129–39.

Scatton, B., Javoy-Agid, F., Rouquier, L., and Agid, Y. (1983). Reduction of cortical dopamine, noradrenaline, serotonin and that metabolites in Parkinson's disease. *Brain Res.* **275**, 321–8.

Teräväinen, H. and Calne, D. B. (1983). Motor system in normal aging and Parkinson's disease. In *The neurology of aging* (ed. R. Katzman and R. D. Terry), pp. 85–109. F. A. Davis Company, Philadelphia.

Terry, R. D. and Peña, C. (1965). Experimental production of neurofibrillary degeneration. *J. Neuropath. exp. Neurol.* **24**, 200.

Tomlinson, B. E., Irving, D., and Blessed, G. (1981). Cell loss in the locus coeruleus in senile dementia of Alzheimer-type. *J. Neurol. Sci.* **49**, 419–28.

Whitehouse, P. J., Hedreen, J. C., White, C. L., and Price, D. L. (1983). Basal forebrain neurons in dementia of Parkinson's disease. *Ann. Neurol.* **13**, 243–8.

13

Central nervous system patterns of neurochemical abnormality in cognitive disorders

M. ROSSOR

Many neurotransmitters, receptors, and related enzymes are sufficiently stable after death to permit reliable determination, and autopsy studies are now well-established in the neurochemical analysis of neuropsychiatric disorders (for review see Bird and Iversen 1982). Post-mortem neurochemical studies have provided information on the regional distribution of neurotransmitter markers in normal human brain and of alterations in a variety of nervous system disorders. The classic example is that of Parkinson's disease, in which a profound loss of striatal dopamine can be related to a loss of nigro–striatal neurones. However, information is now available on neurochemical changes in a variety of neuropsychiatric disorders which includes Alzheimer's, Huntington's, and motor neurone disease, spinocerebellar degenerations, and schizophrenia.

Consistent changes have been found in these disorders, but considerable care has to be taken before attributing differences between a control and disease group to the disease process itself, since many non-specific factors such as drug therapy, agonal state, and autopsy delay can influence the neurochemical profile. Moreover, post-mortem studies cannot readily distinguish between changes due to alterations in turnover and those due to loss of neuronal integrity. The most reliable interpretation has been in degenerative disorders in which loss of neurotransmitter may be related to cell damage by the use of concomitant classical histology and immunohistochemistry.

The technique can then be used to assess the selectivity of neuronal damage, although with the increase in available data it has become apparent that single neurotransmitter deficits are uncommon, if they exist at all, and that the changes are usually part of a more complex pattern of deficit. With neurochemical studies as an adjunct to classical neuropathology, it may be possible to relate specific clinical deficits to dysfunction within a defined neurotransmitter system, which may provide additional information to that derived from anatomical–clinical correlates. Although such an aim has yet to be realized for cognitive disorders, characteristic patterns of neurochemical abnormality are discerned in certain diseases associated with cognitive impairment. The main example is that of Alzheimer's disease and related abnormalities of normal ageing, but in addition, the basal ganglia disorders, Huntington's and Parkinson's disease have associated cognitive deficits and characteristic neurochemical abnormalities. The neurochemistry of schizophrenia is discussed in Chapters 18 and 19.

ALZHEIMER'S DISEASE AND NORMAL AGEING

Reduction in cortical activity of the cholinergic marker enzyme choline acetyl-transferase (ChAT) has been a consistent finding in autopsy (Perry and Perry 1980; Bowen, Allen, Benton, Goodhardt, Haan, Palmer, Sims, Smith, Spillane, Esiri, Neary, Snowdon, Wilcock, and Davison 1983; Rossor, Garrett, Johnson, Mountjoy, Roth, and Iversen 1982; Bird, Stranahan, Sumi, and Raskind 1983; Wilcock, Esiri, Bowen, and Smith 1982) and biopsy studies (Sims, Bowen, Allen, Smith, Neary, Thomas, and Davison 1983). The majority of cortical ChAT activity is found within the axon terminals of an ascending projection from the nucleus basalis in the basal forebrain (Wenk, Bigl, and Meyer 1980; Johnston, McKinney, and Coyle 1981) although intrinsic cortical cholinergic neurons contribute about 30 per cent of total ChAT activity (Johnston *et al.* 1981).

The loss of ChAT activity in Alzheimer's disease is thought to relate predominantly to damage to the ascending projection since a reduction in large neurones within the nucleus basalis has been reported (Whitehouse, Price, Struble, Clark, Coyle, and DeLong 1982) and a similar loss observed using ChAT immunostaining (Nagai, McGeer, Peng, McGeer, and Dolman 1983), and determinations of ChAT activity (Rossor *et al.* 1982). However, shrinkage of basalis neurons can occur following cortical damage, and the extent to which changes in the ascending cholinergic system reflect such retrograde damage is unclear (Pearson, Sofroniew, Cuello, Powell, Eckenstein, Esiri, and Wilcock 1983). Similarly, the contribution of intrinsic cortical damage is unknown. It is of interest to note, however, that the losses of ChAT activity which are maximal in the temporal cortex rarely exceed 70 per cent, and the concentration of vasoactive intestinal polypeptide (VIP), which has been reported to coexist within cortical cholinergic neurons (Eckenstein and Baughman 1984), is un-altered (Rossor 1982).

The cholinergic deficit has been found to correlate with the severity of histological change (Perry, Tomlinson, Blessed, Bergmann, Gibson, and Perry 1978; Wilcock, Esiri, Bowen, and Smith 1982; Mountjoy, Rossor, Iversen, and Roth 1984) and with the severity of dementia at the time of death (Perry *et al.* 1978). An association between the cholinergic abnormality and the severity of disease need not indicate a causal relationship although both animal and human (Drachman 1977) studies have implicated central cholinergic systems in cognitive function. Recently, specific lesioning of the ascending projection from basal forebrain in animals has revealed a variety of cognitive deficits (Flicker, Dean, Watkins, Fisher, and Bartus 1983).

Despite the consistent cholinergic abnormality, it is clear that a single neurotransmitter deficit is not found in Alzheimer's disease, and in particular, there is evidence of abnormalities in other ascending projections to cerebral cortex. Cortical concentrations of noradrenaline and metabolite MHPG are low (Adolfsson, Gottfries, Roos, and Winblad 1979; Cross, Crow, Johnson, Joseph, E. K. Perry, R. H. Perry, Blessed, and Tomlinson 1982) which reflects a loss of locus coeruleus cells (Bondareff, Mountjoy, and Roth 1982; Iversen, Rossor, Reynolds, Hills, Roth, Mountjoy, Foote, Morrison, and Bloom 1983); the noradrenergic deficit is found predominantly in younger cases (Bondareff *et al.* 1982; Rossor *et al.* 1984). Concentrations of 5-hydroxytryptamine and of post-synpatic receptors are also reduced in cerebral cortex (Bowen, Spillane, Curzon, Meier-Ruge, White, Goodhardt, Iwangoff, and Davison 1983; Reynolds, Arnold, Rossor, Iversen, Mountjoy, and Roth 1984).

In contrast to the biochemical evidence of damage to ascending projection systems, the histopathological features are found predominantly within the cerebral cortex. It is not known if the cortical neurons which are lost in Alzheimer's disease (Terry, Peck, DeTeresa, Schechter, and Horoupian 1981; Mountjoy, Roth, Evans, and Evans 1983), and those which contain neurofibrillary tangles, constitute a distinct neurotransmitter category, although a number of intrinsic chemical markers have been studied. Variable reductions in glutamic acid decarboxylase activity may relate to the agonal state, but changes of *c*.30 per cent in GABA concentration are found in the temporal lobe (Rossor *et al.* 1982). The concentrations of cholecystokinin and VIP are unchanged (Perry, Dockray, Dimaline, Perry, Blessed, and Tomlinson 1981; Rossor 1982) but there is a loss of somatostatin immunoreactivity, particularly from the temporal lobe (Davies *et al.* 1980; Rossor, Emson, Mountjoy, Roth, and Iversen 1980; Perry, Candy, and Perry 1983). The reduction in somatostatin has been found to correlate with the density of senile plaques and peptide immunostaining can be demonstrated within their vicinity (Perry *et al.* 1983). However, neither the functional role of somatostatin within the cerebral cortex, nor the contribution of such a deficit to the cognitive treatment in Alzheimer's disease is known.

AGEING

The decreased cognition seen with progression from maturity to senescence has been compared to that of Alzheimer's disease. Moreover, the impairment resulting from cholinergic blockade by scopolamine in young adults mimics that seen in the elderly, suggesting that, as with Alzheimer's disease, impaired cholinergic function may be important in normal ageing (Bartus *et al.* 1982). To what extent does the neurochemical profile of ageing resemble that of Alzheimer's disease?

The results from neurotransmitter analyses of normal ageing are variable. This may relate to the different age groups examined, and some of the substantial changes observed are more properly associated with maturation than senescence. The pharmacological evidence for a cholinergic-related cognitive decline (Bartus *et al.* 1982) can, to some extent, find a correlate in neurochemical changes in that reduced activity of ChAT with age is found in the frontal cortex (Rossor *et al.* 1982) and more prominently in the caudate nucleus (Allen *et al.* 1983). There is evidence that the number of muscarinic receptors also declines with age (Bartus *et al.* 1982). Cell counts of the locus coeruleus are reported to change with age but clear biochemical evidence for changes in noradrenaline and in 5-hydroxytrytamine is lacking (Cross *et al.* 1983; Allen *et al.* 1983).

γ-Aminobutyric acid concentrations, which are reduced in some cases of Alzheimer's disease, also decline with normal ageing (Rossor *et al.* 1982; Allen *et al.* 1983). In contrast, there is no change in somatostatin with age (Davies *et al.* 1980; Rossor *et al.* 1984). The neurochemical profile of normal ageing and Alzheimer's disease are compared in Table 13.1.

In addition to the neurotransmitter changes in normal senescence, age itself can have an important influence on the neurochemical profile of Alzheimer's disease. In general, young-at-death cases of Alzheimer's disease show more severe clinical and histological features than older patients, and this also applies to cholinergic and somatostatin abnormalities which are both more severe and widespread in the younger age group (Bowen *et al.* 1979; Bird *et al.* 1983;

TABLE 13.1. *Comparison of neurochemical changes in cortex in ageing and Alzheimer's disease*

	Ageing	Alzheimer's
Choline acetyltransferase	Modest reduction in frontal cortex.	Widespread reduction greatest in temporal cortex.
Muscarinic receptors	Reduced/unchanged.	Unchanged.
Noradrenaline	Slight reduction/ unchanged.	Reduced in younger cases.
Dopamine	Limited data.	Unchanged.
5-Hydroxytryptamine	Slight reduction/ no change.	Modest reduction.
GABA	Reduced.	Reduced in younger cases.
Somatostatin	No change.	Reduced especially in temporal cortex.

Data derived from Adolfsson *et al.* (1979); Allen *et al.* (1983); Bartus *et al.* (1982); Bird *et al.* (1983); Davies *et al.* (1980); Perry and Perry (1980); Reynolds *et al.* (1984); Rossor *et al.* (1982, 1984).

Rossor *et al*. 1984). The reductions in GABA and noradrenaline are found in those patients dying below 79 y but are not apparent in older patients (Rossor *et al*. 1984). The neurochemical profile in young cases of Alzheimer's disease is distinct from that found in 80- and 90-year-old controls implying that the changes seen are not simply the consequence of accelerated ageing (Rossor *et al*. 1984).

PARKINSON'S DISEASE AND HUNTINGTON'S DISEASE

Although neuropathological changes may be widespread, the brunt of the damage in these diseases is found in the basal ganglia with degeneration of the nigro-striatal projection in Parkinson's disease and degeneration of the striatum in Huntington's disease. The neurochemical correlate of the histological changes in Parkinson's disease is the loss of dopamine from the corpus striatum and substantia nigra together with a loss of cholecystokinin immunoreactivity which coexists in some mesencephalic dopamine neurones. This can be contrasted with the striatal changes in Huntington's disease in that dopamine concentrations are increased due to preservation of the nigro-striatal dopamine system but striopallidal neuronal loss leads to reductions in GABA, met-enkephalin, substance P, and cholecystokinin (Spokes 1980; Emson, Arregui, Clement-Jones, Sandberg, and Rossor 1980).

Although Parkinson's and Huntington's disease are characterized by motor abnormalities, the latter is usually associated with additional features of dementia. Moreover, there is now evidence that up to a third of patients with Parkinson's disease may also have impaired cognitive function (Mayeux and Stern 1983); some of these have the histological features of Alzheimer's disease. Since the major histological and biochemical abnormalities are found in the basal ganglia, it is possible that these changes contribute directly to the observed cognitive deficits, although there have been few attempts to correlate the clinical features with striatal neurotransmitter abnormalities. In a recent study by Brown, Marsden, Quinn, and Wyke (1984) it was found that patients who had severe 'on-off' fluctuations in motor performance with treatment did not show corresponding fluctuations in cognitive function.

In addition to the degenerative changes in the basal ganglia, there are abnormalities within the cerebral cortex which may be of greater importance in determining the cognitive impairment. Reduced cortical thickness is commonly found in the frontal lobe in Huntington's disease, although the concentrations of cortical markers GABA, VIP, cholecystokinin, and somatostatin are unchanged. Similarly, neocortical ChAT activity is normal, although reduced activity is found in the hippocampus (Spokes 1980).

The histological abnormalities of Alzheimer's disease may be found in some Parkinsonian patients but cannot explain all cases with coincident dementia. Although cortical pathology is not otherwise a feature of Parkinson's disease, degenerative changes in the nucleus basalia occur with a concomitant reduction in ChAT activity. This, together with an increase in muscaric receptor binding using ^{3}HQNB as ligand, is reported in the frontal cortex and is most prominent in those patients with dementia (Dubois, Ruberg, Javoy-Agid, Ploska, and Agid 1983). In addition, the patients with dementia also have reduced concentrations of somatostatin immunoreactivity which is most marked in the frontal cortex (Epelbaum, Ruberg, Moyse, Javoy-Agid, Dubois, and Agid 1983).

CORTICAL AND SUB-CORTICAL DEMENTIAS

Albert (1978) has proposed that a characteristic cognitive deficit, 'subcortical dementia', occurs in progressive supranuclear palsy, and this concept has been extended to other diseases with pathology of subcortical nuclear structures such as Parkinson's disease, Huntington's disease, and Korsakoff's psychosis. Clinically, the syndrome is characterized by emotional and personality changes, typically inertia or apathy, whch may be seen in frontal lobe syndromes.

The term 'subcortical dementia' may now be confusing since it is clear that Alzheimer's disease demonstrates additional subcortical pathology, and that Parkinson's and Huntington's disease share cortical changes. If the clinical differences in the cognitive dysfunction cannot be attributed to the anatomical dissociation between cortical and subcortical pathologies, it may be related to the difference in cortical abnormalities. Since the clinical features of inertia and apathy are frequently seen in frontal lobe disease, it is of interest that the biochemical changes in Alzheimer's disease are most marked in the temporal cortex whereas those of Parkinson's disease are prominent in the frontal cortex, although regional studies of the latter are limited. In addition, cognitive tasks which have been found to decline in early untreated Parkinson's disease include the Wisconsin Card Sorting Test and the Benton's Word Fluency Test, both of which are impaired in frontal lobe disease (Lees and Smith 1983).

In conclusion, it is clear that the dopaminergic and cholinergic deficits found in Parkinson's and Alzheimer's disease are part of a complex pattern of neurotransmitter abnormalities and these have not yet been related to distinct patterns of cognitive impairment. Although a single neurotransmitter system may not underlie a specific cognitive process, it is possible that diffuse systems such as the cholinergic projection which modulate the level of response of other neurones can have a profound effect on complex functions such as cognition.

REFERENCES

Adolfsson, R., Gottfries, C. G., Roos, B. E., and Winblad, B. (1979). Changes in brain catecholamines in patients with dementia of Alzheimer type. *Br. J. Psychiat.* **135**, 216–23.

Albert, M. L. (1978). Subcortical dementia. In Alzheimer's disease; senile dementia and related disorders. (Aging, Vol. 7). (ed. R. Katzman, R. D. Terry, and K. L. Bick), pp. 173–80. Raven Press, New York.

Allen, S. J., Benton, J. S., Goodhardt, M. J., Haan, E. A., Sims, N. R., Smith, C. C. T., Spillane, J. A., Bowen, D. M., and Davison, A. N. (1983). Biochemical evidence of selective nerve cell changes in normal ageing human and rat brain. *J. Neurochem.* **41**, 256–65.

Bartus, R. T., Dean, R. L., Beer, B., and Lippa, A. S. (1982). The cholinergic hypothesis of geriatric memory dysfunction. *Science* **217**, 408–17.

Bird, E. and Iversen, L. L. (1982). Human brain post-mortem studies of neurotransmitters and related markers. In *Handbook of Neurochemistry* (ed. A. Lajtha), Vol. 2, pp. 225–51. Plenum Press, New York.

Bird, T. D., Stranahan, S., Sumi, S. M., and Raskind, M. (1983). Alzheimer's disease: choline acetyltransferase activity in brain tissue from clinical and pathological subgroups. *Ann. Neurol.* **14**, 284–93.

Bondareff, W., Mountjoy, C. Q., and Roth, M. (1982). Loss of neurons of origin of the adrenergic projection in cerebral cortex (nucleus locus ceruleus) in senile dementia. *Neurology* **32**, 164–8.

Bowen, D. M., Spillane, J. A., Curzon, G., Meier-Ruge, W., White, P., Goodhardt, M. J., Iwangoff, P., and Davison, A. N. (1979). Accelerated ageing or selective neuronal loss as an important cause of dementia. *Lancet* i, 11–14.

——, Allen, S. J. Benton, J. S., Goodhardt, M. J., Haan, E. A., Palmer, A. M., Sims, N. R., Smith, C. C. T., Spillane, J. A., Esiri, M. M., Neary, D., Snowdon, J. S., Wilcock, G. K., and Davison, A. N. (1983). Biochemical assessment of serotonergic and cholinergic dysfunction and cerebral atrophy in Alzheimer's disease. *J. Neurochem.* **41**, 266–72.

Brown, R. G , Marsden, C. D., Quinn, N., and Wyke, M. A. (1984). Alterations in cognitive performance and affect-arousal state during fluctuations in motor function in Parkinson's disease. *J. Neurol. Neurosurg. Psychiat.* **47**, 454–65.

Cross, A. J., Crow, T. J., Johnson, J. A., Joseph, M. H., Perry, E. K., Perry, R. H., Blessed, G., and Tomlinson, B. E. (1983). Monoamine metabolism in senile dementia of Alzheimer type. *J. Neurol. Sci.* **60**, 383–92.

Davies, P., Katzman, R., and Terry, R. D. (1980). Reduced somatostatin-like immunoreactivity in cerebral cortex from cases of Alzheimer's disease and Alzheimer senile dementia. *Nature, Lond.* **288**, 279–80.

Drachman, D. (1977). Memory and cognitive function in man: Does the cholinergic system have a specific role? *Neurology* **27**, 783–90.

Dubois, B., Ruberg, M., Javoy-Agid, F., Ploska, A., and Agid, Y. (1983). A subcortico-cortical cholinergic system is affected in Parkinson's disease. *Brain Res.* **288**, 213–18.

Eckenstein, F. and Baughman, R. W. (1984). Two types of cholinergic innervation in cortex, one co-localised with vasoactive intestinal polypeptide. *Nature. Lond.* **309**, 153–5.

Epelbaum, J., Ruberg, M., Moyse, E., Javoy-Agid, F., Dubois, B., and Agid, Y. (1983). Somatostatin and dementia in Parkinson's disease. *Brain Res.* **278**, 376–9.

Emson, P. C., Arregui, A., Clement-Jones, V., Sandberg, B. E. B., and Rossor, M. (1980). Regional distribution of methionine-enkephalin and substance P-like immunoreactivity in normal human brain and in Huntington's disease. *Brain Res.* **199**, 147–60.

Flicker, C., Dean, R. L., Watkins, D. L., Fisher, S. K., and Bartus, R. T. (1983). Behavioural and neurochemical effects following neurotoxic lesions of a major cholinergic input to the cerebral cortex in the rat. *Pharmac. Biochem. & Behav.* **18**, 973–81.

Iversen, L. L., Rossor, M. N., Reynolds, G. P., Hills, R., Roth, M., Mountjoy, C. Q., Foote, S. L., Morrison, J. H., and Bloom, F. E. (1983). Loss of pigmented dopamine-β-hydroxylase positive cells from locus coeruleus in senile dementia of Alzheimer's type. *Neurosci. Lett.* **39**, 95-100.

Johnston, M. V., McKinney, M., and Coyle, J. T. (1981). Neocortical cholinergic innervation: a description of extrinsic and intrinsic components in the rat. *Exp. Brain. Res.* **43**, 159-72.

Lees, A. J. and Smith, E. (1983). Cognitive deficits in early stages of Parkinson's disease. *Brain* **106**, 257-70.

Mayeux, R. and Stern, Y. (1983). Intellectual dysfunction and dementia in Parkinson's disease. In *The dementias Advances in neurology* (ed. R. Mayeux and W. G. Rosen), Vol. 38, pp. 211-27. Raven Press, New York.

Mountjoy, C. Q., Roth, M., Evans, N. J. R., and Evans, H. M. (1983). Cortical neuronal counts in normal elderly controls and demented patients. *Neurobiol. Aging* **4**, 1-11.

—, Rossor, M. N., Iversen, L. L., and Roth, M. (1984). Correlation of cortical cholinergic and GABA deficits with quantitative neuropathological findings in senile dementia. *Brain* **107**, 507-18.

Nagai, R., McGeer, P. L., Peng, J. H., McGeer, E. G., and Dolman, C. E. (1983). Choline acetyltransferase immunohistochemistry in brains of Alzheimer's disease patients and controls. *Neurosci. Lett.* **36**, 195-9.

Pearson, R. C. A., Sofroniew, M. V., Cuello, A. C., Powell, T. P. S., Eckenstein, F., Esiri, M. M., and Wilcock, G. K. (1983). Persistence of cholinergic neurons in the basal nucleus in a brain with senile dementia of the Alzheimer's type demonstrated by immunohistochemical staining for choline acetyltransferase. *Brain Res.* **289**, 375-9.

Perry, E. K., Tomlinson, B. E., Blessed, G., Bergmann, K., Gibson, P. H., and Perry, R. H. (1978). Correlation of cholinergic abnormalities with senile plaques and mental test scores in senile dementia. *Br. med. J.* ii, 1457-9.

— and Perry, R. H. (1980). The cholinergic system in Alzheimer's disease. In *Biochemistry of dementia* (ed. P. J. Roberts), pp. 135-83. John Wiley, Chichester.

Perry, R. H., Dockray, G. J., Dimaline, R., Perry, E. K., Blessed, G., and Tomlinson, B. E. (1981). Neuropeptides in Alzheimer's disease, depression and schizophrenia: a post mortem analysis of vasoactive intestinal polypeptide and cholecystokinin in cerebral cortex. *J. Neurol. Sci.* **51**, 465-72.

—, Candy, J. M., and Perry, E. K. (1983). Some observations and speculations concerning the cholinergic system and neuropeptides in Alzheimer's disease. In *Banbury Report 15. Biological aspects of Alzheimer's disease* (ed. R. Katzman), pp. 351-61. Cold Spring Harbor Laboratory.

Reynolds, G. P., Arnold, L., Rossor, M. N., Iversen, L. L., Mountjoy, C. Q., and Roth, M. (1984). Reduced binding of (^{3}H) ketanserin to cortical 5-HT$_2$ receptors in senile dementia of the Alzheimer type. *Neurosci. Lett.* **44**, 47-51.

Rossor, M. N. (1982). Neurotransmitters and CNS disease: dementia. *Lancet* ii, 1200-4.

—, Emson, P. C., Mountjoy, C. Q., Roth, M., and Iversen, L. L. (1980). Reduced amounts of immunoreactive somatostatin in the temporal cortex in senile dementia of Alzheimer's type. *Neurosci. Lett.* **20**, 373-7.

—, Garrett, N. J., Johnson, A. L., Mountjoy, C. Q., Roth, M., and Iversen, L. L. (1982). A post mortem study of the cholinergic and GABA systems in senile dementia. *Brain* **105**, 313-30.

—, Iversen, L. L., Reynolds, G. P., Mountjoy, C. Q., and Roth, M. (1984).

Neurochemical characteristics of early and late onset types of Alzheimer's disease. *Br. med. J.* **288**, 961–4.

Sims, N. R., Bowen, D. M., Allen, S. J., Smith, C. C. T., Neary, D., Thomas, D. J., and Davison, A. N. (1983). Presynaptic cholinergic dysfunction in patients with dementia. *J. Neurochem.* **40**, 503–9.

Spokes, E. G. S. (1980). Neurochemical alterations in Huntington's chorea. *Brain* **103**, 179–210.

Terry, R. D., Peck, A., DeTeresa, R., Schechter, R., and Horoupian, D. S. (1981). Some morphometric aspects of the brain in senile dementia of the Alzheimer's type. *Ann. Neurol.* **10**, 184–92.

Wenk, H., Bigl, V., and Meyer, U. (1980). Cholinergic projections from magnocellular nuclei of the basal forebrain to cortical areas in rats. *Brain Res. Rev.* **2**, 295–316.

Whitehouse, P. J., Price, D. L., Struble, R. G., Clark, A. W., Coyle, J. T., and DeLong, M. R. (1982). Alzheimer's disease and senile dementia: loss of neurons in the basal forebrain. *Science* **215**, 1237–9.

Wilcock, G. K., Esiri, M. M., Bowen, D. M., and Smith, C. C. T. (1982). Alzheimer's disease: correlation of cortical choline acetyltransferase activity with the severity of dementia and histological abnormalities. *J. Neurol. Sci.* **57**, 407–17.

14

Neuropsychological evaluation of higher cognitive function in animals and man: can psychopharmacology contribute to neuropsychological theory?

T. W. ROBBINS

INTRODUCTION

Recent advances in understanding the neurochemical basis of conditions such as Parkinson's disease, senile dementia of the Alzheimer's type (SDAT), Huntingdon's chorea, schizophrenia and Korsakoff's psychosis (Rossor 1981; Mair and McEntee 1983) have enhanced the relevance of psychopharmacological studies to neuropsychology, for a number of reasons. First, drugs such as L-DOPA, clonidine cholinomimetics and neuroleptics are now being used to treat psychological symptoms occurring in these conditions. Secondly, many of these psychoactive drugs alter neurotransmission in specific pathways of subcortical origin which innervate diverse forebrain regions having discrete psychological functions. These pathways include, for example, not only the major monoaminergic transmitters, namely the coeruleo–cortical noradrenergic (NA) projection, the mesotelencephalic dopamine (DA) projection, and the ascending 5-HT pathways, but also the recently characterized cholinergic inputs to neocortex from the basal nucleus of Meynert (nbM) and the medial septal projections to the hippocampus. Thirdly, these pathways probably mediate non-specific processes akin to arousal, optimal levels of which are necessary for these specific psychological functions. Lastly, these different neurotransmitter systems may be responsible for rather different aspects of arousal-like processes. These points will be illustrated mainly by considering the function of the central DA projections, as revealed by animal studies, while some consideration will be given to the modulatory effects of NA and ACh systems innervating neocortex and hippocampus, with special respect to mnemonic function.

IS AROUSAL A USEFUL CONCEPT IN PSYCHOPHARMACOLOGY?

The concept of arousal has a chequered history partly because of its many connotations. Thus, it can be linked with the concept of drive or activation, as a general energizer of behaviour, or as a process linked with the reticular formation which provides a suitable, tonic background of cortical activity for efficient synaptic operations, or as a relatively undifferentiated source of visceral feedback which could have dual functions of providing either specific information about bodily function or modulating non-specific central arousal. Its measurement has involved behavioural indices, such as simple and choice reaction time, electrophysiological indices such as the EEG and autonomic indices such as pulse and respiratory rate. Frequently, these measures fail to intercorrelate to a high degree, are idiosyncratic for individual subjects, dissociate both pharmacologically and neurally and are affected by psychological variables in a way suggestive of much more complex functional interactions. For example, stressors assumed to act in opposite ways upon arousal fail to interact in a way that would be expected for a unidimensional process. Thus, for example, combining incentives with alcohol in an attentional task in man further worsens performance rather than improving it (see Eysenck 1982).

All of these considerations leads to the rejection of a single arousal process and encourages the search for independent, though probably related, mechanisms to account for the results. Indeed, Broadbent (1971) postulated two related arousal processes with an 'upper mechanism' compensating for sub- or supra-optimal activity of a 'lower' one, and Robbins (1984) and Sahgal and Wright (1983) have considered the possible application of similar models to account for patterns of psychopharmacological results. Indeed, there are good reasons for believing that at least some of the neurotransmitter systems described above mediate different forms of arousal. For example, electrophysiological data indicate that the cell bodies of the coeruleo–cortical NA projection respond to a variety of sensory events in a relatively undifferentiated fashion and the neurochemical activity of this pathway is elevated by a variety of stressors. Moreover, the neuroanatomical organization of the so-called dorsal NA bundle (DNAB) suggests that it is capable of simultaneously altering processing in regions having diverse functions, ranging from movement to memory and neuroendocrine regulation (see Robbins and Everitt 1982).

Similarly, evidence of electrophysiological recording from DA cells, of the behavioural effects of dopamine depletion in animals and of the neurochemical effects of stress (see Robbins and Everitt 1982, and Bannon and Roth 1983, for reviews), again suggests that the forebrain DA systems play rather general roles in behavioural output. Recently, similar questions have begun to be asked about the functions of the newly-characterized forebrain ACh projections, psychopharmacological evidence suggesting that these projections also affect a broad range of cognitive processes, including attention as well as memory (see Drachman and Sahakian 1979).

Despite the evidently non-specific, modulatory nature of these forebrain projections, they probably mediate radically different functions. For example, it has been suggested that the coeruleo–cortical NA projection enhances the signal-to-noise (S/N) ratios of evoked neuronal firing in hippocampal and neocortical regions, thus perhaps affecting cortical desynchrony and enhancing the processing of salient exteroceptive (or interoceptive) events. On the other hand, the DA projections appear to amplify the probability and speed of behavioural output following response selection (see Robbins and Everitt 1982). Therefore, in one sense, these ascending projections represent a functional differentiation of the old reticular formation (and of structures afferent to it), in a way corresponding to the psychological dissection of different arousal processes.

One guiding principle for understanding how these neurotransmitter pathways contribute to performance rests on what is already known about the functions of the forebrain regions to which they project. However, this approach does not in itself specify *how* either hyperactivity or hypoactivity in a given pathway affects the process in question. Nor has it been sufficiently considered how the various 'arousal systems' interact to affect performance in the way mooted, for example, by Broadbent's psychological theorizing.

To answer some of these questions, it is worth listing a few important general results which have been established from previous work on arousal processes in man and other animals (see Eysenck 1982).

1. Performance is often an inverted-U-shaped function of arousal level, with an intermediate level for optimal performance.
2. Therefore, equal levels of degraded performance can result from different levels of arousal.
3. Different tasks (and functions) have different optima of arousal level: in particular, 'easy' tasks are performed better at higher levels of arousal than 'difficult' tasks, as embodied in the Yerkes–Dodson principle.
4. Compensatory mechanisms appear to minimize deleterious effects of stressors and changes in endogenous arousal.

With these considerations in mind, it is now timely to reconsider how the various notions of arousal can help us to explain the impaired functions of those ascending neurotransmitters in Parkinson's disease, senile dementia of the Alzheimer's type, Korsakoff's psychosis, and possibly even schizophrenia.

DOPAMINE, ACTIVATION AND PARKINSON'S DISEASE

Degeneration of the nigro-striatal dopamine (DA) projection causes the motor symptoms of Parkinson's disease, but the precise nature of the deficit, as well as its relationship to the depression or cognitive impairments which sometimes accompany the motor symptoms is unclear (see Marsden and Fahn 1982). Studies in rats of the effects of unilateral DA depletion (using the neurotoxin 6-hydroxydopamine (6-OHDA)) have produced evidence of postural bias and paw preference ipsilateral to the lesion as well as a syndrome subjectively assessed as 'sensory neglect' (Marshall and Teitelbaum 1977). In recent studies, we have attempted to define further the nature of this impairment by measuring the accuracy and reaction times of rats with unilateral DA depletion in detecting a brief visual target (a light) presented to either side of the head in an unpredictable manner, whilst the rat is responding in a central location (Carli, Evenden, and Robbins, 1985). One group of rats had to respond in the hole where the light occurred, the other group in the opposite hole, to gain food. Unilateral DA depletion produced a response bias towards the side of the lesion regardless of where the target occurred. This bias was enhanced on probe trials by simultaneous targets at both locations and reduced by omitting the target. Reaction time measures showed that rats were slower to withdraw their heads from the central hole to make responses contralateral to the lesion but not, from this point, to execute the required head movement. These data are interpreted as showing that the striatal DA innervation facilitates the initiation of motor programs, perhaps by mediating the activational (as distinct from the discriminative) impact of salient events.

This conclusion agrees quite well with a recent analysis of performance of Parkinsonian subjects in simple- and choice-reaction time tasks (Bloxham, Mindel and Frith 1984). These authors found that Parkinsonian patients failed to show the usual improvement in reaction time produced by providing an informative warning signal in advance of the required reaction, as also observed by Evarts, Teräväinen and Calne (1981). These data too could be interpreted as showing no major deficit in response selection, but one instead in the *initiation* of a selected plan. This response initiation problem could also be linked to one of motor execution, although it is entirely possible that apparent deficiencies in execution result from problems of initiating new elements in a response sequence.

DA depletion from other regions, such as nucleus accumbens, also reduces the speed and probability of movement as distinct from discrimination of visual events in a 5-choice serial reaction task (Robbins, Everitt, Fray, Gaskin, Carli, and de la Riva 1982). By contrast, drugs such as amphetamine, which release DA and thus enhance dopaminergic neurotransmission, increase the speed of responding (if this is slow) and the probability of premature responding in the same task, without affecting discrimination *per se* (Robbins and Sahakian 1983). At higher doses, the drug produces hyperactivity and stereotyped responding which parallel increases in response switching and perseveration (reminiscent of those seen in certain types of schizophrenia (see Frith and Done 1983) and disrupt co-ordinated responding. These data are consistent with the Lyon and Robbins (1975) hypothesis that amphetamine-like drugs increase the probability of initiation of all responses exceeding some minimal tendency, with resultant impairments of sequencing due to behavioural competition. Overall, the hypothesis is advanced that there exist optimal levels of DA release (or activation) for efficient response initiation and sequencing, with the more complicated sequences requiring lower optimal levels, in keeping with the Yerkes–Dodson principle.

THE INTELLECTUAL DEFICIT IN PARKINSON'S DISEASE: FRONTAL-STRIATAL INTERACTIONS

Although an activational impairment resulting from forebrain dopamine depletion accounts quite well for the predominant symptoms of Parkinsonism, there are growing indications that additional dementia is a late feature of Parkinson's disease and this immediately raises two questions: (1) are such deficits correlated with DA depletion, if not from striatum, then from other DA projections such as prefrontal cortex? or (2) do the deficits depend upon additional damage to other systems such as the locus coeruleus NA, or to the ACh cells of nbM, which are known to be reduced in Parkinson's disease as well as in SDAT (Rossor 1981)?

One obvious way to tackle this question is to analyse the psychological nature of the dementias presented in Parkinsonism and SDAT. Thus, it is salient to note first, that demented subjects seem to have different problems to the normal Parkinsonian subject in response output. For example, Miller (1974) using a 5-choice serial reaction-time task reported deficits in response selection (and also execution) rather than in response initiation in demented subjects. Secondly, the Parkinsonian cognitive impairment resembles deficits produced by frontal lobe injury, shown for example by deficits in visuospatial ability, as measured by subtests of the Wechsler Adult Intelligence Scale (WAIS) (Mortimer, Pirozzolo, Hansch, and Webster 1982) and perseveration as measured by the Wisconsin Card Sorting Test (e.g. Lees and Smith 1983).

Although patients with SDAT can show comparable frontal lobe impairments, this syndrome is usually characterized by a much broader range of impairments, including signs of temporal lobe pathology, as shown in the diminished ability to acquire new information and form new memories (e.g. Weingartner, Grafman, Boutelle, Kaye, and Martin 1983) and also of parietal lobe dysfunction (impaired drawing, apraxia and retrieval of semantically related information) (McDonald 1969; Weingartner *et al.* 1983).

If the pattern of cognitive impairment in Parkinsonism is indeed akin to frontal lobe impairment, then there are, of course, several ways in which this could arise – (1) from specific cell loss in that structure, (2) from damage to DA, NA, or ACh projections to that area, (3) from dysfunction of those portions of the striatum to which prefrontal cortex projects, perhaps caused by nigro-striatal DA depletion.

There is evidence that relatively specific lesions of mesocortical dopamine in the rat or rhesus monkey impair performance in 'delayed alternation', a task particularly sensitive to the effects of frontal lobe lesions in animals (Brozoski, Brown, Rosvold, and Goldman 1979; Simon 1981), thus providing a plausible mechanism for the cognitive deficits in Parkinsonism. However, these animal studies pose major problems of interpretation. First, it is by no means clear which behavioural processes contribute to the delayed alternation deficit (or to the related frontal impairment of 'delayed response'). Both the delayed alternation and delayed response procedures are behaviourally 'impure' in that they involve both spatial and short-term memory factors. Furthermore, they are susceptible to non-specific disruption by other sequelae of frontal lobe lesions such as distractibility and perseveration (although it is also unclear to what extent the latter arises from the inability to perform the task rather than as a primary effect of the lesion). Indeed, it is generally thought that both spatial impairment and disinhibition contribute to the decline in performance (Mishkin 1964). Which of all of these factors is the primary effect of the mesocortical DA lesion is unclear. Secondly, it is likely that 'disinhibitory' effects of frontal lesions result from a reduced modulation of subcortical function; for example, of the striatum. Indeed, in a recent cognitive theory of action control, Norman and Shallice (1980) suggest that the frontal cortex acts as a 'supervisory' mechanism mediating among lower order schema or routines selected by the striatum. Therefore, the activating influence of the nigro–striatal DA pathway (which increases the speed and probability of responding) could be opposed by the inhibitory frontal influence, which keeps these automatic response tendencies in check. This, of course, is reminiscent of Broadbent's 'upper' and 'lower' mechanisms, and is also consistent with the potentiating effects of frontal cortex lesions upon the behavioural response to amphetamine, which mainly depends upon subcortical DA mechanisms (e.g. Iversen 1971). However, it is by no means clear how or why mesocortical DA depletion should cause similar effects to those of frontal cortex lesions.

A third complication concerns the effects of d-amphetamine upon delayed response and delayed alternation. As noted by Ridley and colleagues, this drug mimicks the effects of frontal lobe lesions, in both the rat (Kesner, Bierley, and Pebbles 1981) and the marmoset (Weight, Ridley, and Baker 1980). Furthermore, some of these disruptive effects have recently been shown by Koek and Slangen (1984) to be paralleled by increases in the tendency to repeat the most recent response (i.e. to perseverate), suggesting that they result from disruptive activating effects of the drug rather than because of specific effects on spatial or mnemonic function. Presumably, these indirect effects themselves result from over-activation of the subcortical DA systems. This type of mechanism might also account for the increased alternation and perseveration seen in the response strategies of chronic schizophrenics (Frith and Done 1983), and such effects would be exacerbated by additional frontal cortical damage. In the case of Parkinsonian subjects, the perseveration expected to result from a diminished frontal cortical influence would be offset by reduced subcortical DA activity. However, the simple notion of opposed effects of frontal cortex output and striatal DA activation is complicated by the fact that underactivity, as well as overactivity of the nigro–striatal DA projection also apparently impairs delayed alternation. Thus, DA depletion from the anterior striatum is reported to impair delayed alternation (Simon 1981), suggesting that there is an optimal level of DA activation in striatum for this behaviour, as well as for more simple forms.

Lastly, mesocortical DA turnover is increased by stress (Bannon and Roth 1983), but it is difficult to reconcile this with the facilitating influence of meso-cortical DA on cognition unless either: (1) elevated cortical DA activity some-how regulates potentially disruptive effects of overactivity in other subcortical DA systems. While some studies have reported disinhibiting effects of meso-cortical DA depletion on subcortical DA processes and locomotor activity (see Bannon and Roth 1983) the latter results have proven difficult to replicate (Joyce, Stinus, and Iversen 1983). Or (2) in fact, elevated as well as reduced cortical DA activity impairs performance, there being an intermediate level of cortical DA activity for optimal performance. Recent unpublished work of Sahakian, Curzon, Jackson, Sarna, Hutson, and Kantamaneni may support this view. In a group of normal, albino rats ($n = 17$), individual DA levels in cortex, but not in striatum or nucleus accumbens showed a significant, negative relationship with errors made in delayed alternation ($R_s = -0.635$, $p < 0.001$; $R_s = -0.192$ and $R_s = 0.149$, respectively). Although this relationship at first sight seems to agree with the evidence of lesions showing impairment of delayed alternation following mesocortical DA depletion, it is quite likely for normal rats that errors in delayed alternation are associated with increased rather than decreased DA turnover, because small reductions in neurotransmitter level or store are commonly associated with increased activity within the system. Indeed, a crude index of turnover (DOPAC + HVA/DA) was positively correlated with errors made for both cortex ($R_s = 0.668$; $p < 0.001$) and striatum ($R_s = 0.414$; $p < 0.5$), but not nucleus accumbens. Therefore, these results may indicate that there are intermediate, optimal levels of DA activity and behavioural activation for effective performance for at least two levels in the hierarchy of neural mechanisms controlling response output.

AROUSAL AND MEMORY

From the above discussion of delayed alternation, it is apparent that (1) disrup-tions in this task are not necessarily indicative of specific impairments of short-term memory (STM), and (2) increments (as well as decrements) in activation can impair STM. But need this necessarily lead to *long-term* memory deficits? The answer is apparently not, because treatments which disrupt STM tasks, can lead to *enhanced* LTM retrieval under certain conditions — for example in the case of d-amphetamine and midbrain reticular stimulation (see Kesner *et al.* 1981). This evidence integrates well with that from human studies showing how high levels of arousal, produced for example, by white noise or emotional material impair short-term recall, but can actually benefit long-term retention (Eysenck 1982). This dissociation, of course, suggests the possibility of partially independent memory processes (Kesner *et al.* 1981), and leads us to ask which types of arousal process affect memory consolidation and retrieval and which neurotransmitter systems mediate these processes.

VISCERAL AROUSAL AS A COMPONENT OF MEMORY RETRIEVAL

The most commonly-used memory paradigm in animals is one-trial passive avoidance, in which post-trial treatments are administered which cannot affect performance, but which can alter the way in which the memory trace becomes more permanent (see Gold and Zornetzer 1983). Retention is generally tested after 24h, rather than in the very short term. A bewilderingly large number of treatments including drugs, ECS and disruptive intracranial stimulation can produce retrograde 'amnesic' effects (see Table 14.1), although STM has generally been found to be left unaffected on the few occasions it has been tested. A straightforward interpretation of many of these effects in terms of impaired consolidation of traces is difficult, because all too few experiments have examined the possibility of state-dependent learning — that the drug or manipulation becomes a necessary part of the memory trace for retrieval.

Facilitatory effects on memory can likewise result from effects on motivation by boosting a weak motivational state. Thus, post-trial adrenaline and ACTH can both facilitate retention of one trial passive avoidance, but only at low doses and with weak footshocks which produce low endogenous plasma levels of these two hormones (see Gold and Zornetzer 1983). Recently, the memory-enhancing effects of arginine vasopressin have been explained in similar terms, as resulting indirectly from the pressor action of this hormone (Le Moal, Koob, Koda, Bloom, Manning, Sawyer, and Rivers 1981).

However, there are several findings suggesting that the action of these hormones can be more complex than acting simply as peripheral components of the mnemonic context provided by motivational state. First, high doses of adrenaline and ACTH, or low doses combined with a strong footshock actually impair retention (see Gold and Zornetzer 1983). In addition, post-trial AVP impairs as well as improves memory at the same dose in different rats (Sahgal and Wright 1983). Therefore, there appears to be optimal levels of neuroendocrine activity for memory-trace formation. Secondly, there is some recent evidence for dissociation between the peripheral and central effects of AVP upon memory (de Wied, Gaffori, van Ree, and de Jong 1984). The central effects of the peptide could be modulating arousal directly rather than via peripheral visceral cues. Furthermore, these memory facilitation effects can be mimicked by post-trial events such as white noise, flashing lights, or midbrain reticular stimulation (see Emmerson and DeVietti 1982). Therefore, it is likely that these stimuli are affecting memory by changing overall arousal state rather than by directly affecting motivation, and this possibility obviously also holds for the central actions of neuropeptides.

It is appropriate to ask whether such diverse effects could be acting through the same neurotransmitter system or systems and available evidence in fact suggests that both the amnesic and facilitatory effects of many of these treatments work through the agency of changes in central NA activity.

TABLE 14.1. *Effects of post-trial treatments on 'long-term' retention*

I. HORMONES, OPIATE PEPTIDES, OPIATES

Retrograde amnesia

Adrenaline (high doses = H)
ACTH (H)
AVP

γ-endorphin
Morphine (L)
Met-enkephalin (H)

Oxytocin
Intra-nigral substance P
Intra-amygdaloid substance P
Intra-caudate-angiotensin II

Facilitation

Adrenaline (low doses = L)
ACTH (L)
AVP
Intra-caudate ACTH
α-endorphin
β-endorphin
Morphine (H), ivt morphine
Met-enkephalin (L)
Leu-enkephalin
Naloxone
Intra-amygdaloid naloxone

Intra-hypothalmic substance P

II. CATECHOLAMINE MANIPULATIONS

d-Amphetamine (H)
Clonidine
DDC
Reserpine
Intra-amygdaloid propanolol

d-Amphetamine (L)
Intra-caudate amphetamine
Noradrenaline
Caffeine
Intra-amygdaloid phentolamine

III. ACETYLCHOLINE

Scopolamine
Intra-caudate scopolamine
Atropine

Nicotine
Oxotremorine
Atropine (L)
Physostigmine

IV. MISCELLANEOUS PHARMACOLOGICAL TREATMENTS

Protein synthesis inhibition
Intra-nigral picrotoxin

Strychnine
Pentylenetetrazol

V. ELECTRICAL STIMULATION

Hippocampus
Substantia nigra
Medial nucleus of amygdala
Frontal cortex

Reticular formation
Lateral hypothalamus

Table 14.1 (*cont.*)

VI. MISCELLANEOUS

REM sleep deprivation   Flashing lights
ECT   White noise
Hypothermia

(For sources, see Gold and Zornetzer 1973; Emmerson and De Vietti 1982; Martinez, Jensen, Messing Rigter, and McGaugh 1981.)

AROUSAL, MEMORY, AND THE COERULEO-CORTICAL NA SYSTEMS

A previous article (Robbins 1984) summarized evidence that the coeruleo-cortical NA projection is involved in mechanisms of arousal and attention. It was specifically suggested that activity in this system produced by high levels of stress or arousal, leads to increases in S/N ratio of environmental events evoking activity in terminal regions such as hippocampus and neocortex, and hence affects stimulus selection processes upon which response choice ultimately depends, rather than the overall speed or rate of output.

In a sense then, this NA activity could 'protect' the memory trace from the disruptive effects of distractors during rehearsal and encoding and allow the beneficial effects of arousal to facilitate consolidation (by processes at present unknown). If the facilitatory effects themselves also depend directly upon NA mechanisms, then this would be compatible with Crow's and Kety's original suggestions about the role of NA in learning (see Robbins and Everitt 1982), though without making these processes necessary conditions for learning. These interpretations are consistent with evidence that:

(1) Central NA depletion using a DβH inhibitor can produce an amnesia which is reversible with intraventricular NA (see Gold and Zornetzer 1983).

(2) 6-Hydroxydopamine lesions of the DNAB can retard the acquisition of certain forms of appetitive, as well as aversive discrimination tasks (see Robbins *et al.* 1982; Mair and McEntee 1983).

(3) The amnesic effects of a number of post-trial agents including adrenaline and ECT are attenuated by the protection of central NA from depletion (Gold and Zornetzer 1983).

(4) The facilitatory effects of AVP are reported to depend upon the integrity of the DNAB (Kovacs, Bohus, and Versteeg 1979).

(5) There are reduced levels of CSF MOPEG in patients with Korsakoff's psychosis, which may reflect reduced central NA turnover. Moreover, some success has been reported in alleviating the memory impairments of these subjects with clonidine, an α_1/α_2-agonist (although the precise mode of action of this drug is very unclear in this case) — further strengthening the argument for NA involvement in memory (Mair and McEntee 1983). However, it should be emphasized that any explanation of anterograde amnesia by alterations in

central NA must be integrated into a scheme including damage to limbic and diencephalic structures, such as. medial thalamus. The NA influence may well promote superior memory without being a necessary link in the synaptic interaction in these terminal regions by which memory traces becomes more permanent.

CHOLINERGIC CONTRIBUTIONS TO COGNITION

The recent discoveries associating SDAT and Parkinson's disease with cell loss of ACh cells in nbM have reopened the debate about the ACh contribution to memory and learning. Of all the neurotransmitters, ACh has been linked most frequently to memory processes, principally because of the diverse amnesic effects of the anti-muscarinic drug scopolamine which probably arise from muscarinic receptor blockade in widespread regions of neocortex and hippocampus (e.g. Drachman and Sahakian 1979; Bartus 1980). Scopolamine has also been shown to disrupt performance in difficult perceptual tasks having minimal mnemonic involvement. For example, human performance on a divided attention, dichotic listening task is markedly impaired by this drug (Drachman and Sahakian 1979). This is reinforced by animal studies showing that scopolamine can produce reductions in d' in signal detection tasks, whereas the anticholinesterase, physostigmine has opposite effects (Warburton 1972). The significance of these results is that a blockade of ACh transmission may lead to general impairments in discrimination, rather than to specific effects on memory.

This interpretation is compatible with evidence that ACh mechanisms modulate memory trace retrieval. Deutsch (1983) has reviewed evidence that whereas cholinesterase inhibition impairs the recall of relatively recent, quite well-established memories, it facilitates recall of poorly-remembered associations, when produced by physostigmine injected prior to retention testing. This result can readily be explained if the ACh treatment increases S/N ratio of weak memories (Drachman and Sahakian 1979) because this strengthening of weak traces may interfere with the retrieval of stronger ones. Thus, it is unnecessary to postulate that 'supra-optimal' ACh activity impairs retrieval because of depolarization blockade, as Deutsch suggests. Rather, increased strengthening of weak signals will necessarily lead to impaired retrieval, except where there is a general impairment of memory retrieval as occurs in SDAT. Even then, it is plain that non-specific strengthening of memory traces above noise will still leave the problem of appropriate selection among the different traces.

Specific cholinergic contributions to performance by the distinct ACh inputs to neocortex and hippocampus remain to be defined. Preliminary reports have suggested that learning and memory impairments result from specific destruction of the ACh cells in nbM in the rat (Flicker *et al.* 1983). These findings encourage the view that damage to the extrinsic cortical ACh system can produce functional deficits in animals even in the absence of cortical cell loss. However, the precise relevance of these deficits to those seen in SDAT is, at present, unclear.

INTERACTIONS AMONG THE AROUSAL MECHANISMS

The functional significance of the extrinsic NA and ACh innervations of cortex is problematic, although it is evident that manipulations of these systems produce effects on processes more related to discrimination of signals and response selection than rate of behavioural output. The notion that each transmitter acts to increase S/N ratios of evoked responses to signals is consistent with some published results, but should not prevent us from being critical of the vagueness of this proposal and of the fact that it fails to separate the different processes with which each neurotransmitter is presumably involved. One obvious untested possibility is that these systems achieve enhanced S/N ratios in different ways — in the case of NA, perhaps by reducing the effect of 'neural noise', but in the case of ACh, perhaps by enhancing the evoked response to the signal itself. Another salient consideration is that whereas the NA mechanism might be engaged in times of stress to preserve attentional selectivity, the ACh mechanism might function to maintain alertness at times when arousal is low.

If NA, ACh, and DA contribute to distinct, but interactive arousal mechanisms along the lines suggested, then their interactions should also be studied, especially given the possibility of mutual compensation and when it is realized that for Parkinson's disease and SDAT at least, more than one of these neurotransmitter systems is generally affected. There are, indeed, some indications in the literature that this will prove to be a useful approach — the deleterious effects of scopolamine on WAIS performance for example are markedly increased by d-amphetamine at a dose which by itself has little effect (Drachman and Sahakian 1979). This parallels the synergistic deficits on choice accuracy in a delayed matching-to-sample task in monkeys of these two drugs, even though their effects on rate of performance counteracted one another (Glick and Jarvik 1969). Furthermore, the effects of DNAB lesions in rats on choice accuracy in a 5-choice task occur mainly when the rats are exposed to distracting bursts of white noise which greatly increase premature responding and activate responding in a way analogous to that produced by amphetamine (Carli, Robbins, Evenden, and Everitt 1983). In each of these cases one could infer the existence of mechanisms modulated perhaps by NA or ACh input which compensate for the impairments of response selection resulting from impulsive responding produced by elevated striatal DA activity.

A promising model system to study the precise function of cortical NA, ACh, and DA projections is in prefrontal cortex, where each of these neurotransmitters is represented and where there is a clear interface with response output mechanisms. However, it is significant, in the context of 'upper' and 'lower' arousal mechanisms, that subcortical DA projections contribute not only to the prefrontal cortex, but also to striatal function. The upper and lower arousal mechanisms may be useful heuristic notions, but they do not entail a feudal neurochemical phrenology.

REFERENCES

Bannon, M. J. and Roth, R. H. (1963). Pharmacology of mesocortical dopamine. *Pharmac. Rev.* **35**, 53-67.

Bartus, R. F. T. (1980). In *Aging in the 1980s: psychological issues* (ed. L. W. Poon), pp. 163-80. American Psychological Association, Washington.

Bloxham, C. A., Mindel, T. A., and Frith, C. D. (1984). Initiation and execution of predictable and unpredictable movements in Parkinson's disease. *Brain* **107**, 371-84.

Broadbent, D. E. (1971). *Decision and stress*. Academic Press, London.

Brozoski, T. J., Brown, R. M., Rosvold, H. E., and Goldman, P. S. (1979). Cognitive deficit caused by regional depletion of dopamine in prefrontal cortex of rhesus monkey. *Science* **205**, 929-31.

Carli, M., Evenden, J. L., and Robbins, T. W. (1985). Depletion of unilateral striatal dopamine impairs initiation of contralateral actions and not sensory attention. *Nature* **313**, 679-82.

—, Robbins, T. W., Evenden, J. L., and Everitt, B. J. (1983). Effects of lesions to ascending noradrenergic neurones on performance of a 5-choice serial reaction task in rats: implications for theories of dorsal noradrenergic bundle function based on selective attention and arousal. *Behav. & Brain Res.* **9**, 361-80.

Deutsch, J. A. (1983). The cholinergic synapse and the site of memory. In *The Physiological Basis of Memory*, 2nd edn (ed. J. A. Deutsch), pp. 367-86. Academic Press, London.

Drachman, D. A. and Sahakian, B. J. (1979). The effects of cholinergic agents on human learning and memory. In *Nutrition and the brain*, Vol. 5 (ed. A. Barbeau, J. Growdon, and R. J. Wiertman), pp. 351-66. Raven Press, New York.

Emmerson, R. Y. and DeVietti, T. L. (1982). Presentation of a flashing light following one trial fear conditioning enhances retention. *Animal Learn. & Behav.* **10**, 325-9.

Evarts, E. V., Terävainen, H., and Calne, D. B. (1981). Reaction time in Parkinson's disease. *Brain* **104**, 167-86.

Eysenck, M. W. (1982). *Attention and arousal*. Springer-Verlag, Berlin.

Flicker, C., Dean, R. L., Watkins, D. L., Fisher, S. K., and Bartus, R. T. (1983). Behavioral and neurochemical effects following neurotoxic lesions of a major cholinergic input to the cerebral cortex in the rat. *Pharmac. Biochem. & Behav.* **18**, 973-81.

Frith, C. D. and Done, D. J. (1983). Stereotyped responding by schizophrenic patients on a two-choice guessing task. *Psychol. Med.* **13**, 779-86.

Glick, S. D. and Jarvik, M. (1969). Amphetamine, scopolamine and chlorpromazine interactions on delayed matching performance in monkeys. *Psychopharmacologia* **16**, 147-55.

Gold, P. E. and Zornetzer, S. F. (1983). The Mnemon and its juices: Neuromodulation of memory processes. *Behav. & Neural Biol.* **38**, 151-89.

Iversen, S. D. (1971). The effect of surgical lesions to frontal cortex and substantia nigra on amphetamine responses in rats. *Brain Res.* **31**, 295-311.

Joyce, E. M., Stinus, L., and Iversen, S. D. (1983). Effect of injections of 6-OHDA into either nucleus accumbens septi or frontal cortex on spontaneous motor activity. *Neuropharmacology* **22**, 1141-5.

Kesner, R. P., Bierley, R. A., and Pebbles, P. (1981). Short term memory: The role of d-amphetamine. *Pharmac. Biochem. & Behav.* **15**, 673-6.

Koek, W. and Slangen, J. (1984). Effects of d-amphetamine and morphine on delayed discrimination: signal detection analysis and assessment of response repetition in the performance deficits. *Psychopharmacology* **83**, 346–50.

Kovacs, G. L., Bohus, B., and Versteeg, D. H. G. (1979). The effects of vasopressin on memory processes: the role of noradrenergic neurotransmission. *Neuroscience* **4**, 1529–37.

Lees, A. J. and Smith, E. (1983). Cognitive deficits in the early stages of Parkinson's disease. *Brain* **106**, 257–70.

Le Moal, M., Koob, G. F., Koda, L. Y., Bloom, F. E., Manning, M., Sawyer, W. H., and River, J. (1981). Vasopressor receptor antagonist prevents behavioural effects of vasopressin. *Nature (Lond.)* **291**, 491–3.

Lyon, M. and Robbins, T. W. (1975). The action of central nervous system stimulant drugs: A general theory concerning amphetamine effects. In *Current developments in psychopharmacology*, Vol. 2 (ed. W. B. Essman and L. Valzelli), pp. 79–163. Spectrum, New York.

Mair, R. G. and McEntee, W. J. (1983). Korsakoff's psychosis: noradrenergic systems and cognitive improvement. *Behav. & Brain Res.* **9**, 1–32.

Marsden, C. D. and Fahn S. (eds.) (1982). *Movement disorders*. Butterworth, London.

Marshall, J. F. and Teitelbaum, P. (1977). The neuropsychology of motivated behavior. In *Handbook of psychopharmacology*, Vol. 7 (ed. L. L. Iversen, S. D. Iversen, and S. H. Snyder), pp. 201–29. Plenum Press, New York.

Martinez, J. L. Jr., Jensen, R. A., Messing, R. B., Rigter, H., and McGaugh, J. L. (1981). *Endogenous peptides and learning and memory processes*. Academic Press, New York.

McDonald, C. (1969). Clinical heterogeneity in senile dementia. *Br. J. Psychiat.* **115**, 267–71.

Miller, E. G. (1974). Psychomotor performance in presenile dementia. *Psychol. Med.* **4**, 65–8.

Mishkin, M. (1964). Perseveration of central sets after frontal lobe lesions in monkeys. In *The frontal granular cortex and behavior* (ed. J. M. Warren and K. Akert), pp. 219–45. McGraw-Hill, New York.

Mortimer, J. A., Pirozzolo, F. J., Hansch, E. C., and Webster, D. D. (1982). Relationship of motor symptoms to intellectual deficits in Parkinson's disease. *Neurology* **32**, 133–7.

Norman, D. A. and Shallice, T. (1980). Attention to action: willed and automatic control of behavior. *Center for Human Information Processing, Techn. Rep. No. 99*. University of California, San Diego.

Robbins, T. W. (1984). Cortical noradrenaline, attention and arousal. *Psychol. Med.* **14**, 13–21.

— and Everitt, B. J. (1982). Functional studies of the central catecholamines. *Int. Rev. Neurobiol.* **23**, 303–65.

— and Sahakian, B. J. (1983). Behavioural effects of psychomotor stimulant drugs: clinical and neuropsychological implications. In *Stimulants: neurochemical, behavioral and clinical perspectives* (ed. I. Creese), pp. 301–338. Raven Press, New York.

—, Everitt, B. J., Fray, P. J., Gaskin, M., Carli, M., and de la Riva, C. (1982). The roles of the central catecholamines in attention and learning. In *Behavioral models and the analysis of drug action*, Proc. 27th OHOLO Conference, Zichron Ya'acov, Israel 28–31 March 1982 (ed. M. Y. Spiegelstein and A. Levy), pp. 109–34. Elsevier, Amsterdam.

Rossor, M. N. (1981). Parkinson's disease and Alzheimer's disease as disorders of the isodendritic core. *Br. med. J.* **283**, 1588-90.

Sahgal, A. and Wright, C. (1983). A comparison of the effects of vasopressin and oxytocin with amphetamine and chlordiazepoxide on passive avoidance behaviour in rats. *Psychopharmacology* **80**, 88-92.

Simon, H. (1981). Neurones dopaminergiques A10 et systeme frontal. *J. Physiol. (Paris)* **77**, 81-95.

Warburton, D. M. (1972). The cholinergic basis of internal inhibition. In *Inhibition and Learning* (ed. R. Boakes and M. Halliday), pp. 431-60. Academic Press, London.

Weight, M. L., Ridley, R. M., and Baker, H. F. (1980). The effect of amphetamine on delayed response performance in the monkey. *Pharmac. Biochem. & Behav.* **12**, 861-4.

de Wied, D., Gaffori, O., van Ree, J. M., and de Jong, W. (1984). Central target for the behavioural effects of vasopressin neuropeptides. *Nature (Lond.)* **308**, 276-8.

Weingartner, H., Grafman, J., Boutelle, W., Kaye, W., and Martin, P. R. (1983). Forms of memory failure. *Science* **221**, 380-2.

15

The study of cholinomimetics in Alzheimer's disease and animal models

VAHRAM HAROUTUNIAN, KENNETH L. DAVIS,
BONNIE M. DAVIS, THOMAS B. HORVATH, CELESTE A. JOHNS,
AND RICHARD C. MOHS

INTRODUCTION

Alzheimer's disease (AD) has been demonstrated to be associated with a marked cortical and hippocampal reduction of choline acetyl transferase (CAT) activity (for review, see Bartus et al. 1982) and a profound degeneration of cholinergic neurons originating in the nucleus basalis of Meynert (nbM) (Price et al. 1982; Whitehouse et al. 1982; Wilcock et al. 1983). Evidence that this cholinergic deficit is specifically implicated in the cognitive symptoms of AD is provided both by studies that have shown a direct correlation between severity of dementia and CAT deficiency (Perry et al. 1978) and by pharmacologic studies in healthy young adults in which manipulation of the cholinergic system by anticholinergic or cholinergic drugs has produced memory deficits (Drachman and Leavitt 1974; Drachman 1977) or enhancement (Davis et al. 1978; Sitaram et al. 1978), respectively, in patterns that are typical of AD (Torak 1978). While changes in other neurotransmitters have also been observed in AD (Perry et al. 1981), none correlate with the histopathological lesions and clinical presentation of AD or are as ubiquitous as the cholinergic deficit. Thus, pharmacologic enhancement of cholinergic activity might be a rational treatment approach in AD. Low doses of intravenous physostigmine have been administered to AD patients, and results suggesting that intravenous physostigmine does enhance memory in AD encouraged trials of the clinically more practical oral route of physostigmine administration.

Further exploration of the cholinergic hypothesis of cognitive impairment in AD and of pharmacologic treatment possibilities would be facilitated by the development of a animal model of cholinergic deficiency. Of the two cholinergic pathways of particular interest to AD — the septohippocampal system and the nbM cortical projection system — only the interaction of the septohippocampal pathway with learning and memory has been verified experimentally in animals (Olton et al. 1979). However, the recognition that cholinergic dysfunction in AD may result from selective degeneration of neurons originating in the nbM suggests that a more appropriate animal model might be one in which the nbM is lesioned. The effects of nbM lesions on learning and memory could then be examined, as could the potential of various cholinomimetic agents to reverse lesion-induced deficits.

INTRAVENOUS PHYSOSTIGMINE IN AD

The effect of intravenous (i.v.) physostigmine on cognition was tested in 20 patients with AD. All patients met research criteria previously presented (Davis and Mohs 1982). Three patients with moderate dementias whose MIT or DRS (Kay 1977) were within three points of cut-off scores with histopathological justification were also studied but were classified as 'equivocal AD'.

Intravenous physostigmine was tested in two-phase protocol. In the first, or dose-response phase, subjects were each given 0.0 mg, 0.125 mg, 0.25 mg, and 0.5 mg of physostigmine delivered in 100 cc of saline over 30 min, in random order under double-blind conditions. Each infusion was preceded by 2.5 mg Probanthine, a peripheral anticholinergic, given i.v. For the last six subjects, the 0.125 mg dose was replaced by a testing day on 0.0 mg physostigmine and 0.0 mg Probanthine to provide a control condition for the saline/Probanthine day of testing in order to rule out untoward effects of the anti-cholinergic drug on memory testing. In the second, or replication phase, the dose of psysostigmine associated with the subject's best performance was repeated as was a placebo infusion, again randomly and under double-blind conditions, preceded by 2.5mg of i.v. Probanthine. Trials were separated by two to four days and were done at the same time each day. This study design was adopted because animal and human studies have shown that intravenously-administered physostigmine has an extremely narrow therapeutic window, with an optimal dose that varies from individual to individual (Bartus 1979; Bartus *et al.* 1980; Davis *et al.* 1979).

Cognitive testing consisted of (1) Famous Faces Test (LTM retrieval), (2) Digit Span Task (STM), and (3) Recognition Memory Task (RMT). The RMT consists of showing patients 12 pictures or words which they are asked to describe or read. These are then shown to the patient again intermixed with 12 unfamiliar words or pictures and the patient is asked to state whether or not he recognizes each item. Three trials are completed.

In all except two of the seventeen 'definite AD' patients and two of the three 'equivocal AD' patients, the best response on RMT was seen on some dose of physostigmine rather than placebo, although the optimum dose of physostigmine varied from patient to patient. No adverse effect of Probanthine was noted in those patients who were tested on two placebo days with and without Probanthine. These sixteen patients (fifteen definite AD and one equivocal AD) who demonstrated a best response to physostigmine in the dose-finding phase were then entered in the replication phase. In this phase of the study, mean total correct responses over all three trials was better on i.v. physostigmine than on placebo ($p = 0.02$, paired t = test, two tailed). When the equivocal AD patient, who responded to physostigmine, was eliminated from statistical analysis, differences remained significant at $p = 0.02$. However, four patients showed no improvement. The degree of improvement of the twelve patients who responded to i.v. physostigmine ranged from 1.3 per cent to 18.1 per cent (mean 9.4 per cent) (Davis and Mohs 1982).

There was a trend for all definite AD patients who demonstrated a response to physostigmine in the dose-finding phase to have more correct responses on physostigmine than on placebo on each of the three RMT trials during the replication phase. Patients made significantly fewer false positive errors on physostigmine ($p = 0.02$, ANOVA). In contrast to its effect on RMT, i.v. physostigmine did not alter performance on either Digit Span or Famous Faces Tasks.

ORAL PHYSOSTIGMINE IN AD

Demonstration of improved cognition during intravenous physostigmine infusions led to trials of oral physostigmine in AD patients, to test the hypothesis that more chronic enhancement of central cholinergic activity might lead to sustained cognitive improvement. Sixteen patients (eleven males and five females), ten of whom met MIT or DRS criteria for 'definite AD', and six of whom were designated 'equivocal AD', have been studied thus far in a two-phase protocol as outlined for the intravenous physostigmine study. In the dose-finding phase patients were given 0.5mg, 1.0mg, 1.5mg, and 2.0mg of physostigmine and placebo, each dose for four days, every two hours from 7a.m. to 11p.m. The replication phase consisted of four days of best dose administration randomized with four days of placebo. Cognitive testing was done on the final day of each dose trial. On the last night of each drug condition in the replication phase, patients participated in an all-night sleep study during which blood was drawn every half-hour and assayed for cortisol. To ensure that drug effects on early morning changes in this hormone could be detected, administration of oral physostigmine or placebo was continued until 1100 hours on the morning following the sleep study. Valid sleep studies were obtained in seven patients.

The first four patients (three definite AD and one equivocal AD) were given physostigmine in dosages of 0.0mg, 0.25mg, 0.5mg, 0.75mg and 1.0mg every two hours. This low maximum dose was chosen in order that any potential adverse reaction might be demonstrated before higher doses were administered in subsequent trials to examine effects on cognition. Testing consisted of a visual memory task. Three of the four patients had their best performance on a dose of physostigmine; the one who did not was the one 'equivocal AD' patient. These same three patients again performed better on physostigmine than on placebo during the replication phase; the improvement ranged from 6 per cent to 12 per cent.

As no patients experienced significant side effects to physostigmine at these doses, the maximum dose was raised to 2.0mg for the next twelve patients, seven of whom had 'definite AD'. Methodology of drug administration remained the same; doses of 0.0mg, 0.5mg, 1.0mg, 1.5mg and 2.0mg were now given. The procedure was further modified by expanding cognitive testing to the Alzheimer's Disease Assessment Scale (ADAS), which measures behavioural disorders, mood states, and cognitive functions such as language, praxis, and memory, and was designed specifically for use in AD. Test re-test reliability is Wilcoxin r = 0.97 (p < 0.01), interrater reliability is Spearman 0.99 order (p < 0.001) and the total ADAS score is significantly correct with the Sandoz Clinical Assessment Geriatric (SCAG) score (r = 0.89, p < 0.01) (Rosen *et al.*, in press).

All 'definite AD' patients and all but one 'equivocal AD' patient had their best performance on a dose of physostigmine; this best dose varied from patient to patient. During the replication phase, given to those eleven patients who demonstrated a response to physostigmine in the dose-finding phase, six of the seven 'definite AD' patients again showed improvement on physostigmine; this ranged from 3.5–20.8 per cent improvement over placebo.

One of the four 'equivocal AD' patients showed a mild improvement on physostigmine; two others had worsenings of performance, particularly on depression/irritability and cognitive/language scores. The fourth patient became delusional and reported visual hallucinations while receiving the 0.5mg dose of physostigmine.

When overnight cortisol measurements were analysed, a significant positive correlation was found (r = 0.87, p = 0.01) between percentage increase in cortisol and symptom improvement. This suggests that the patients' symptoms were improved to the extent that physostigmine enhanced central cholinergic transmission.

nbM-LESIONED RATS

The effects of nbM lesions on learning and memory were examined in 72 male Sprague–Dawley rats, half of whom received excitotoxic lesions of the nbM area using $6\mu g/\mu l$ of ibotenic acid (Regis) and half of whom were sham-operated. Habituation and passive avoidance tasks were chosen as indices of learning and memory, as both have been shown to have validity as measures of learning and retention across a wide range of experimental conditions (Bammer 1982; Bartus *et al.* 1980; Bartus and Dean 1981; Bignami and Michalen 1978; Black *et al.* 1977; Brizzee and Ordy 1979; Campbell and Coulter 1976; Deutsch 1973; Gold and McGaugh 1975; Jeffrey 1976; Kandel 1976; Karczman and Dunn 1981; Strong *et al.* 1980; Thompson and Spencer 1966; Wishart and Mogenson 1970).

Ten to fourteen days after lesions or sham operations were performed, rats were exposed to a novel environment — a large polypropylene cage trisected with light beams to allow quantification of activity — for two 15-min intervals separated by 24h in a home cage. Short-term habituation was determined by measuring activity in the first and last minutes of each 15-min exposure to the novel apparatus. Behaviour in the apparatus during the second exposure relative to the first exposure was quantified to assess long-term habituation.

During the first test exposure, the two groups of animals had comparable levels of activity both in total and during the first and last minutes of exposure. During the second test exposure, however, animals with nbM lesions were significantly more active than sham-operated controls during the first minute of the test and throughout the 15-min exposure period (Table 15.1). ANOVA of the first minute activity of the two groups on the two test-days showed a significant main effect of tests (F $1/70$ = 15.5, $p < 0.001$) as well as a significant test-days-by-treatment groups interaction (F $1/70$ = 15.0, $p < 0.001$). Newman–Keuls analysis of the first minute of activity showed that nbM lesioned rats did not differ in their activity levels on the two test days ($p < 0.05$); these lesioned animals were more active than sham-operated animals on second exposure to the apparatus ($p < 0.01$). Sham-operated animals, in contrast, were significantly less active on the second exposure than they had been during the first exposure ($p < 0.01$). ANOVA performed on the total activity scores of the two animal groups revealed identical results: a significant main effect of lesions (F $1/70$ = 6.8, $p < 0.05$), significant main effect of tests (F $1/70$ = 7.7, $p < 0.01$) and a significant treatment-group-by-test-days interaction (F $1/70$ = 10.9, $p < 0.005$). Newman–Keuls analysis showed that these significant effects were due to a decrease in activity of the sham-operated animals from first to second exposure ($p < 0.01$) while the lesioned animals maintained the same level of activity during the two tests.

The effect of physostigmine on the retention of passive avoidance in nbM lesioned animals and sham-operated controls was investigated using a post-acquisition drug treatment paradigm. The same two groups of thirty-six animals were divided into three subgroups of twelve rats each, matched on the basis of their activity scores in the habituation study. Subgroup 1 was assigned to the saline condition, subgroup 2 to the 0.03mg/kg physostigmine condition, and subgroup 3 to the 0.06 mg/kg physostigmine condition.

Each rat was given one training session in a standard passive avoidance apparatus (Bartus *et al.* 1980). Doses of physostigmine salicylate dissolved in

TABLE 15.1. *Twenty-four-hour retention of habituation*
(*Test 1-Test 2*)

	1st min	15-min total
Sham-lesioned	12.2 (±1.6)	26.3 (±8.1)
nbM-lesioned	3.5 (±1.2)*	2.8 (±1.8)*

*vs. sham $p < 0.01$.

saline or saline placebo were administered intraperitoneally (IP) 60s after termination of the shock given at the end of the training procedure. Rats were then placed in a holding cage for 15–25min before being returned to the home cage. Retention of one-trial passive avoidance was determined 72h later in a procedure identical to that used during training.

Seventy-two-hour retention was strongly influenced by sham or nbM lesion conditions as well as by physostigmine administration (Table 15.2). When performance was analysed by ANOVA of lesion condition and physostigmine dose, a main effect of lesion was revealed (F $1/66 = 8.0, p < 0.01$) as was a significant lesion by physostigmine interaction (F $2/66 = 8.5, p < 0.001$). Newman-Keuls analysis showed that, in the subgroups of rats treated with saline injections, nbM-lesioned rats crossed into the shock compartment significantly faster than sham-operated controls ($p < 0.05$). The performance of both sham-operated and nbM-lesioned rats improved with a dose of physostigmine ($p < 0.05$), although the sham-operated animals had their best performance on 0.03mg/kg physostigmine, while a 0.06mg/kg dose was required to improve significantly the performance of the nbM-lesioned rats.

All 72 animals were sacrificed by decapitation within ten days of the last behavioural test so that cortical CAT activity could be determined. Cortices were quickly dissected over ice and were assayed for CAT activity (Fonnum 1975). Excitotoxic lesion of the nbM area resulted in approximately a 20 per cent decrement of CAT activity ($t = 2.8, p < 0.01$). Since the nbM is thought to contribute 45–55 per cent of total cortical CAT activity (Johnston *et al.* 1979) the ibotenic acid-induced lesions destroyed approximately 50 per cent of the nbM cells. Histologic examinations of the lesion site showed a lesion diameter of approximately 0.75mm, sparing the caudal and rostral extensions of the nbM.

DISCUSSION

Cognitive and global functioning has been shown to improve when the cholinergic drug physostigmine is administered to patients with AD, supporting the

TABLE 15.2. *Seventy-two-hour retention of passive avoidance learning* (*mean crossthrough latency in seconds*)

	Saline	Physostigmine 0.03mg/kg	Physostigmine 0.06mg/kg
Sham-lesioned	270.2 (±77)	449.6 (±90)*	100.2 (±31)
nbM-lesioned	66.8 (±18)	110.0 (±32)	234.7 (±78)*

*vs. saline $p < 0.05$.

hypothesis that clinical symptoms of AD, particularly those in the sphere of learning, are due in part to the cholinergic deficit documented in numerous studies of autopsied AD brains. Specifically, patients given physostigmine intravenously demonstrated significant improvement in their ability to store information in LTM. This was demonstrated both in the patients' overall performance in RMT testing and in the number of false positive responses per trial. Patients with Alzheimer's disease had significantly fewer false positive responses on RMT during physostigmine infusions than during placebo infusions. Signal detection analysis of the data indicates that patients were better able to discriminate old from new items on physostigmine (Mohs and Davis 1982). The most likely explanation is that physostigmine enhanced a patient's ability to learn information about old items and store this in LTM, making the old items more familiar to them. Patients with AD tend to 'recall' information incorrectly to a significantly greater extent than patients with dementia of other etiologies, and a significant association between the presence of such errors and both decreased CAT activity and increased number of senile plaques on autopsy has been demonstrated (Fuld *et al.* 1982). This suggests that decreased cholinergic activity is a possible causative factor in false positive responses in AD patients. Thus, pharmacological evidence in patients with AD suggests that specific cognitive symptoms of AD, particularly those of storage into LTM, are a result of cholinergic deficits.

While i.v. physostigmine produces improvements in AD patients that are of theoretical importance, practical pharmacological treatment agents should be longer-acting, safe, and be suitable for oral administration. Cholinesterase inhibitors can produce chronic enhancement of cholinergic systems without requiring presynaptic neurons to make compensatory increases in ACh production, and their mechanism of action may be closer to the physiological activity of cholinergic systems than direct long-acting pharmacological receptor agonists. Physostigmine, a competitive inhibitor of acetylcholinesterase, is relatively safe when given orally. Despite its short half-life, in multiple small doses it produces chronic enhancement of cholinergic systems. In doses up to 2.0mg given orally every 2h, physostigmine was relatively free of side-effects and did yield modest improvements both in specific cognitive areas and overall functioning in six of our seven 'definite AD' patients. The variability of response to oral physostigmine, ranging from no response to a 21 per cent improvement over placebo, suggests that there may be a subgroup of patients who would benefit from this cholinomimetic therapy.

Since cholinomimetics can enhance cortisol release the extent to which oral physostigmine increased mean cortisol levels can be regarded as one measure of the extent to which physostigmine actually increased central cholinergic activity. Patients with the largest physostigmine enhancement of cortisol, also displayed the greatest physostigmine-induced cognitive improvement. A similar result was reached by Thal who found that oral physostigmine's enhancement of memory in patients with AD was highly correlated with percentage cholinesterase inhibition in CSF (Thal *et al.* 1983). Given that the efficacy of physostigmine is dependent upon the integrity of the cholinergic neuron, a neuron that is degenerating, physostigmine should not benefit all AD patients. Thus, a biological measure like cortisol concentrations, that establishes an independent central nervous system effect of physostigmine, provides an additional support for the notion that the physostigmine-related changes in the cognition of AD patients is the result of increased central cholinergic activity.

The theoretical rationale of cholinomimetic treatment for AD patients is strengthened by studies of rats with nbM lesions. These rats, with histologically verified lesions of the nbM and 20 per cent decrements of cortical CAT activity, had poor retention of two different experimental tasks which can be likened to the LTM deficits seen in human subjects with AD. When learning was tested via a habituation paradigm, nbM-lesioned rats did not differ from sham-operated controls, nbM rats re-exposed to the testing apparatus 24h after their within-session habituation of activity; however, 24h later, they showed no evidence of retention or long-term habituation of activity. In contrast to sham-operated controls, nbM rate re-exposed to the testing apparatus 24h after their initial exposure, behaved as though they had never seen the testing apparatus. Rats injected with scopolamine have similar deficits in the retention of exploratory behaviour, as do weanling rats (Bishop and Kimmel 1969; Horsburgh and Hughes 1981; Hughes 1982; O'Brien and Corman 1970; Parsons *et al.* 1973; Platel and Porsolt 1982), who, because of ontogenic constraints, have a cholinergic deficit (Coyle and Yamamura 1976).

nbM-lesioned rats also showed poorer 72-h-retention of a one-trial passive avoidance task than sham-operated controls. This study, when reviewed in light of the similar results seen in the investigation of habituation, suggests that memory deficits occur as a result of nbM lesion which are general, not task-specific, phenomena. Both groups of rats learned a passive avoidance response to shock in the same number of trials, and both demonstrated an equivalent sensitivity to shock, indicating that nbM-lesioned rats have an isolated memory deficit without impairment of pain threshold, locomotion, or short-term learning.

Seventy-two-hour retention of a one-trial passive avoidance task, which was poor in nbM-lesioned rats, improved and approached the retention time of sham-operated animals when nbM-lesioned rats were treated with physostigmine. These results demonstrate that the beneficial effects of cholinergic enhancement on LTM seen in normal human subjects and in AD patients can be extended to a hypocholinergic animal model. However, while physostigmine was markedly efficacious in reversing deficits of retention in nbM-lesioned rats, it has thus far proven to be only modestly effective in enhancing the cognitive performance of a subgroup of AD patients. This disparity is not unexpected, as a nbM-lesioned rat does not provide an animal model that is completely analogous to a human with AD. The rats in these studies were given localized excitotoxic lesions that destroyed approximately 50 per cent of the nbM, while the diagonal band of Broca and septum were preserved. This resulted in a 20 per cent decrement of cortical CAT activity. AD patients, in contrast, have been shown to have far more widespread losses of cholinergic nuclei, and correspondingly greater CAT decrements. In addition, other neurotransmitter system deficits have been identified in AD, particularly but not exclusively involving the locus coeruleus/ noradrenergic system, and these appear to coexist with cholinergic deficits in at least a subgroup of AD patients. Thus, the development of a nbM-lesioned animal is the first of several steps needed to create a realistic animal model of AD. The cholinergic deficiency model in animals would more closely approximate AD if lesions of the nbM could be extended to include the septum as well. Other animal models must then be developed with deficits that mimic other neuropathological features of AD, such as locus coeruleus ablations and somatostatin deficits. The behavioural effects of these lesions could then be studied in combination and singly to ascertain the pertinence of such deficits to the clinical symptomatology of AD. Finally, if all lesions could be combined in a single animal that would remain viable, a working model of AD may be developed, and research in the area of prospective treatments of AD would be greatly expedited.

Alzheimer's disease is a multi-symptom disease that may ultimately prove to be mediated by multiple neurochemical abormalities. The response of some AD patients to physostigmine supports the hypothesis that decreased central cholinergic activity is manifested clinically in specific symptoms of AD, and animal studies support the clinical significance of the nbM degeneration observed in AD brains. Alterations of other neurotransmitter systems, neuropeptides, and receptor sites, may contribute to clinical impairment but have yet to be completely elucidated. Perhaps definitive treatment of AD awaits clarification of these multiple neurochemical variables, delineation of parameters that can predict response, and development of appropriate safe, long acting pharmacological agents. None the less, it is encouraging that the course we are now taking is a rational strategy based on observed neurochemical deficits.

ACKNOWLEDGEMENTS

This work was supported in part by a Grant #AG02219 from the Institute on Aging and NIH Grant #RR-71, Division of Research Resources, General Clinical Research Centers Branch.

REFERENCES

Bammer, G. (1982). Pharmacological investigations of neurotransmitter involvement in passive avoidance responding: A review and some new results. *Neurosci. & Biobehav. Rev.* **6**, 247–96.
Bartus, R. T. (1979). Physostigmine and recent memory effects in young and aged nonhuman primates. *Science* **206**, 1087–9.
— and Dean, R. L. (1981). Age-related memory loss and drug therapy: Possible directions based on animal models. In *Brain neurotransmitters and receptors*

in aging and age-related disorders (ed. S. J. Enna *et al.*), *Aging*, Vol. 17. Raven Press, New York.

—, —, and Beer, R. (1980). Memory deficits in aged cebus monkeys and facilitation with central cholinomimetics. *Neurobiol. Aging* 1, 145-52.

—, —, —, and Lippa, A. S. (1982). The cholinergic hypothesis of geriatric memory dysfunction. *Science* 217, 408-17.

—, —, Goas, J. A., and Lippa, A. S. (1980). Age related changes in passive avoidance retention: Modulation by dietary choline. *Science* 209, 301-3.

Bignami, G. and Michalek, H. (1978). Cholinergic mechanisms and aversively motivated behaviors. In *Psychopharmacology of aversively motivated behavior*, (ed. H. Anisman and G. Bignami). Plenum Press, New York.

Bishop, P. D. and Kimmel, H. R. (1969). Retention of habituation and conditioning. *J. exp. Physchol.* 81, 317-21.

Black, A. H. L., Nadel, L., and O'Keefe, J. (1977). Hippocampal function in avoidance learning and punishment. *Psychol. Bull.* 84, 1107-29.

Brizzee, K. R. and Ordy, J. M. (1979). Age pigment, cell loss, and hippocampal function. *Mechanisms of Aging and Development* 9, 143-63.

Campbell, B. A. and Coulter, X. (1976). Ontogeny of learning and memory. In *Neural mechanisms of learning and memory* (ed. E. L. Bennett and M. R. Rosenzweig), pp. 209-35. MIT Press, Cambridge, Mass.

Coyle, J. T. and Yamamura, H. I. (1976). Neurochemical aspects of the ontogenesis of cholinergic neurons in the rat brain. *Brain Res.* 118, 429-40.

Davis, K. L. and Mohs, R. C. (1982). Enhancement of memory processes in Alzheimer's disease with multiple dose intravenous physostigmine. *Am. J. Psychiat.* 139, 1421-4.

—, Mohs, R. C., and Tinklenberg, J. R. (1979). Enhancement of memory by physostigmine. *New Engl. J. Med.* 301, 946.

—, —, —, Pfefferbaum, A., Hollister, L. E., and Kopell, B. S. (1978). Physostigmine: Improvement of long-term memory processes in normal subjects. *Science* 201, 272-4.

Deutsch, J. A. (1973). The cholinergic synapse and the site of memory. In *The physiological basis of memory* (ed. J. A. Deutsch), pp. 59-77. Academic Press, New York.

Drachman, D. A. (1977). Memory and cognitive function in man: does the cholinergic system have a specific role. *Neurology* 27, 783-90.

— and Leavitt, J. (1974). Human memory and the cholinergic system. *Arch. Neurol.* 30, 113-21.

Fonnum, F. (1975). A rapid radiochemical method for the determination of choline acetyltransferase. *J. Neurochem.* 24, 407-9.

Fuld, P. A., Katzman, R., Davies, P., and Terry, R. D. (1982). Intrusions as a sign of Alzheimer dementia: chemical and pathological verification. *Ann. Neurol.* 11, 155-9.

Gold, P. E., and McGaugh, J. L. (1975). Changes in learning and memory during aging. In *Neurobiology of aging* (ed. J. M. Ordy and K. R. Brizzee), pp. 145-58. Plenum Press, New York.

Horsburgh, R. J. and Hughes, D. L. (1981). Modification of novelty preference in rats by current and prior treatment with scopolamine and methylscopolamine. *Psychopharmacology* 73, 388-90.

Hughes, R. N. (1982). *Behav. & Neural Biol.* 34, 4-41.

Jeffrey, W. E. (1976). Habituation as a mechanism for perceptual development. In *Habituation: perspectives from child development, animal behavior, and neurophysiology* (ed. T. J. Tighe and R. N. Leaton), pp. 279-96. Lawrence Erlbaum Assoc., Hillsdale, New Jersey.

Johnston, M. V., McKinney, M., and Coyle, J. T. (1979). Evidence for a cholinergic projection to the neocortex from neurons in basal forebrain. *Proc. natn Acad. Sci. U.S.A.* **76**, 5392–6.

Kandel, E. R. (1976). *Cellular basis of behavior*. Freeman, San Francisco.

Karczman, A. G. and Dunn, N. J. (1981). Cholinergic synapses: Physiological, pharmacological and behavioral considerations. In *Psychopharmacology: a generation of progress* (ed. M. A. Lipton, A. D. DiMascio, and K. F. Killman). Raven Press, New York.

Kay, D. W. K. (1977). The epidemiology and identification of brain deficit in the elderly. In *Cognitive and emotional disturbance in the elderly* (ed. C. Eisdorfer and R. O. Friedel), pp. 11–26. Year Book Medical Publishers, Chicago.

Mohs, R. C. and Davis, K. L. (1982). A signal detectability analysis of the effect of physostigmine on memory in patients with Alzheimer's disease. *Neurobiol. Aging* **3**, 105–9.

O'Brien, R. M. and Corman, C. D. (1970). Retention of exploratory behavior. *Psychonomic Science* **18**, 23–4.

Olton, D. S., Becker, J. T., and Handelsman, G. C. (1979). Hippocampus, space and memory. *Behav. & Brain Sci.* **2**, 313–22.

Parsons, P. J., Fagan, T., and Spear, N. E. (1973). Short-term retention of habituation in the rat: A developmental study from infancy to old age. *J. comp. Physiol. Psychol.* **84**, 545–53.

Perry, E. K., Blessed, G., and Tomlinson, B. E. (1981). Neurochemical activities in human temporal lobe related to aging and Alzheimer-type changes. *Neurobiol. Aging* **2**, 251.

—, Tomlinson, B. E., Blessed, G., Bergman, K., Gibson, P. H., and Perry, R. H. (1978). Correlation of cholinergic abnormalities with senile plaques and mental test scores in senile dementia. *Brt. med. J.* **2**, 1457–9.

Platel, A. and Porsolt, R. D. (1982). Habituation of exploratory activity in mice: A screening test for memory enhancing drugs. *Psychopharmacology* **78**, 346–52.

Price, D. L., Whitehouse, P. J., Struble, R. G., Clark, A. W., Coyle, J. T., DeLong, M. R., and Hedreen, J. C. (1982). Basal forebrain cholinergic systems in Alzheimer's disease and related dementias. *Neurosci. comment.* **1**, 84–5.

Rosen, W. G., Mohs, R. C., and Davis, K. L. A new rating scale for Alzheimer's disease. *Am. J. Psychiat.* (in press).

Sitaram, N., Weingartner, H., and Gillin, J. C. (1978). Human serial learning: enhancement with arecholine and impairment with scopolamine correlated with performance on placebo. *Science* **201**, 274–6.

Strong, R., Hicks, P., Hsu, L., Bartus, R. T., and Enna, S. J. (1980). Age-related alterations in the rodent brain cholinergic system and behavior. *Neurobiol. Aging* **1**, 59–63.

Thal, L. J., Fuld, P. A., Masur, D. M., and Sharpless, N. S. (1983). Oral physostigmine and lecithin improve memory in Alzheimer's disease. *Ann. Neurol.* **13**, 491–6.

Thompson, R. F. and Spencer, W. A. (1966). Habituation: A model phenomenon for the study of neuronal substrates of behavior. *Psychol. Rev.* **73**, 16–43.

Torack, R. M. (1978). *The pathological physiology of dementia*, pp. 17–25. Springer-Verlag, Berlin.

Whitehouse, P. J., Price, D. L., Struble, R. G., Clark, A. W., Coyle, J. T., and DeLong, M. R. (1982). Alzheimer's disease and senile dementia: loss of neurons in the basal forebrain. *Science* **215**, 1237–9.

Wilcock, G. K. Esiri, M. M., Bowen, D. M., and Smith, C. C. T. (1983). The nucleus basalis in Alzheimer's disease: cell counts and cortical biochemistry. *Neuropath. & appl. Neurobiol.* **9**, 175-9.
Wishart, T. and Mogenson, G. (1970). Effects of lesions of the hippocampus and septum before and after passive avoidance training. *Physiol. & Behav.* **5**, 32-4.

PART 4
Schizophrenia

16

Schizophrenia: genetics and environment

FINI SCHULSINGER

ADOPTION STUDIES

The traditional methods in psychiatric genetics have been twin-studies and pedigree studies. The twin-studies provide evidence for a possible genetic liability, whereas the pedigree studies serve the purpose of illustrating a possible genetic mode: Mendelian or polygenetic.

The critique of the classical pedigree studies, because they represent a possible infiltration of genetic and environmental influences, could be counteracted if it were possible to study persons who shortly after birth were placed in adoptive − or foster − families with whom they were not at all biologically related. This method was proposed more than fifty years ago by Reiter (1930) from East Prussia, who then published the first assessment of a group of boys placed in foster homes, with the intention of a later follow-up (although this never happened, perhaps because Reiter did not want to submit to the eugenics of the Third Reich). Newkirk (1957), Skeels (1936), Skodak and Skeels (1949), and Ann Roe (1945) published studies of personality disorders, mental retardation, and alcoholism in foster-home-placed probands and their foster relatives. These studies were not methodologically sufficient. Either they were based on only a few cases, or the probands were not entirely unrelated to the foster families.

The same weakness occurred to a minor degree in Heston's (1966) pioneering study of the offspring of psychotic mothers, born at a mental hospital in Oregon, and either placed in foster families or in orphanages. They were matched with children with the same types of placement, but without psychotic mothers. The study showed 10 per cent psychosis, and 35 per cent other mental abnormalities in the offspring of psychotic mothers, no matter what kind of placement they were subjected to. The control subjects, whose mothers were not psychotic did not exhibit psychotic or other serious mental abnormalities.

Simultaneously with Heston's study, Seymour Kety and his co-workers (Rosenthal, Wender, Schulsinger, and Jacobsen), had collected in Denmark a pool of all individuals, who from 1924 to 1947 were adopted away during early childhood to non-biologically-related adoptive parents, a total of 14 500 subjects. More than half of them were placed in the adoptive homes less than one month after birth, whereas the remainder spent more or less time (up to a total of two years) with biological relatives or in children's homes before the adoptive placement. The sample exhibited social selection to a minor degree, inasmuch as the children from biological parents of the very lowest social class had a tendency towards placement in the lowest class adoptive families. At the other extreme, in the very highest social classes, the same trend was found.

It is obvious that such a sample represents a unique source for studies of genetics and environment in all diseases or conditions, where this dichotomy is still unsettled.

So far we have hosted studies in the following areas (one major reference for each):

Schizophrenia (Kety *et al.* 1975)
Affective disorders (in preparation)
Psychopathy (Schulsinger 1972)
Criminality (Mednick and Christiansen 1977)
Alcoholism (Goodwin *et al.* 1973)
Suicide (Schulsinger *et al.* 1979)
Intelligence and education (Teasdale and Owen 1984)
Obesity (body mass index) (in preparation)
Premature death (in preparation)
Breast cancer in women (in preparation)

The schizophrenia studies were carried out by two different methodological approaches. Rosenthal *et al.* (1968, 1974) and Wender *et al.* (1974) carried out a series of studies using the adoptee's design, i.e. studying adoptees who were selected on the basis of schizophrenia or non-schizophrenia in one of their biological parents or schizophrenia in their adoptive parents. A supplementary study of individuals reared with their biological parents, of which one was schizophrenic, permitted an approximation of a cross-breeding study.

The classification of parents, based on their hospital records, and of probands based on intensive free interviews does not meet the rigid methodological requirements of today, but was based on DSM–II traditions. In spite of this, the overall results of these studies demonstrate that genetic as well as environmental influences are present in the transmission of schizophrenia. The adoptees without schizophrenia in their biological and adoptive families showed the least schrizophrenia-like psychopathology, whereas the non-adopted children of a biological parent with schizophrenia showed the most. The adoptees with a biological, or an adoptive schizophrenic parent were placed in the middle, and were not too different from each other with regard to schizophrenia-like manifestations (Rosenthal *et al.* 1975; Wender *et al.* 1974).

Kety *et al.* (1968, 1975) carried out studies based on the so-called family study design, in which the types and prevalence of mental illness in the biological and adoptive relatives of schizophrenic adopted away probands and their matched, healthy controls. The first study (Kety *et al.* 1968) was based only on hospital records, and showed a significant surplus of schizophrenia spectrum

TABLE 16.1. *Schizophrenia spectrum disorders in the biological and adoptive relatives of adoptees who became schizophrenic*

Probands	No. of probands	Relatives	
		Biological	Adoptive
Index	34	13/150	2/74
Control	34	3/156	3/83
p		0.007	

disorders in the biological relatives of the schizophrenic adoptees (Table 16.1). A later study (Kety *et al.* 1975) was based on interviews with relatives and control probands, and thus yielded many more cases with psychopathology. The overall results were substantial. In addition, it was demonstrated that the harder parts of the schizophrenia spectrum (schizophrenia, borderline schizophrenia, and possible cases of these two classes) were valid, whereas softer parts of a spectrum (schizoid or paranoid personality, inadequate personality (DSM-II)) produced a certain amount of 'noise', in so far as they did not discriminate very well between index and control probands.

HIGH-RISK STUDIES

The most efficient way of studying etiological factors in schizophrenia seems to be to make use of the longitudinal, prospective study of children at a high genetic risk for schizophrenia. The American psychologist, Sarnoff A. Mednick and the present author began such a study in Copenhagen in 1962. We studied 207 children between 10 and 20 years of age, whose mothers were severely schizophrenic, and a matched control group of 104 children, whose parents and grandparents had never been hospitalized for mental illness (Mednick and Schulsinger 1973).

Table 16.2 shows the major assessment years in our study. In addition we received information on the subjects from various sources.

In what follows, results from four sub-studies on the same sample will be described:

1. An analysis of pregnancy and birth complications distributed over diagnostic outcome in 1972–4.
2. An analysis of institutional care during the first five years of life — and the diagnostic outcome in 1972–4.
3. An analysis of premorbid behaviour until the 1962 assessment, and diagnostic outcome in 1972–4.
4. Data from a study carried out 1979–80 in order to test a hypothesis on the nature of what is genetically transmitted, and what is not.

TABLE 16.2. *Design of the project*

High-risk children *n* = 207
Low-risk children *n* = 104
x̄ age 15,1 years

1962	→	1967	→	1972	→	1980
INITIAL ASSESSMENT		5-year follow-up		10-year diagnostic follow-up		subsample follow-up

Obstetrical data

Detailed midwife reports were rated on a 0-4 weighted rating scale for specific complications. This scale was developed with the assistance of Professor Frits Fuchs of the Department of Gynaecological Obstetrics at Cornell University Medical School. The individual scores could be utilized to create three different global scores of pregnancy and birth complications.

1. Frequency score
2. Severity score
3. Total score

The total score was derived by adding all the individual weighted scores, and the total score correlated highly with the other scores. Figure 16.1 shows the total scale scores for the four diagnostic groups: schizophrenia, borderline schizophrenia, other diagnoses, 'no mental illness' or well. The schizophrenic group had significantly higher complication scores than the borderline group. The mean values for the 'no mental illness' group did not differ significantly from either those of the schizophrenics or those of the borderlines. In fact, the

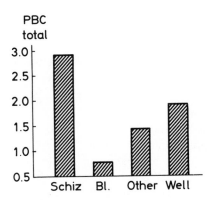

Fig. 16.1. Pregnancy and birth complications in high-risk group.

mean values for the 'no mental illness' group lay close to the midpoint between these two pathological groups. The majority of the schizoprenics (67 per cent) experienced some form of complication; i.e. our results do not come from very few schizophrenics suffering a tremendous amount of severe complications. These results are reported by Parnas, F. Schulsinger, Rasdale, H. Schulsinger, Feldman, and Mednick (1982).

Behavioural precursors of schizophrenia spectrum

During the first assessment of our subjects from 1962-4 we collected information on the subjects' behaviour from infancy up to the time of assessment. We interviewed their rearing parents or rearing agencies. All the subjects were interviewed during the assessment, and all the investigators involved completed an adjective checklist on the subjects. Finally, we got very detailed information from their teachers about the subjects' achievements and behaviour in school. Table 16.3 demonstrates the overall results from the study of premorbid behavioural characteristics within the schizophrenia spectrum. Part of the information is retrospective, as for example the early childhood factors where we find that schizophrenia spectrum, i.e. schizophrenia and borderline schizophrenia, exhibited passivity and poor attention according to parental descriptions. School behaviour was retrospective to some extent, but for the majority of the subjects the information was actually current. We found, that schizophrenia spectrum subjects in school were more isolated and rejected by others, and they were more sensitive. In addition, they were characterized by poor affect control, they got more easily upset, and more liable to contain their upset state for a longer time than the comparison groups. With regard to this item, the schizophrenics were significantly worse than the borderlines which was the only significant difference between these two parts of the schizophrenia spectrum. The clinical assessment items were non-retrospective, and they comprised cognitive as well as emotional items as premorbid discriminators.

As a preliminary conclusion of the behavioural precursor study which is

TABLE 16.3. *Behavioural precursors of*
Schizophrenia spectrum

Early childhood	passivity
	poor concentration
School behaviour	rejected by others
	poor affect control*
Clinical assessment	formal thought disorder
(15 years of age)	defective emotional rapport

*This item discriminated schizophrenics from borderline schizophrenics.

described in detail in Parnas, F. Schulsinger, H. Schulsinger, Mednick and Teasdale (1982) we can state that our results seem to point toward a basic behavioural relationship between schizophrenia and borderline schizophrenia. Both disorders were characterized by premorbidly defective emotional rapport, and formally disturbed cognition. Pre-schizophrenics, however, tended to display more attention deficit, and exhibited poor affective control. In their psychopathological picture, both disorders exhibit fundamental schizophrenic symptoms but, of course, to a different degree. The distinction between them, however, relies mainly on the intensity of such accessory psychotic symptoms as hallucinations and delusions. This study of behavioural precursors substantiates Eugen Bleuler's concept of schizophrenia as a disorder essentially characterized by formally disturbed cognition and defective emotional rapport: 'The disease is characterized by a specific type of alteration of thinking, feeling, and relation to the external world which appears nowhere else in this particular fashion . . . Hallucinations and delusions are partial phenomena of the most varied disease. Their presence is often helpful in making the diagnosis of a psychosis, but not in diagnosing the presence of schizophrenia.'

As the fundamental symptoms can be traced premorbidly, we find that Bleuler's concept of schizophrenia as a development rather than a disease process hitting a healthy person, is also substantiated by our results.

Institutionalization

The basic advantage of the prospective, high-risk design is that it makes it possible to find out which environmental factors might be correlated to the differences in clinical outcome. Michael Rutter (1981) concluded his review of the consequences of deprivation in childhood by endorsing Caldwell's recommendation that future studies should fulfil three criteria, namely: (1) genetic factors should be taken into account, (2) stringently defined measures of stress should be employed, and (3) they should focus upon specific psythopathological outcome variables. We have tried to analyse the history of institutionalization in relation to the clinical outcome within and outside the schizophrenia spectrum in our sample of children of severely schizophrenic mothers. We proposed, with respect to genetic loading, that schizophrenics and borderline schizophrenics share a similar genetic predisposition that is more severe than that of those high-risk individuals who remain mentally healthy. Operationally, this means that we hypothesize that age of onset of maternal schizophrenia should be lower among schizophrenics and borderline schizophrenics than among high-risk individuals who remain healthy. With respect to the environmental factors we have suggested that it is the schizophrenics themselves, in particular, rather than borderlines who have premorbidly experienced the most stressful conditions. Operationally, this means that schizophrenics should have spent more time in institutions during the first five years of life than did other diagnostic outcome groups. Table 16.4 presents means and standard deviations for each of the three independent variables as a function of diagnoses in the high-risk group. In this

TABLE 16.4. *Predictor variables as a function of diagnosis (high-risk group only)*

	Schizophrenics $n = 13$		Borderline schizophrenics $n = 29$		Other diagnoses $n = 79$		'No mental illness' $n = 55$		ANOVA		p
	mean	s.d.	mean	s.d.	mean	s.d.	mean	s.d.	F		
MAH (age)	27.7	5.4	29.5	8.3	32.1	8.2	34.5	8.3	3.86		0.011
INS (months)	22.2	22.8	10.8	16.0	4.1	10.6	2.4	7.6	11.33		<0.001*
CM (months)	32.5	23.5	41.6	21.0	50.1	17.2	50.3	18.1	4.66		0.004*

*In view of the skewness of these two variables we have repeated the analyses using a non-parametric test (Kruskal-Wallis).
For INS the corresponding probability is <0.001 and for CM 0.003.

study we have also included a group of all the other diagnoses apart from schizophrenia, borderline schizophrenia, and 'no mental illness'. The three variables are: mother's age at first hospitalization (MAH), the number of months spent in institution during the first five years of life (INS), and finally, the number of months spent with the schizophrenic mother during the first five years of life (CM). Both the schizophrenics and borderlines have mothers whose age at first hospitalization was significantly lower than those of the 'no mental illness' group. The 'other diagnoses' group occupied a middle position.

With respect to institutionalization (INS) the schizophrenics experienced significantly more through the first five years of life than did the borderlines, who in turn lie significantly above the 'other diagnoses' as well as the 'no mental illness' group on this variable. In the case of contact with the mother (CM) the schizophrenics had significantly less contact with the mothers during the first five years of life than had both the 'other diagnoses' and 'no mental illness' groups which do not differ significantly from each other. These three variables can be expected to be heavily intercorrelated, and this is also what was found.

An analysis of co-variance of institutionalization, corrected for mother's age at first hospitalization and for contact with the mother, showed that institutionalization significantly keeps its effect. If we entered mother's age at hospitalization and institutionalization as co-variates for contact with the mother, the four diagnostic groups did not differ significantly. Thus, contact with the mother may only have significance for later psychopathology in the child to the extent that it indirectly reflects the degree of genetic loading the child has inherited and/or the amount of time spent in institutions. A detailed report on institutionalization has been published (Parnas, Teasdale, and Schulsinger, in press).

Cerebral ventricular size within the schizophrenia spectrum

A number of studies over the last three decades indicate that chronic schizophrenia is associated with cerebral ventricular enlargement. The NIMH studies of twins discordant for schizophrenia showed that the schizophrenic twins had more soft neurological signs than had the healthy co-twins. Other studies, for example by Max Pollock and co-workers, have shown that siblings of schizophrenics have less neurological deficit than had the schizophrenics themselves. As described above, we, and many others, have shown that schizophrenics have suffered more pregnancy and birth complications than the other high-risk children. Taking into consideration also that the American–Danish adoption studies (Kety *et al.* 1975) have demonstrated that schizophrenia and borderline schizophrenia appears among the biological relatives of the same schizophrenic index probands, we put forward the hypothesis that the genetically transmitted condition is not schizophrenia itself, but borderline schizophrenia. Real schizophrenia then is a complicated (frequently neurologically complicated) form of borderline schizophrenia. Our concept of borderline schizophrenia corresponds with the DSM–III schizotypal personality disorder.

In order to test this bold hypothesis we studied from 1979–80 a subgroup of the total high-risk sample consisting of ten schizophrenics, ten borderlines, and sixteen 'no mental illness' cases, as diagnosed in our 1972 assessment during which diagnoses were made as a consensus between two of three diagnostic instruments: a clinical diagnosis, the Current And Past Psychopathology Scale (CAPPS), or the Present State Examination (PSE), 9th edition. In 1979–80, these 36 subjects were clinically reassessed by the same clinical interviewer, and the subjects were also examined with a 1010 EMI-scanner. We used the same method of measurement as reported by Weinberger and his colleagues from the United States.

There were no significant differences in the third ventricle width or the ventricular brain ratio (VBR) as a function of the 1972 consensus or even the 1972 clinical diagnoses. However, the clinical diagnoses made in 1980 had changed to some extent from the clinical diagnoses in 1972. Two of the schizophrenias had turned into borderlines, one of the borderlines had turned into schizophrenia, one into 'no mental illness', and one into 'other psychiatric disorders'. Comparisons based on the 1980 diagnoses showed that schizophrenics had the largest third ventricles. Figure 16.2 shows that ventricular size as measured by the VBR was the largest for the schizophrenics and the smallest for the borderlines, with the 'no mental illness' group in between. No relationship was found between ventricular size and the age of the subject, length of psychiatric hospitalization, drug treatment, or electroconvulsive treatment.

We examined the relationship between ventricular size in 1980 and the pregnancy–birth complication data obtained as part of the initial 1962 assessment. We found significant associations between enlarged ventricles in adulthood

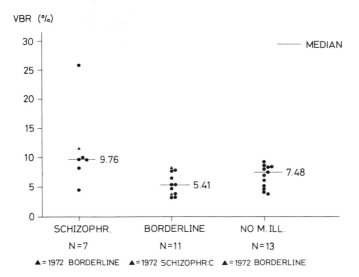

Fig. 16.2. Ventricular brain ratio by 1980 diagnosis

and signs of prematurity at birth. There was also a modest correlation between the width of the third ventricle and a global rating of perinatal complications (F. Schulsinger, Parnas, Petersen, H. Schulsinger, Teasdale, Mednick, and Møller 1984).

CONCLUSION

It is an almost insuperable task to report results from more than twenty years of prospective work with this group of children of schizophrenic mothers and their controls. In the references detailed descriptions of and discussions about methodology, and about the concepts of the various parts of the schizophrenia spectrum may be found. What we have tried to show is *one* development within the genetics of schizophrenia: the utilization of genetic knowledge to facilitate the study of environmental effects. We have seen, that the clinical outcome of the children of severely schizophrenic mothers may depend to some extent on obstetrical complications, and on institutional care. We have seen that pre-morbidly there is a great overlap between the components of the schizophrenia spectrum. We have also seen, that differences in ventricular size might be to some extent a reflection of differences in environment.

We believe that prospective studies of populations at a high risk for schizophrenia is the most powerful way of studying the interactions between heredity and environment.

First, it is not too burdened by the doubtful reliability of retrospective information.

Second, the value of following the same specific individuals over time is a strong advantage, as demonstrated with the diagnostic changes over time in the cerebral ventricle study.

The high-risk design provides us with the best possible controls: those high-risk subjects who do not become schizophrenics in spite of the genetic risk. ·

REFERENCES

Goodwin, D. W., Schulsinger, F., Hermansen, L., Guze, S. B., and Winokur, G. (1973). Alcohol problems in adoptees raised apart from alcoholic biological parents. *Arch. gen. Psychiat.* **28**, 238–43.

Heston, L. L. (1966). Psychiatric disorders in foster home reared children of schizophrenic mothers. *Br. J. Psychiat.* **112**, 819–35.

Kety, S. S., Rosenthal, D., Wender, P. H., and Schulsinger, F. (1968). The types and prevalence of mental illness in the biological and adoptive relatives of adopted schizophrenics. In *The transmission of schizophrenia* (ed. D. Rosenthal and S. S. Kety), pp. 345–62. Pergamon Press, London.

—, —, —, —, and Jacobsen, B. (1975). Mental illness in the biological and adoptive relatives of adopted individuals who became schizophrenic. In *Genetic research in psychiatry* (ed. R. Fieve, D. Rosenthal, and H. Brill), pp. 147–65. John Hopkins University Press.

Mednick, S. A. and Schulsinger, F. (1973). Studies of children at high risk for

continuously for more than one year. This population was suitable for an examination of the issue of whether or not ventricular enlargement resulted from past physical treatment because treatment policies which had been practised in that hospital in the past had been variable so that while some patients had received a full range of physical treatment others had received little or none. It was possible to find groups of patients who had received no ECT insulin or neuroleptic treatment and to compare them with groups matched for age, sex, and length of illness who had been heavily treated by these methods. Comparison was also made between similarly matched samples who had not been treated and who had been heavily treated with each modality, the exposure of these samples to treatments other than the one under consideration being equal. The results of these comparisons show that treatment with insulin or ECT or neuroleptic drugs – and/or the degree of treatment with each was unrelated to present lateral ventricular size (Table 17.1). Furthermore, the combination of past physical treatments did not correlate with VBR in that no differences in ventricle size were found between those with no history of physical treatment and matched subjects heavily treated. Thus, it can be concluded that the past physical methods of treatment are not the cause of the ventricular enlargement associated with schizophrenia. If indeed the features of schizophrenia which tend to be associated with increased lateral ventricular size result from some

TABLE 17.1. *Comparisons of VBRs of matched groups of chronic schizophrenic inpatients*

Comparison group (all matched for age, sex and length of illness)	Numbers	VBR	Significance
No physical treatments	9	13.13 SD 3.68	
vs.			NS
Heavy physical treatments	7	11.46 SD 3.68	
No insulin	8	13.36 SD 2.0	
vs.			NS
Much insulin (matched for ECT and neuroleptics)	8	11.36 SD 2.0	
No ECT	8	12.56 SD 2.12	
vs.			NS
Much ECT (matched for insulin and neuroleptics)	8	13.01 SD 3.28	
No neuroleptic	8	14.48 SD 3.97	
vs.			NS
Much neuroleptic (matched for insulin and ECT)	8	12.97 SD 3.5	

form of cerebral injury, that injury is not the result of the treatment of the schizophrenia.

It must be emphasized that lateral ventricular enlargement does not occur in all or even the majority of schizophrenics, and that indeed it does not occur in all patients manifesting profound neuropsychological impairments, behavioural deterioration, negative features, etc. There are patients in whom these abnormalities have unquestionably been present for years who have entirely normal CT appearances (Owens *et al.* 1985). None the less, of the many CT scan studies of lateral ventricular appearances there are few which do not show enlargement more frequently in schizophrenic patients than in the control sample used. It is possible to explain the occasional negative findings on the basis that as by no means all schizophrenic patients share the finding of lateral ventricular enlargement, some study samples will, by chance alone, include none who do.

The pneumoencephalographic, echoencephalographic, and computed tomographic studies of schizophrenia would appear to indicate that in some patients, there is a degree of enlargement of the ventricular system and that where clinical correlates are demonstrated there tend to be those of deterioration and defect. Such findings raise a number of questions.

The first of these is whether or not these apparent abnormalities are really present at all. There are very many examples in the literature of apparent biological correlates of psychiatric disorders which have appeared convincing and important at one time but which have not been sustained by subsequent experiments and have faded away 'like elephants' footprints in the mud' (Editorial 1978). The numerous confirmations of the finding of ventricular enlargement in schizophrenia mean that oblivion seems an unlikely fate for this result but it is not an impossible one. If it is accepted that ventricular enlargement occurs in schizophrenia more often than in controls and that it is not due to treatment, the relationship between the schizophrenic illness and the structural abnormality must be considered. It has been established that ventricular enlargement is not a necessary concomitant of schizophrenia even in its most severe and most chronic forms. Nor indeed is ventricular enlargement sufficient for the development of schizophrenia as it has been noted in manic-depressive illness, e.g. (Rieder, Mann, Weinberger, van Kammen, and Post 1983), in long term benzodiazepine users (Lader, Ron, and Petursson 1984) and as a phenomenon which may be reversible in association with alcoholism (Carlen, Wortzman, Holgate, Wilkinson, and Rankin 1978) and anorexia nervosa (Heinz, Martinez, and Haenggli 1977). These latter two results suggest the possibility that changes in ventricular size may reflect fluid electrolyte and nutritional status. It is implausible that such factors underlie the consistent findings in schizophrenic patients as these have been demonstrated in out-patients as well as in the institutionalized (Owens *et al.* 1985) and in young patients in their first episodes or who had not been ill for long (Weinberger *et al.* 1983).

Lateral ventricular enlargement is therefore a non-specific finding which, more frequently than would be expected by chance, occurs in schizophrenia.

Its temporal relationship to the development of the disease is an important question. The clinical correlates of ventricular enlargement tend to be those characteristic of relatively chronic and advanced disease. There are no satisfactory studies correlating CT scan appearances and the process of schizophrenic disease over a period of years. Clearly, these are desirable, but there were ethical difficulties concerning repeated scans when earlier machines were used and there are difficulties in comparing images taken at different times using different machines. In some pneumoencephalographic studies (e.g. Haug 1962) repeat examinations were done and there were a few instances of apparent deterioration. Such a deterioration if it were replicable would suggest that increase in ventricular enlargement occurred with and perhaps as a result of the schizophrenia disease process. On the other hand the fact that ventricular enlargement may be present in first-episode schizophrenics suggests not that the enlargement results from schizophrenia but rather that it may be a predisposing factor to this disorder. This important question has yet to be resolved.

We are left with the finding that non-specific structural abnormalities have repeatedly been demonstrated in schizophrenia and appear to be associated with the disease rather than its treatment. Whether they are a result of the schizophrenic disease process or represent a predisposing factor to that condition is unclear. Presumably these structural abnormalities have a basis in pathology of some cerebral cells, but the size and nature of these changes remains obscure (Owens *et al.* 1985). It is not particularly difficult to accept that the cellular pathology underlying the relatively gross structural changes implied by the results of imaging studies may remain unclear, but the implication from the imaging studies is merely that the ventricles are larger because the brain substance has become less. Without confirmation of this reduction of brain substance at post-mortem, the conclusion that there are technical and other difficulties with all imaging studies and that these have misled us could seem very reasonable. At Northwick Park, however, a recent post-mortem study of brain weights and of photographs of slices of brains of patients who died in Runwell Hospital has shown that schizophrenics have reduced brain weights and enlarged lateral cerebral ventricles (Brown, Colter, Corsellis, Crow, Frith, Jagoe, Johnstone, and Marsh 1985), by comparison with the affectively ill. Direct support for the evidence of structural change shown by the imaging studies has thus been provided.

In conclusion, many years have passed since Griesinger and Kraepelin stated their belief that brain pathology was the basis of psychiatric illness and of the disease that is now called schizophrenia. The results of these various studies of structural brain changes suggest that at least in some cases there is now evidence that they were correct.

REFERENCES

American Roentgen Ray Society (1929). Report of Committee on Standardization of Encephalography. *Am. J. Roentgenol.* 22, 474-80.

Andreasen, N. C., Olsen, S. A., Dennert, J. W., and Smith, M. R. (1982). Ventricular enlargement in schizophrenia: relationship to positive and negative symptoms. *Am. J. Psychiat.* 139, 297-302.

Asano, N. (1967). Pneumoencephalographic study of schizophrenia. In *Clinical genetics in psychiatry* (ed. N. Mitsuda), pp. 209-19. Igaku-Shoin, Tokyo.

Barron, S. A., Jacobs, L., and Kinkel, W. R. (1976). Changes in size of normal lateral ventricles during aging determined by computerized tomography. *Neurology (Minneap.)* 26, 1011-13.

Benes, F., Sunderland, P., Jones, B. D., Le May, M., Cohen, B. M., and Lipinski, J. F. (1982). Normal ventricles in young schizophrenics. *Br. J. Psychiat.* 141, 90-3.

Brown, R., Colter, N., Corsellis, J. A. N., Crow, T. J., Frith, C. D., Jagoe, R., Johnstone, E. C., and Marsh, L. (1985). Brain weight and parahippocampal cortical thickness are decreased and temporal horn is increased in schizophrenia by comparison with affective disorder. *Arch. gen. Psychiat.* (in press).

Carlen, P. L., Wortzman, G., Holgate, R. C., Wilkinson, D. A., and Rankin, J. C. (1978). Reversible cerebral atrophy in recently abstinent chronic alcoholics measured by computed tomography scans. *Science* 200, 1076-8.

Dandy, W. E. (1919). Roentgenography of the brain after injection of air into the cerebral ventricles. *Am. J. Roentgenol.* 6, 26.

Daum, C. H., McKinney, W. M., Proctor, R. C., Barnes, R. W., and Potter, P. (1976). Echoencephographs of 100 consecutive acute psychiatric admissions. *J. clin. Ultrasound* 4, 329-33.

Donnelly, E. F., Weinberger, D. R., Waldrum, I. N., and Wyatt, R. J. (1980). Cognitive impairment associated with morphological main abnormalities on computed tomography in chronic schizophrenic patients. *J. nerv. ment. Dis.* 168, 305-8.

Editorial (1978). The biochemistry of depression. *Lancet* i, 422-3.

Griesinger, W. (1857). *Mental pathology and therapeutics* (Transl. C. Lockhart Robertson and J. Rutherford). New Sydenham Society, London.

Gross, G., Huber, G., and Schuttler, R. (1982). Computerised tomography studies in schizophrenic disease. *Arch. Psychiat. u. Nervenkr.* 231, 519-26.

Haug, J. O. (1962). Pneumoencephalographic studies in mental disease. *Acta psychiat. scand.*, suppl. 165, 38, 1-114.

Heinz, R., Martinez, J., and Haenggli, A. (1977). Reversibility of cerebral atrophy in anorexia nervosa and Cushing's syndrome. *J. comp. assis. Tomogr.* 1, 415-18.

Holden, J. M. C., Forno, G., Itil, T., and Hsu, W. (1973). Echoencephalographic patterns in chronic schizophrenia. *Biol. Psychiat.* 6, 129-41.

Hounsfield, G. N. (1973). Computerised transverse axial scanning (tomography). Part I: Description of the system. *Br. J. Radiol.* 46, 1016-22.

Huber, G. (1957). *Pneumoencephalographische und Psychopathologische Bilder bei Endogen Psychosen.* Springer Verlag, Berlin.

Huber, G. (1979). Pure defect and its meaning for a somatosis hypothesis of schizophrenia. In *Biological psychiatry today* (ed. J. Obiols, C. Ballus, E. Gonzales, and J. Pugol), pp. 345-50. Elsevier/North Holland, Amsterdam.

Jacobi, W. and Winkler, H. (1927). Encephalographische studien an chronisch schizophrenen. *Arch. Psychiat. u. Nervenkr.* 81, 299-332.

Jernigan, T. L., Zatz, L. M., Moses, J. A., and Berger, P. A. (1982). Computed tomography in schizophrenics and normal volunteers. *Arch. gen. Psychiat.* **39**, 765–70.

Johnstone, E. C., Crow, T. J., Frith, C. D., Husband, J., and Kreel, L. (1976). Cerebral ventricular size and cognitive impairment in chronic schizophrenia. *Lancet* ii, 924–6.

—, —, —, Stevens, M., Kreel, L., and Husband, J. (1978). The dementia of dementia praecox. *Acta psychiat. scand.* **57**, 305–24.

Kraepelin, E. (1896). *Psychiatrie*, 5th edn. Barth, Leipzig.

Lader, M. H., Ron, M., and Petursson, H. (1984). Computed axial brain tomography in long term benzodiazepine users. *Psychol. Med.* **14**, 203–6.

LeMay, M. (1967). Changes in ventricular size during and after pneumoencephalography. *Radiology* **88**, 57–63.

Levi, C., Gray, J. E., McCullough, E. C., and Hattery, R. R. (1982). The unreliability of CT numbers as absolute values. *Am. J. Radiol.* **139**, 443–7.

Mundt, C. H., Radii, W., and Gluck, E. (1980). Computertomographische untersuchungen der liquorraume an chronish schizophrenen patienten. *Nervenarzt* **51**, 743–8.

Nagy, K. (1963). Pneumoencephalographische befunde bei endogen psychosen. *Nervenarzt* **34**, 543–8.

Nyback, H., Berggren, B. M., and Hindmarsh, T. (1982). Computed tomography of the brain in patients with acute psychosis and in healthy volunteers. *Acta psychiat. scand.* **65**, 403–14.

Okasha, A. and Madkour, O. (1982). Cortical and central atrophy in chronic schizophrenia. A controlled study. *Acta psychiat. scand.* **65**, 29–34.

Owens, D. G. C., Johnstone, E. C., Crow, T. J., Frith, C. D., Jagoe, J. R., and Kreel, L. (1985). Lateral ventricular size in schizophrenia: relationship to the disease process and its clinical manifestations. *Psychol. Med.* **15**, 27–41.

Penn, R. D., Belanger, M. G., and Yasnoff, W. A. (1978). Ventricular volume in man computed from CAT scans. *Ann. Neurol.* **3**, 216–23.

Rieder, R. O., Mann, L. S., Weinberger, D. R., van Kammen, D. P., and Post, R. M. (1983). Computed tomographic scans in patients with schizophrenia, schizoaffective and bipolar affective disorder. *Arch. gen. Psychiat.* **40**, 735–9.

Storey, P. B. (1966). Lumbar air encephalography in chronic schizophrenia: a controlled experiment. *Br. J. Psychiat.* **112**, 135–44.

Takahashi, R., Inaba, Y., Inanaga, K., Kato, N., Kumashiro, H., Nishimura, T., Okuma, T., Otsuki, S., Sakai, T., Sato, T., and Shimazono, Y. (1981). CT scanning and the investigation of schizophrenia. In *Biological Psychiatry* (ed. C. Perris, G. Struwe, and B. Jansson), pp. 259–68. Elsevier/North Holland, Amsterdam.

Tanaka, T., Hazama, H., Kawahara, R., and Kobayashi, K. (1981). Computerized tomography of the brain in schizophrenic patients. *Acta psychiat. scand.* **63**, 191–7.

Weinberger, D. R., Torrey, E. F., and Wyatt, R. J. (1979*a*). Cerebellar atrophy in chronic schizophrenia. *Lancet* i, 718–19.

—, —, Neophytides, A., and Wyatt, R. J. (1979*b*). Structural abnormalities of the cerebral cortex in chronic schizophrenia. *Arch. gen. Psychiat.* **36**, 935–9.

—, Wagner, R. L., and Wyatt, R. J. (1983). Neuropathological studies of schizophrenia: A selective review. *Schizophrenia Bull.* **9**, 193–212.

18

Mechanism of action of antipsychotic drugs: retrospect and prospect

LESLIE L. IVERSEN

INTRODUCTION

The introduction of chlorpromazine for the treatment of schizophrenia by Delay and Deniker in 1952 revolutionized the management of the illness, and radically altered the character of mental hospitals (for review see Deniker 1970). Although Delay and Deniker were convinced that chlorpromazine was truly antischizophrenic and not simply a supersedative, this idea was slow to become widely accepted. It was not until the late 1950s in the United States that large-scale trials showed clearly that barbiturate sedatives were no more effective than placebo in relieving schizophrenic symptoms, whereas phenothiazines were consistently efficacious (Klein and Davis 1969). Similar studies showed that anti-anxiety drugs of the benzodiazepine class were also no more effective than placebo. The discovery of a new class of drugs which relieve the fundamental symptoms of schizophrenia: thought disorder, abnormalities of affect, withdrawal, and autism, is one of the most significant events in the short history of psychopharmacology. It is not surprising that a large research effort has subsequently been devoted to understanding how the phenothiazines and related antischizophrenic drugs act in the brain. Such knowledge might lead not only to a more rational basis for the development of new drugs, but also perhaps give some clue as to the nature of the abnormalities which underly schizophrenic illness. This has been on the one hand a great success story — as it is now widely accepted that the mechanism of action of antipsychotic drugs is understood — on the other hand, this understanding has not necessarily led us much nearer to the riddle of schizophrenia in neurobiological terms.

EARLY EVIDENCE FOR THE 'DOPAMINE HYPOTHESIS'

Many different lines of research lead to the conclusion that antischizophrenic drugs act by blocking dopamine receptors in brain. An important empirical discovery was made by Paul Janssen and colleagues in the early 1960s from their systematic studies of potential new drugs in animal tests, from which emerged a large and potent new family of drugs, the butyrophenones (for review see Janssen and Van Bever 1978). Among the many animal tests used, two turned out to be highly predictive of antipsychotic activity — the ability of drugs to block the behavioural stimulation and repetitive movements (stereotypy) elicited by d-amphetamine in laboratory animals, and their ability to block the behavioural stimulation and emesis induced by apomorphine. Both amphetamine and apomorphine act in these tests by activating dopamine mechanisms in brain. A further intriguing link was provided by the observation that amphetamines at high doses can reliably induce a form of schizophrenia-like psychosis in man, and that this 'amphetamine psychosis' is consistently reversed by phenothiazines and other antipsychotic drugs (Angrist, Sathamanthan, Wilk, and Gershon 1974). Clinically, it also became clear that the ability of antipsychotics to relieve schizophrenic symptoms was invariably accompanied by the induction of extrapyramidal symptoms resembling those of Parkinson's disease, a dopamine deficiency state (Deniker 1970).

A crucial advance was made by Carlsson and Lindqvist (1963) who first proposed that phenothiazines might act specifically to block dopamine receptors in brain. This conclusion was drawn from their observation that haloperiodol and chlorpromazine stimulated the rate of dopamine turnover in rat brain. This was measured biochemically as an increase in the brain concentration of the dopamine metabolite 3-methoxytyramine, although the levels of dopamine itself were unchanged. Carlsson and Lindqvist reasoned that the increased rate of dopamine turnover might reflect a compensation in response to blockade of dopamine receptors. Such studies were systematically pursued using a variety of other methods to assess dopamine turnover (see Sedvall 1975), and it was established that all effective antipsychotic drugs affect brain dopamine metabolism in this way, while having variable effects on the rate of turnover of noradrenaline in brain. Direct electrophysiological recordings have since shown that intravenously infused neuroleptics cause an acceleration in the firing rate of dopamine neurones in rat midbrain, presumably by activating reflex compensatory mechanisms subsequent to receptor blockade (Bunney, Walters, Roth, and Aghajanian 1973).

BIOCHEMICAL STUDIES OF DOPAMINE RECEPTORS

D1 receptors

By the early 1970s it was clear that what was needed to test the 'dopamine hypothesis' was the ability to assess the potencies of a wide range of antipsychotic drugs as antagonists at dopamine receptors in mammalian brain. This was not easy to do, as such receptors have no obvious counterpart in peripheral tissues, and assessing drug actions in the intact brain is very difficult, as drug potency may be affected by metabolism or inadequate penetration into CNS. It was, thus, a major step forward when a simple biochemical model became available. The discovery by Kebabian, Petzgold, and Greengard (1972) that dopamine-rich areas of brain contained a dopamine-stimulated adenylate cyclase seemed to offer a means of testing the 'dopamine hypothesis' *in vitro*. Initial studies by Greengard and colleagues (Clement-Cormier, Kebabian, Petzgold, and Greengard 1974) and in our own laboratory (Miller, Horn, and Iversen 1974) seemed to offer promising results. The ability of phenothiazines to block the dopamine-stimulated formation of cyclic AMP in homogenates of rat striatum parallelled the antipsychotic potencies of these drugs, with fluphenazine being most potent (K_i approx 1 nM) and chlorpromazine weakest, and clinically inactive compounds such as promazine and promethazine were also inactive in this test. Furthermore, the blockade of dopamine-cyclase was specific for the active *cis*-isomers of the thioxanthenes, such as cis-flupenthixol, whereas the pharmacologically inactive *trans*-isomers were inactive or only weakly active (Miller *et al.* 1974). Similarly, the pharmacologically-active stereoisomer (+)butaclamol was effective, while the inert (−)isomer was inactive. It was quickly recognized, however, that one important group of drugs, the butyrophenones, did not fit into this model. Compounds such as haloperidol were very potent antischizophrenic drugs, many times more potent than chlorpromazine in animal test predictive of antipsychotic activity, but were only weakly active in blocking the dopamine–cyclase response (see Iversen 1975).

It is now recognized that the dopamine receptors which are coupled to cyclic AMP formation in brain, retina, and autonomic ganglia represent a particular pharmacological class − the D1 receptors. Their function remains unknown, and they do not appear to be of crucial importance in the mechanism of action of antipsychotic drugs. Nevertheless, some classes of antipsychotics, especially the thioxanthenes, are particularly potent antagonists of the D1 receptors, and some of these, e.g. flupenthixol and piflutixol can be used as radioligands to identify D1 sites in receptor binding experiments (Hyttel 1981). Whether blockade of D1 receptors by such drugs contributes in any important way to their pharmacological profile is not clear.

D2 receptors

The second class of dopamine receptors is the D2 type, characterized by the fact that they are not linked to stimulation of adenylate cyclase activity. Indeed, the D2 receptors in some tissues exert inhibitory effects on adenylate cyclase activity (see Creese, Hamblin, Leff, and Sibley 1983). In anterior pituitary, dopamine inhibits prolactin secretion, and the receptor type involved is of the D2 type, perhaps involving a decrease in intracellular cyclic AMP concentrations; in the intermediate lobe of pituitary, Kebabian and colleagues have shown that activation of D2 receptors inhibits the increase in cyclic AMP and the secretory response elicited by β-adrenoceptor agonists such as isoprenaline; in the striatum the same group provided evidence that activation of D2 receptors inhibited the cyclic AMP response elicited by D1 agonists. The D2 receptors have a quite different specificity for agonists and antagonists from the D1 sites. They are potently stimulated by apomorphine and by various ergolines, such as bromocriptine, which are inactive on D1 receptors. In their antagonist profile the D2 receptors respond very sensitively to butyrophenones, and to all other known classes of antipsychotic drugs. They are easily studied *in vitro* by using potent butyrophenones such as spiperone as radioligands, which bind with nanomolar affinities (Creese, Burt, and Snyder 1978, Creese *et al.* 1983; Seeman 1980). The most convincing evidence that the D2 receptors represent the key site of action of antipsychotic drugs comes from studies in which the potencies of many different compounds were assessed *in vitro*, and shown to correlate well with the known clinical potencies of the same drugs when used in treating the symptoms of schizophrenia (Fig. 18.1). When the same drugs were tested in other *in vitro* receptor binding assays, to assess their potencies as H1 histamine antagonists, α-adrenoceptor blockers, serotonin antagonists, or anticholinergics, no such correlations were found (Peroutka and Snyder 1980) (Table 18.1). Nevertheless, among the antipsychotic drugs individual compounds may possess potent activities at one or more of these receptors, in addition to their D2 activity, a fact which has lead to considerable confusion in studies in which only limited

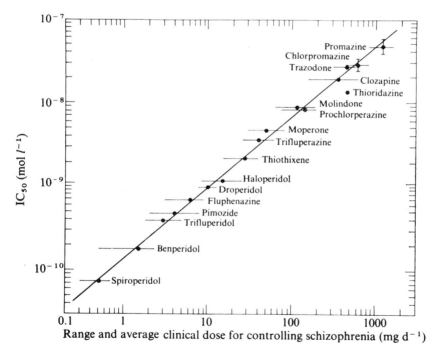

Fig. 18.1. Comparison of the clinical potencies of neuroleptic drugs, measured as average daily dose in treating schizophrenia with potencies of the same drugs in displacing ^{3}H-haloperidol from dopamine receptor binding sites *in vitro* (IC_{50} = concentration of drug required to displace 50 per cent of specific haloperidol binding). (From Seeman, Lee, Chau-Wong, and Wong 1976.)

TABLE 18.1. *Average clinical daily dose for neuroleptics and in vitro potency at neurotransmitter receptors*

Neuroleptic	Average clinical dose (mg/day)	INHIBITION OF ^{3}H-LIGAND BINDING K_i (nM)			
		At dopamine D2 receptors ^{3}H-spiroperidol (caudate)	At 5-HT$_2$ receptors ^{3}H-spiroperidol (cortex)	^{3}H-WB-4101 at α_1-adrenergic receptors	^{3}H-mepyramine histamine H$_1$ receptors
Phenothiazines					
Fluphenazine	15.0	3.7	25.0	13.0	58
Trifluoperazine	25.0	4.4	24.0	67.0	135
Chlorpromazine	600.0	25.0	19.0	4.3	28
Thioridazine	625.0	63.0	16.0	7.1	25
Promazine	660.0	280.0	130.0	9.4	25
Butyrophenones					
Spiroperidol	1.5	0.68	0.59	14.0	550
Benperidol	1.6	1.4	3.7	7.1	200

Clofluperol	2.4	4.2	42.0	56.0	300
Trifluoperidol	3.0	2.7	6.8	8.4	2,100
Bromperidol	4.0	3.7	26.0	100.0	700
Droperidol	8.0	3.0	4.6	1.4	2,500
Haloperidol	12.0	4.4	45.0	14.0	2,600
Moperone	22.0	9.3	52.0	22.0	22,000
Fluanisone	100.0	16.0	36.0	1.8	150
Pipamperone	450.0	360.0	6.1	100.0	450
Others					
Fluspirilene	2.0	2.6	5.9	240.0	1,700
α-Flupenthixol	4.0	3.0	13.0	8.2	39
Pimozide	4.0	3.6	25.0	20.0	1,100
(+)-Butaclamol	6.0	3.8	2.6	20.0	470
cis-Thiothixene	30.0	4.5	36.0	11.0	37
Penfluridol	30.0	7.8	150.0	280.0	3,400
Clozapine	725.0	380.0	29.0	17.0	20

Data from Peroutka and Snyder (1980).

numbers of compounds are examined. The ancillary pharmacological actions of antipsychotics may contribute importantly to their overall profiles, as discussed below, but it seems clear that dopamine receptor blockade at the D2 sites is the only action common to all effective compounds. Indeed, this conclusion about the mechanism of action of this important group of psychopharmacological agents, covering diverse chemical classes, is probably the most unambiguous demonstration of a mechanism of action for any class of centrally-acting drugs.

Other categories of dopamine receptors, apart from the D1 and D2 types may exist. A D3 type has been proposed, characterized by *in vitro* binding studies as having a high affinity for agonist ligands, but being only weakly affected by neuroleptics (Seeman 1980; Creese *et al.* 1983). Whether these represent a real pharmacological class, or merely an *in vitro* artefact, however, remains unclear, and in any case they seem of little relevance to understanding the mechanism of action of antipsychotic drugs.

PROSPECTS FOR THE FUTURE

Disadvantages of present drugs

Present-generation antipsychotic drugs are very effective in relieving many of the symptoms of schizophrenic illness, but they can certainly be improved. Major disadvantages are associated with the extrapyramidal motor dysfunction caused by dopamine receptor blockade. This includes the liability to cause Parkinsonian symptoms initially, and the more serious danger of tardive dyskinesia, the development of involuntary movements, after prolonged use. As these symptoms arise because of blockade of dopamine receptors in basal ganglia it would be desirable to develop antipsychotic drugs which worked only on forebrain limbic dopamine pathways (the probable target for antipsychotic actions) and not on basal ganglia (for review see Bannon and Roth 1983). However, despite some claims to the contrary, there is no evidence that the dopamine receptors in forebrain regions are any different from the D1 and D2 types found in basal ganglia, so there seems little prospect of achieving this objective by means of dopamine receptor blockade. Many antipsychotic drugs are heavily sedating, and while this may be a desirable feature in the initial treatment of agitated and severely ill patients, it may be highly undesirable in drugs used for long-term treatment. A possibly related feature is that current drugs appear most effective in treating the 'positive' symptoms of schizophrenic illness, and are less effective in relieving the 'negative' symptoms — withdrawal, negative effect, apathy — characteristic of the long-term patient, with the 'Type II' schizophrenia syndrome described by Crow (1980).

Prospect for dopamine blockade

While D2 dopamine receptor blockade remains the key feature for antipsychotic activity, there is still considerable scope for manipulation of the profile of individual drugs by combining other ancillary pharmacological activities with dopamine blockade in the same molecule. As outlined above, many existing antipsychotic drugs possess a variety of other potent pharmacological activities. Some possibilities which have not yet been fully explored are as follows:

Altering the ratio of D1/D2 antagonism

Most existing drugs possess some activity at both D1 and D2 sites; this may vary from somewhat higher D1 to D2 potency in some of the thioxanthes (flupenthixol, piflutixol) to butyrophenones which may be several hundred times more potent at D2 than at D1 sites. Is the combination of potent activity at both dopamine receptors a desirable feature? Might it have some relation to the well-documented antidepressant properties of flupenthixol? What would the profile of a pure D1 antagonist be? An experimental drug SCH 23390 with pure D1 antagonist properties has been described (Iorio, Barnett, Leitz, Houser, and Korduba 1983). At the other extreme are the substituted benzamides, of which sulpiride is the prototype. These are pure D2 antagonists, virtually devoid of any action at D1 sites. There are many new drugs of this class under development as antipsychotics, most of which are many times more potent than sulpiride. Sulpiride was at first thought to be devoid of antipsychotic activity, but has become widely used and appears efficacious. It is hoped that the substituted benzamides will have a lower liability to cause extrapyramidal side effects and tardive dyskinesia, but there seems little reason a priori to believe that this will prove to be the case. The relative lack of such side-effects with sulpiride may merely reflect the fact that it penetrates only poorly into the CNS and is a very weak compound — thus, in the doses used clinically, it may cause only partial blockade of basal ganglia dopaminergic mechanisms. Newer compounds in this class will be far more potent, and hence more liable to the usual spectrum of undesirable extrapyramidal side-effects.

Combining dopamine blockade with anticholinergic properties

Some antipsychotic drugs possess potent antimuscarinic activity in addition to their actions on dopamine receptors (Iversen 1975). Interestingly, the two compounds which are most potent in this respect, thioridazine and clozapine, do not exhibit the extrapyramidal effects normally associated with dopamine receptor blockade in animal tests. As dopamine and acetylcholine have long been known to exert mutually opposite effects on basal ganglia function, it is logical to suppose that combining dopamine and acetylcholine antagonism might be desirable in limiting motor side-effects. Although these compounds cause less Parkinsonian side-effects, clinically, it is not clear that this necessarily limits their liability to cause tardive dyskinesia. It has also been argued that the anticholinergic property of such compounds may actually limit their effectiveness as antipsychotics. Although clozapine was withdrawn because of other undesirable haematological side-effects, other compounds of this type are in development, and this may still represent a fruitful field for the future.

Which properties contribute to sedative actions?

Peroutka and Snyder (1980) suggested that the ability of some antipsychotic drugs to block α-adrenoceptors in brain may contribute importantly to their sedative properties. Classical α-blockers such as phenoxybenzamine are known to possess sedative actions. Many antipsychotic drugs are also potent H1 anti-histamines, and such compounds are also well known to cause sedation and drowsiness; this may be another important feature, which could be exaggerated or removed if sedating or non-sedating antipsychotics were to be designed. The importance of serotonin receptor blockade in this context remains unclear.

Calcium channel blockade in neuroleptics

The recent finding by Gould *et al.* (1983) that antipsychotic drugs of the diphenylbutylpiperidine class (e.g. pimozide, fluspirilene) possess unexpectedly high potency as calcium channel blockers is intriguing. These drugs act in a manner similar to verapamil on calcium channels in brain. Although the functional significance of these channels in CNS is not known, Gould, Murphy, Reynolds, and Snyder (1983) argue that this property might help to explain the unusual efficacy of this group of drugs in treating 'negative' symptoms in long-term schizophrenic patients. If this is correct, this could prove a very important finding.

In summary, dopamine blockade remains the only mechanism currently known which can be used reliably to predict new antipsychotic drugs. By combining this with other pharmacological features, however, a wide range of possibilities may exist for improving present-day antipsychotics.

Other possible routes to novel antipsychotic drugs

Autoreceptor agonists

It is known that dopamine neurones possess on their surface 'autoreceptors' at which dopamine can act both to inhibit cell firing and to inhibit dopamine release. Thus, when given in very low doses dopamine agonists, such as apomorphine, can paradoxically *inhibit* dopaminergic function by suppressing dopamine release in brain — leading to behavioural sedation rather than the usual signs of excitation seen at higher doses (Carlsson 1975). If it were possible to develop dopamine agonist drugs which acted specifically at such auto-receptors, this might offer a novel means of developing antipsychotic drugs which suppressed central dopaminergic function without blocking dopamine postsynaptic receptors. The compound (+)(3-(3-hydroxyphenyl)-*N-n*-propyl-piperidine, (3-PPP) at first appeared to represent such a drug (Clark, Carlsson, Hjorth, Svensson, Engel, and Sanchez 1982). It blocked amphetamine-induced hyperactivity in rats, but did not disrupt conditioned avoidance behaviour; it suppressed dopamine turnover in rat brain and exerted sedative actions on behaviour. However, subsequent studies using the resolved isomers of the racemic compound used initially have failed to support the simple hypothesis that 3-PPP is an autoreceptor agonist. Its effects appear to be due to a complex mixture of receptor antagonist and agonist actions combined with an amphetamine-like dopamine releasing property (Hjorth, Carlsson, Clark, Svensson, Wikstrom, Sanchez, Lindberg, Hacksell, Arvidsson, Johansson, and Nilsson 1983). It remains unclear whether autoreceptors represent a separate pharmacological class, or whether they are simply D2 receptors in an unusual location. If this were correct, then the prospect for developing selective autoreceptor agonists would not seem encouraging.

Neuropeptide agonists/antagonists

The possibility of manipulating dopaminergic function in particular regions of brain by means of dopamine receptor agonists or antagonists may not be good, but this objective might still be achieved by indirect approaches. The most promising line of research here lies with the neuropeptides. There is good evidence that several different neuropeptide systems impinge upon central dopaminergic pathways (see Iversen 1983). Neurotensin and neurotensin receptors, for example, are highly concentrated in dopamine-rich areas, including substantia nigra and limbic forebrain areas such as nucleus accumbens. Neurotensin when administered intracerebrally can exert actions resembling those of neuroleptics — inhibiting arousal caused by amphetamine, and inhibiting dopaminergic activity (Nemeroff, Luttinger, and Prange 1983). The development of neurotensin agonists might lead to novel antipsychotic agents.

Similarly, cholecystokinin octapeptide (CCK-8) is present with dopamine in some but not all dopamine neurones in brain. It is restricted to some of the dopaminergic neurones of the limbic forebrain projection (for review see Emson and Marley 1983). Its functions in these neurones is not known, but drugs based on CCK might represent a novel means of manipulating central dopaminergic mechanisms. CCK-8 and related peptides have some neuroleptic-like properties in animal tests (Van Ree, Gaffori, and de Wied 1983; Zetler 1983).

Substance P is also known to be present in relative abundance in regions of brain which contain dopaminergic neurones. Substance P when microinjected near the ventral tegmentum A10 dopamine cell group causes a behavioural arousal response which appears to be due to excitation of the dopamine neurones (Iversen 1982). A monoclonal antibody to substance P when infused into this brain area can prevent the normal excitation of dopamine cell firing in the A10 group in response to mild footshock stress in the rat (Bannon, Elliott, Alpert, Godert, S. D. Iversen, and L. L. Iversen 1983). It is possible that substance P antagonists might provide a novel means of suppressing dopaminergic activity, and could thus potentially exert antipsychotic actions.

In all of these instances, however, the hypothesis cannot adequately be tested until suitable agonists/antagonists acting at peptide receptors become available. Ideally, these should be non-peptide structures which are well-absorbed and penetrate readily into CNS. It may take some time before such agents are discovered and developed.

HAVE ANTIPSYCHOTIC DRUGS TOLD US ANYTHING ABOUT SCHIZOPHRENIA?

Although understanding the mechanism of action of psychotic drugs represents a great advance, it has perhaps been disappointing in these terms. Although post-mortem human brain studies (see chapter by T. Crow in this volume) have revealed increases in the densities of D2 dopamine receptors in the brains of patients dying with schizophrenic illness, it is not clear whether these are intrinsic to the illness or merely due to drug treatment. The primary chemical abnormality in schizophrenia remains elusive, although it may well lie in some neurochemical system which is normally in functional balance with dopaminergic mechanisms in brain.

REFERENCES

Angrist, B., Sathananthan, G., Wilk, S., and Gershon, S. (1974). Amphetamine psychosis; behavioural and biochemical aspects. *J. Psychiat. Res.* **11**, 13–23.

Bannon, M. J. and Roth, R. H. (1983). Pharmacology of mesocortical dopamine neurons. *Pharm. Rev.* **35**, 53–68.

—, Elliott, P. J., Alpert, J. E., Goedert, M., Iversen, S. D., and Iversen, L. L. (1983). Role of endogenous substance P in stress-induced activation of mesocortical dopamine neurones. *Nature, Lond.* **306**, 791–2.

Bunney, B. S., Walters, J. R., Roth, R. H., and Aghanjanian, G. K. (1973). Effects of antipsychotic drugs and amphetamine on single cell activity. *J. Pharmac. exp. Ther.* **185**, 560–71.

Carlsson, A. (1975). Dopaminergic autoreceptors. In *Chemical tools in catecholamine research* (ed. O. Almgren, A. Carlsson, and J. Engel), Vol. II, pp. 219–25. North-Holland, Amsterdam.

— and Lindqvist, J. (1963). Effect of chlorpromazine and haloperidol on formation of 3-methoxytryamine and normetanephrine in mouse brain. *Acta pharmac. & tox.* **20**, 140–4.

Clark, D., Carlsson, A., Hjorth, S., Svensson, K., Engel, J., and Sanchez, D. (1982). Is 3-PPP a potential antipsychotic agent? Evidence from animal behavioural studies. *Eur. J. Pharmac.* **83**, 131–4.

Clement-Cormier, Y. C., Kebabian, J. W., Petzold, G. L., and Greengard P. (1974). Dopamine-sensitive adenylate cyclase in mammalian brain: a possible site of action of antipsychotic drugs. *Proc. natn Acad. Sci. U.S.A.* **71**, 1113–17.

Creese, I., Burt, D. R., and Snyder, S. H. (1978). Biochemical actions of neuroleptic drugs: focus on the dopamine receptor. In *Handbook of psychopharmacology* (ed. L. L. Iversen, S. D. Iversen, and S. H. Synder), Vol. 10, pp. 37–89. Plenum Press, New York.

—, Hamblin, M. W., Leff, S. E., and Sibley, D. R. (1983). CNS dopamine receptors. ibid., Vol. 17, pp. 81–138.

Crow, T. J. (1980). Two syndromes in schizophrenia. *Br. med. J.* **280**, 66–8.

Deniker, P. (1970). Introduction of neuroleptic chemotherapy into psychiatry. In *Discoveries in biological psychiatry* (ed. F. J. Ayd and B. Blackwell), pp. 155–64. Lippincott, Philadelphia.

Emson, P. C. and Marley, P. D. (1983). Cholecystokinin and vasoactive intestinal polypeptide. In *Handbook of psychopharmacology* (ed. L. L. Iversen, S. D. Iversen, and S. H. Snyder), Vol. 16, pp. 255–306. Plenum Press, New York.

Gould, R. J., Murphy, K. M. M., Reynolds, I. J., and Snyder, S. H. (1983). Antischizophrenic drugs of the diphenylbutypiperidine type act as calcium channel antagonists. *Proc. natn Acad. Sci. U.S.A.* **80**, 5122–5.

Hjorth, S., Carlsson, A., Clark, D., Svensson, K., Wikstrom, H., Sanchez, D., Lindberg, P., Hacksell, U., Arvidsson, L. E., Johansson, A., and Nilsson, L. G. (1983). Central dopamine receptor agonist and antagonist actions of the enantiomers of 3-PPP. *Psychopharmacology* **81**, 89–99.

Hyttel, J. (1981). Similarities between the binding of [^{3}H]-piflutixol and [^{3}H]-flupenthixol to rat striatal dopamine receptors *in vitro*. *Life Sci.* **28**, 563–9.

Iorio, L. C., Barnett, A., Leitz, H., Houser, V. P., and Korduba, C. A. (1983). SCH 23390, a potential benzodiazepine antipsychotic with unique interactions on dopaminergic systems. *J. Pharmac. exp. Ther.* **226**, 462–8.

Iversen, L. L. (1975). Dopamine receptors in the brain. *Science* **188**, 1084–9.

— (1983). Non-opioid neuropeptides. *A. Rev. Pharmac.* **23**, 1–27.

Iversen, S. D. (1982). Behavioural effects of substance P through dopaminergic pathways in the brain. In *Substance P in the nervous system*, CIBA Foundation Symposium No. 91, pp. 307–19. Pitman, London.

Janssen, P. A. J. and Van Bever, W. F. M. (1978). Structure-activity relationships of the butyrophenones and diphenylbutylpiperidines. In *Handbook of psychopharmacology* (ed. L. L. Iversen, S. D. Iversen, and S. H. Snyder), Vol. 10, pp. 1–35. Plenum Press, New York.

Kebabian, J. W., Petzgold, G. L., and Greengard, P. (1972). Dopamine-sensitive adenylate cyclase in caudate nucleus and its similarity to the 'dopamine receptor'. *Proc. natn Acad. Sci. U.S.A.* **79**, 2145–9.

Klein, D. F. and Davis, J. M. (1969). *Diagnosis and drug treatment of psychiatric disorders*. Williams & Wilkins, Baltimore.

Miller, R. J., Horn, A. S., and Iversen, L. L. (1974). The action of neuroleptic drugs on dopamine stimulated adenosine cyclic 3''5''-monophosphate production in rat neostriatum and limbic forebrain. *Mol. Pharmac.* **10**, 759–66.

Nemeroff, C. B., Luttinger, D., and Prange, A. J. (1983). Neurotensin and bombesin. In *Handbook of psychopharmacology* (ed. L. L. Iversen, S. D. Iversen, and S. H. Snyder), Vol. 16, pp. 363–466. Plenum Press, New York.

Peroutka, S. J. and Snyder, S. H. (1980). Relationship of neuroleptic drug effects at brain dopamine, serotonin, α-adrenergic, and histamine receptors to clinical potency. *Am. J. Psychiat.* **137**, 1518–22.

Sedvall, G. (1975). Receptor feedback and dopamine turnover in CNS. In *Handbook of psychopharmacology* (ed. L. L. Iversen, S. D. Iversen, and S. H. Snyder), Vol. 6, pp. 127–77. Plenum Press, New York.

Seeman, P. (1980). Brain dopamine receptors. *Pharmac. Rev.* **32**, 229–313.

—, Lee, T., Chau-Wong, M., and Wong, K. (1976). Antipsychotic drug doses and neuroleptic/dopamine receptors. *Nature, Lond.* **261**, 717–19.

Van Ree, J. M., Gaffori, O., and de Wied, D. (1983). In rats, the behavioural profile of CCK-8 related peptides resembles that of antipsychotic agents. *Eur. J. Pharmac.* **93**, 63–78.

Zetler, G. (1983). Neuroleptic-like effects of ceruletide and cholecystokinin octapeptide: interactions with apomorphine, methylphenidate and picrotoxin. *Eur. J. Pharmac.* **94**, 261–70.

19

Dopamine D_2 receptors and schizophrenia

F. OWEN, J. CRAWLEY, A. J. CROSS, T. J. CROW, S. R. OLDLAND, M. POULTER, N. VEALL, AND G. D. ZANELLI

The dopamine hypothesis of schizophrenia, i.e. that schizophrenia is associated with excessive dopaminergic function in the central nervous system, arose from two major lines of evidence. Firstly, it became clear that amphetamine and other dopamine-releasing drugs used by non-psychotic individuals could induce a schizophrenia-like paranoid state (Connell 1958; Griffiths, Cavanaugh, Held, and Oates 1972; Angrist, Sathanathan, Wilk, and Gershon 1974). The second line of evidence emerged from studies on the mode of action of neuroleptic drugs that are effective in the treatment of schizophrenia. Although these drugs belong to several different chemical classes, they have in common the ability to block the dopamine receptor either on the basis of inhibiting dopamine stimulated adenylate cyclase activity (Miller, Horn, and Iversen 1974; Clement-Cormier, Kebabian, Petzgold, and Greengard 1974) or in displacing the high affinity binding of ligands to the dopamine receptor (Seeman, Chau-Wong, Tedesco, and Wong 1975).

However, studies of the concentration of homovanillic acid (HVA), the major end-product of dopamine metabolism in the brain, yielded no evidence of increased dopamine turnover in schizophrenics (Bowers 1974; Post, Fink, Carpenter, and Goodwin 1975). Direct measurement of dopaminergic mechanisms have also been made in post-mortem brains of schizophrenics. Reports of the concentration of dopamine in the brains of schizophrenics have been equivocal. Bird, Spokes, Barnes, Mackay, Iversen, and Shepherd (1977) reported significantly increased dopamine levels in nucleus accumbens but not in putamen of schizophrenics, whereas Owen, Cross, Crow, Longden, Poulter, and Riley (1978) reported a moderate increase in caudate but no difference between controls and schizophrenics in either the putamen or the nucleus accumbens. However, measurements of homovanillic acid concentrations in schizophrenic brains have produced no evidence of increased dopamine turnover (Owen *et al.* 1978; Bird, Crow, Iversen, Longden, Mackay, Riley, and Spokes 1979). In addition, the activity of tyrosine hydroxylase, the rate-limiting enzyme in catecholamine synthesis, has been shown to be similar in controls and schizophrenics (Crow, Baker, Cross, Joseph, Lofthouse, Longden, Owen, Riley, Glover, and Killpack 1979).

Apart from dopaminergic mechanisms, GABA and acetyl choline systems have also been assessed, in order to evaluate suggestions that changes in these systems could result in excessive dopaminergic functions (Roberts 1972; McGeer and McGeer 1977). Glutamate decarboxylase (GAD) catalyses the decarboxylation of glutamate to form GABA and is a marker for GABAergic neurones. An initial promising report by Bird *et al.* (1977) of reduced GAD activity in schizophrenic brains was not confirmed by Cross and Owen (1979), and it became clear, subsequently, that the reduction in enzyme activity reported by Bird *et al.* was the result of a bias of patients dying with bronchopneumonia, which has an adverse effect on GAD activity, in the schizophrenic group (Bird, Spokes, Barnes, Mackay, and Iversen 1978). Choline acetyltransferase (CAT) catalyses the synthesis of acetylcholine from choline and acetyl CoA and is a marker for acetylcholine containing neurones. Bird *et al.* (1977) reported significant decreases in CAT activity in schizophrenic brains. This finding could not be replicated by Cross and Owen (1979). CAT activity has also been reported to be increased (McGeer and McGeer 1977) and normal (Domino, Krause, and Bowers 1973) in schizophrenic brains.

Overall, the studies in cerebrospinal fluid and brains of metabolites and the activities of enzymes involved in the synthesis and inactivation of dopamine, or activities of marker enzymes for neuronal systems indirectly affecting dopaminergic function, did not support the dopamine hypothesis of schizophrenia. However, it had been suggested earlier (Bowers 1974) that the postulated disturbance in dopamine systems in schizophrenic brain might not be in the presynaptic dopamine neurone but at the level of the postsynaptic receptor. The development of high-affinity binding techniques to assess dopamine receptors (Seeman *et al.* 1975) enabled this possibility to be investigated.

DOPAMINE RECEPTORS IN SCHIZOPHRENIA

Kababian and Calne (1979) have categorized dopamine receptors into D1 and D2. Dopamine D1 receptors are linked to adenylate cyclase and do not bind butyrophenones such as spiroperidol (spiperone) or haloperiodol with high affinity. Dopamine D2 receptors are not linked to adenylate cyclase and do bind butyrophenones with high affinity. The majority of studies of dopamine receptors in brains of schizophrenics have been on the dopamine D2 receptor. Owen *et al.* (1978) reported a significant increase in ^{3}H-spiperone binding to D2 receptors in caudate nucleus, putamen, and nucleus accumbens of schizophrenics. A Scatchard analysis (Scatchard 1949) of saturation data in samples of caudate nucleus revealed that the increased binding of ^{3}H-spiperone in schizophrenic brains was due to a greater than 100 per cent increase in maximum binding (B_{max}) or the number of D2 receptors (Fig. 19.1). Similar findings were reported by Lee, Seeman, Tourtellotte, Farley, and Hornykiewicz (1978), and by Lee and Seeman (1980).

Dopamine receptors have also been assessed in schizophrenic brains, using the thioxanthene flupenthixol as ligand (Cross, Crow, and Owen 1981). Tritiated

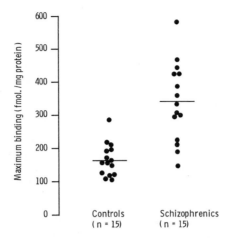

Fig. 19.1. Maximum specific ^{3}H-spiperone binding in caudate nucleus of controls and schizophrenics.

flupenthixol binds with high affinity to both D1 and D2 dopamine receptors. However, by including in the assay procedure the highly-selective D2 antagonist, domperidone, at the appropriate concentration, the binding of ^{3}H-flupenthixol can be resolved into its D1 and D2 components (Cross and Owen 1980). When this technique was applied to brain samples from schizophrenics who had been drug-free for at least one year prior to death only the D2 component of ^{3}H-flupenthixol binding was significantly increased compared with controls (Table 19.1).

Dopamine agonists have also been used to assess dopamine receptors in schizophrenic brains. Owen, Cross, Crow, Lofthouse, and Poulter (1981) used ^{3}H–ADTN (2-amino-6,7-dihydroxy 1,2,3,4-tetrahydronapthalene) as ligand whereas Lee *et al.* (1978) used ^{3}H-apomorphine and both groups observed no differences in agonist binding between controls and schizophrenics.

TABLE 19.1. *D1 and D2 components of ^{3}H-flupenthixol binding in control and schizophrenic caudate samples*

	D1	D2
Controls (*n* = 9)	104 ± 16	57 ± 9
Schizophrenics (*n* = 6) (drug-free)	103 ± 11	109 ± 16*

*$*p < 0.02$ vs. controls. Student's *t*-test (2-tailed) (Results as mean ± SEM; fmol/mg protein).

BINDING OF LIGANDS TO RECEPTORS OTHER THAN DOPAMINE

Several neurotransmitter receptors other than dopamine have now been assessed in schizophrenic brains by high-affinity ligand binding techniques. Owen, Cross, and Crow (1983) found no significant differences between controls and schizophrenics in the binding of ligands to a number of neurotransmitter receptors as outlined in Table 19.2.

There have been two previous reports of receptor changes other than those for dopamine. Bennett, Enna, Bylund, Gillin, Wyatt, and Snyder (1979) reported decreased ^{3}H–LSD binding in frontal cortex of schizophrenics. However, Whitaker, Crow, and Ferrier (1981) were unable to replicate this finding. Likewise, the decrease in opiate receptors in caudate nucleus of schizophrenics reported by Reisine, Rossor, Spokes, Iversen, and Yamamura (1980) could not be replicated by Owen *et al.* (1983*a*). Therefore, of the brain receptors so far studied in schizophrenia, it seems that only the D2 receptor is changed. The outstanding question is whether or not this change is due to the effect of neuroleptic medication.

NEUROLEPTIC MEDICATION AND DOPAMINE RECEPTORS IN SCHIZOPHRENIA

It has been well established in rats that prolonged neuroleptic administration results in an increase (about 30–40 per cent) in striatal D2 receptors. The topic has been thoroughly discussed in a review of brain dopamine receptors by Seeman (1980).

Owen *et al.* (1978) analysed the number of D2 receptors against neuroleptic medication in schizophrenic brains. Schizophrenics who had been neuroleptic-

TABLE 19.2. *Receptors studied in post-mortem brains of schizophrenics*

Receptor	Ligands used
Serotonin	^{3}H-5HT, ^{3}H-LSD
Muscarinic acetylcholine	^{3}H-QNB
β-Noradrenaline	^{3}H-dihydroalprenolol
α-Noradrenaline	^{3}H-clonidine, ^{3}H-WB4101
GABA	^{3}H-GABA
Benzodiazepine	^{3}H-diazepam
Opiate	^{3}H-etorphine

Abbreviations
5-HT = 5-hydroxytryptamine, serotonin; LSD = lysergic acid diethylamide; QNB = quinuclidinyl benzilate; WB4101 = (2,6-dimethyoxyphenoxyethly)aminomethyl-1,4-benzodioxane.

free for at least one year before death had significantly elevated D2 receptors. This was confirmed by Lee and Seeman (1980). However, Mackay, Bird, Spokes, Rosser, and Iversen (1980) reported that the increase in D2 receptors they observed in schizophrenic brains was only present in neuroleptic-treated patients, and that D2 receptor numbers were not significantly different from controls in brains from patients who had not received neuroleptics for at least one month prior to death. It is noteworthy that D2 receptors have been assessed only in small numbers of brain samples from drug-free schizophrenics.

Since the initial report by Owen *et al.* (1978) of increased D2 receptors in schizophrenic brains, a number of other studies of D2 receptors have been carried out in the Division of Psychiatry, at the Clinical Research Centre, Harrow. These are summarized in Fig. 19.2. In the various studies a total of 10 brains from schizophrenics who had been neuroleptic-free for at least one year before death were studied and these are indicated in Fig. 19.2. In each study ^{3}H-spiperone binding (either as a B_{max} value or with ^{3}H-spiperone at 1.2 nM in the assay procedure) was significantly elevated in the schizophrenic group. In addition, in each case, ^{3}H-spiperone binding was significantly elevated in the drug-free schizophrenics compared with controls. Moreover, there was no evidence that the distribution of the ^{3}H-spiperone values in the drug-free groups differed from the values in the respective schizophrenic groups as a whole.

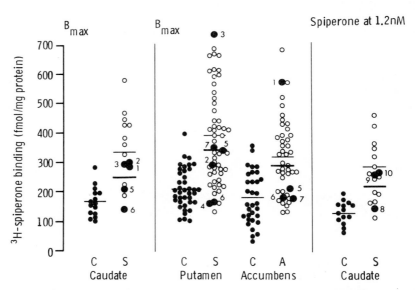

Fig. 19.2. ^{3}H-Spiperone binding in controls, drug-treated, and drug-free schizophrenics.

Drug-free schizophrenics are numbered. The thinner horizontal lines on the scattergrams represent the mean for the individual groups as a whole. The thicker horizontal lines represent the mean of the drug-free schizophrenics in each group.

Apart from analyses of D2 receptors against neuroleptic medication there is other evidence to suggest that the increase in D2 receptors in schizophrenic brains may not be solely due to neuroleptic medication. First, after chronic neuroleptic treatment to rats, ^{3}H–ADTN binding is significantly elevated compared with controls, but ^{3}H–ADTN binding is not increased in schizophrenic brains. Secondly, ^{3}H-spiperone binding is not significantly elevated in brains from patients dying with Huntington's Chorea or Alzheimer's disease who received neuroleptics prior to death (Owen *et al.* 1983*a*), suggesting that the increase in D2 receptors in man, in response to neuroleptic medication, may be small.

RELATIONSHIP BETWEEN D2 RECEPTORS AND SYMPTOMATOLOGY

There is rarely sufficient information in deceased patients' case-notes to assess retrospectively the severity of their schizophrenic symptoms. In order to make a realistic attempt at correlating biochemical changes in post-mortem brains with clinical features it was necessary to collect brains from schizophrenics whose psychoses had been carefully assessed in life. Owen *et al.* (1983*a*) measured D2 receptors in brains from 14 schizophrenics whose symptoms had been rated in life using the rating scale devised by Krawiecka, Goldberg, and Vaughan (1977). Global scores for positive symptoms (defined as hallucinations, delusions, and thought disorder) and negative symptoms (defined as flattening of affect and poverty of speech) were correlated with the number of D2 receptors in caudate nucleus. The result is shown in Table 19.3. There was a significant, positive correlation between positive symptoms and the number of D2 receptors but no significant relationship between D2 receptors and negative symptoms.

TABLE 19.3. *Relationship between D2 receptors and symptomatology in schizophrenics assessed before death*

	'r'	'p'
^{3}H-spiperone binding (B_{max}) vs. positive symptoms	0.698	<0.01
^{3}H-spiperone binding (B_{max}) vs. negative symptoms	−0.369	N.S.
(n= 14)		

DEVELOPMENT OF *IN VIVO* TECHNIQUES FOR ASSESSING D2 RECEPTORS

Recently, considerable energy has been expended in developing *in vivo* techniques for assessing dopamine receptors. Spiperone can be brominated in the para-position on the benzene ring to yield *para*-bromospiperone (BrSp). BrSp has been shown to be a potent displacer of ^{3}H-spiperone binding *in vitro* and to increase plasma prolactin levels in the rat (Huang, Friedman, So, Simonovic, and Meltzer 1980). When [77]bromine is used as the bromine source [77]Br-BrSp is produced (Fig. 19.3) which has a half-life of 56 h. Following tail-vein injection of the radioactive compound into the rat the distribution of radioactivity in the brain is consistent with the known distribution of dopamine receptors, i.e. high in the striatum which is rich in dopamine receptors and low in the cerebellum which is devoid of dopamine receptors (Friedman, Huang, ·Kulmala, Dinerstein, Navone, Brunsden, Gawlas, and Cooper 1982). It has also been reported that after tail-vein injection of [77]Br-BrSp in the rat, striatal [77]Br-BrSp can be stereospecifically displaced by the isomers of α- and β-fluppenthixol consistent with their widely differing potencies *in vitro*. In addition, the increase in striatal D2 receptors induced in the rat by chronic neuroleptic administration can be demonstrated either by ^{3}H-spiperone binding or by specific striatal content of [77]Br-BrSp as illustrated in Fig. 19.4 (Owen, Poulter, Mashal, Crow,

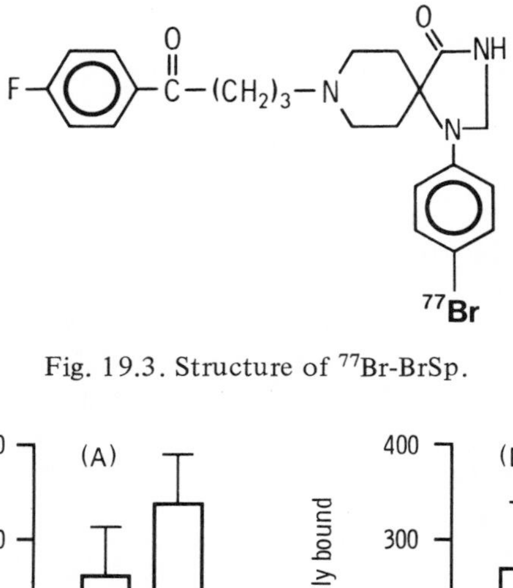

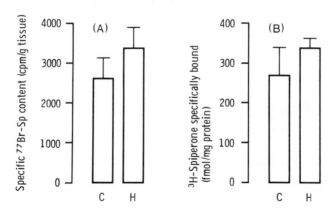

Fig. 19.3. Structure of [77]Br-BrSp.

Fig. 19.4. Rat striatal D2 receptor supersensitivity demonstrated by ^{3}H-spiperone binding (B) and by specific [77]-BrSp content (A).

Specific [77]Br-BrSp content was determined by subtracting the cpm/g tissue of [77]Br-BrSp in the cerebellum from the corresponding cpm/g tissue of [77]Br-BrSp in the striatum.

Veall, and Zanelli 1983*b*). A similar result could be obtained by considering striatum:cerebellum ratios. Although [77]Br-BrSp is not a useful ligand, for *in vitro* characterization of dopamine receptors, due to its high non-specific binding to membranes, there can be little doubt that [77]Br-BrSp is a ligand for D2 receptors *in vivo*. The ratio of striatum:cerebellum content of [77]Br-BrSp after tail-vein injection of the drug in the rat may be as high as 10:1.

After intravenous injection of 6.5 mCi of [77]Br-BrSp into human volunteers, good reconstructed images have been obtained after a one-hour data-acquisition period with single photon-emission computed-tomography using the IGE 400T gamma camera with a Star computer system (Crawley, Smith, Veall, Zanelli, Crow, and Owen 1984). This system allows the radioactivity in coronal, axial, or sagital brain sections to be visualized. An axial section, with the striata clearly visible either side of the mid-line is shown in Fig. 19.5. The striatum: cerebellum ratio of radioactivity in this section was about 7:1.

Quantification of D2 receptors *in vivo*

In order to investigate whether or not a range of striatum:cerebellum ratios in [77]Br-BrSp content could be accurately determined in living subjects experiments were carried out using a 'phantom head' (Fig. 19.6). The phantom head was made of Perspex inside which was an authentic human skull. The whole of

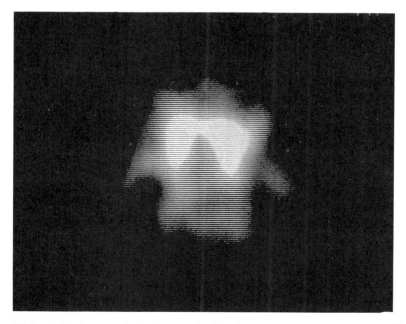

Fig. 19.5. Axial image of the human brain after intravenous injection of [77]Br-BrSp.

the Perspex head was filled with water containing a small quantity of ^{77}Br to simulate background or non-specific ^{77}Br. The amount of ^{77}Br in the inner cylinder was varied by adding ^{77}Br to the reservoir and operating the pump. The known ratio of ^{77}Br in the inner cylinder to that in the Perspex head was then compared with the ratio obtained by tomography of the phantom head. The result is shown in Fig. 19.7. There was a linear relationship between the known ratio and that estimated by tomography. It appears, therefore, that striatum:cerebellum ratios of ^{77}Br-BrSp, an index of the number of D2 receptors, can be accurately determined *in vivo*.

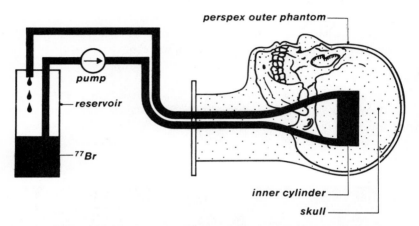

Fig. 19.6. Diagram of phantom head for quantification studies with ^{77}Br.

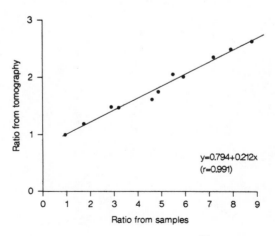

Fig. 19.7. Relationship between known ratio of ^{77}Br and that obtained by tomography.

CONCLUSIONS

(a) There is no evidence of increased dopamine turnover in brains of schizophrenics.

(b) The dopamine hypothesis of schizophrenia can be sustained by postulating increased central dopaminergic function brought about by an increase in dopamine D2 receptors.

(c) The increase in receptors may be specific to dopamine receptors since the binding of ligands to several other neurotransmitter receptors is unchanged in schizophrenic brains.

(d) Neuroleptic induced dopamine receptor supersensitivity, in man, may be small and insufficient to account for the large increases in D2 receptors observed in schizophrenic brains.

(e) There appears to be a relationship between the number of striatal D2 receptors and the positive symptoms of schizophrenia.

(f) The development of techniques using ligands such as [77]Br-BrSp for assessing D2 receptors in living human subjects should lead to a clear demonstration of any relationship between the receptor and schizophrenia.

REFERENCES

Angrist, B., Sathanathan, G., Wilk, S., and Gershon, S. (1974). Amphetamine psychosis: behavioural and biochemical aspects. *J. Psychiat. Res.* **11**, 13–23.

Bennett, J. P., Enna, S. J., Bylund, D. B., Gillin, J. C., Wyatt, R. J., and Snyder, S. H. (1979). Neurotransmitter receptors in frontal cortex of schizophrenics. *Arch. gen. Psychiat.* **36**, 927–34.

Bird, E. D., Spokes, E. G., Barnes, J., Mackay, A. V. P., and Iversen, L. L. (1978). Glutamic-acid decarboxylase in schizophrenia. *Lancet* i, 156.

—, —, —, —, —, and Shepherd, M. (1977). Increased brain dopamine and reduced glutamic acid decarboxylase and choline acetyl transferase in schizophrenia and related psychoses. *Lancet* ii, 1157–9.

—, Crow, T. J., Iversen, L. L., Longden, A., Mackay, A. V. P., Riley, G. J., and Spokes, E. G. (1979). Dopamine and homovanillic acid concentrations in the post-mortem brain in schizophrenia. *J. Physiol.* **293**, 36–37P.

Bowers, M. B. (1974). Central dopamine turnover in schizophrenic syndromes. *Arch. gen. Psychiat.* **31**, 50–4.

Clement-Cormier, Y. C., Kebabian, J. W., Petzgold, G. L., and Greengard, P. (1974). Dopamine-sensitive adenylate cyclase in mammalian brain: a possible site of action of antipsychotic drugs. *Proc. natn Acad. Sci. U.S.A.* **71**, 1113–17.

Connell, P. H. (1958). *Amphetamine psychoses*, Maudsley Monograph No. 5. Chapman & Hall, London.

Crawley, J. C. W., Smith, T., Veall, N., Zanelli, G. D., Crow, T. J., and Owen, F. (1984). Dopamine receptors displayed in living human brain with [77]Br-p.-bromospiperone. *Lancet* ii, 975.

Cross, A. J. and Owen, F. (1979). The activities of glutamic acid decarboxylase and choline acteyltransferase in post-mortem brains of schizophrenics and controls. *Biochem. Soc. Trans.* 145–6.

— and — (1980). Characteristics of ³H-cis-flupenthixol binding to calf brain membranes. *Eur. J. Pharmac.* **65**, 341-7.

—, Crow, T. J., and Owen, F. (1981). ³H-Flupenthixol binding in post-mortem brains of schizophrenics: evidence for a selective increase in dopamine D2 receptors. *Psychopharmacology* **74**, 122-4.

Crow, T. J., Baker, H. F., Cross, A. J., Joseph, M. H., Lofthouse, R., Longden, A., Owen, F., Riley, G. J., Glover, V., and Killpack, W. S. (1979). Monoamine mechanisms in chronic schizophrenia: post-mortem neurochemical findings. *Br. J. Psychiat.* **134**, 249-56.

Domino, E. F. Krause, R. R., and Bowers, J. (1973). Various enzymes involved with putative neurotransmitters. *Arch. gen. Psychiat.* **29**, 195-201.

Friedman, A. M., Huang, C. C., Kulmala, H. A., Dinerstein, R. J., Navone, J., Brunsden, B., Gawlas, D., and Cooper, M. (1982). The use of radiobrominated p-bromospiroperidol for γ-ray imaging of dopamine receptors. *Int. J. nucl. med. Biol.* **9**, 57-61.

Griffiths, J. D., Cavanaugh, J., Held, J., and Oates, J. A. (1972). Dextramphetamine: evaluation of psychomimetic properties in man. *Arch. gen. Psychiat.* **26**, 97-100.

Huang, C. C., Friedman, A. M., So, R., Simonovic, M., and Meltzer, H. Y. (1980). Synthesis and biological evaluation of p-bromospiperone as potential neuroleptic drug. *J. Pharmac. Sci.* **69**, 984-6.

Kebabian, J. W. and Calne, D. B. (1979). Multiple receptors for dopamine. *Nature, Lond.* **277**, 93-6.

Krawiecka, M., Goldberg, D., and Vaughan, M. (1977). A standardised psychiatric assessment for rating chronic psychotic patients. *Acta psychiat. scand.* **55**, 299-308.

Lee, T. and Seeman, P. (1980). Elevation of brain neuroleptic/dopamine receptors in schizophrenia. *Am. J. Psychiat.* **137**, 191-7.

—, Seeman, P., Tourtellotte, W. W., Farley, I. J., and Hornykiewicz, O. (1978). Binding of ³H-neuroleptics and ³H-apomorphine in schizophrenic brains. *Nature, Lond.* **274**, 897-900.

Mackay, A. V. P., Bird, E. D., Spokes, E. G., Rossor, M., and Iversen, L. L. (1980). Dopamine receptors and schizophrenia: drug effect or illness. *Lancet* **ii**, 915-16.

McGeer, P. L. and McGeer, E. G. (1977). Possible changes in striatal and limbic cholinergic systems in schizophrenia. *Arch. gen. Psychiat.* **34**, 1319-23.

Miller, R. J., Horn, A. S., and Iversen, L. L. (1974). The action of neuroleptic drugs on dopamine-stimulated adenosine 3′,5′-monophosphosphate production in neostriatum and limbic forebrain. *Mol. Pharmac.* **10**, 759-66.

Owen, F., Cross, A. J., and Crow, T. J. (1983*a*). Ligand-binding studies in brains of schizophrenics. In *Cell surface receptors* (ed. P. G. Strange), pp. 163-83. Ellis Horwood, Chichester, England.

—, —, —, Lofthouse, R., and Poulter, M. (1981). Neurotransmitter receptors in brain in schizophrenia. *Acta psychiat. scand.* suppl. **62**, 20-6.

—, —, —, Longden, A., Poulter, M., and Riley, G. J. (1978). Increased dopamine-receptor sensitivity in schizophrenia. *Lancet* **ii**, 223-6.

—, Poulter, M., Mashal, R. D., Crow, T. J., Veall, N., and Zanelli, G. D. (1983*b*). ⁷⁷Br-p-Bromospiperone: a ligand for in vivo labelling of dopamine receptors. *Life Sci.* **33**, 765-8.

Post, R. M., Fink, E., Carpenter, W. T., and Goodwin, F. K. (1975). Cerebrospinal fluid amine metabolites in acute schizophrenia. *Arch. gen. Psychiat.* **32**, 1013-69.

Reisine, T. D., Rossor, M., Spokes, E., Iversen, L. L., and Yamamura, H. I. (1980). Opiate and neuroleptic receptor alterations in human schizophrenic brain tissue. *Adv. Biochem. Psychopharmac.* 21, 443–50.

Roberts, E. (1972). An hypothesis suggesting that there is a defect in the GABA system in schizophrenia. *Neurosci. Res. Program Bull.* 10, 468–82.

Scatchard, G. (1949). The attraction of proteins for small molecules and ions. *Ann. N. Y. Acad. Sci.* 51, 660–72.

Seeman, P. (1980). Brain dopamine receptors. *Pharmac. Rev.* 32, 230–87.

—, Chau-Wong, M., Tedesco, J., and Wong, K. (1975). Brain receptors for antipsychotic drugs and dopamine: direct binding assays. *Proc. natn Acad. Sci.* 72, 4376–80.

Whitaker, P. M., Crow, T. J., and Ferrier, I. N. (1981). Tritiated LSD binding in frontal cortex in schizophrenia. *Arch. gen. Psychiat.* 38, 278–80.

20

Integrated viral genes as the cause of schizophrenia: a hypothesis

T. J. CROW

The aetiology of schizophrenia remains obscure. With onset in adult life, and a persistent and fluctuating course the disease resembles such other conditions of unknown aetiology as rheumatoid arthritis and diabetes mellitus. A genetic component is undoubted, but it remains ill-defined and appears insufficient as a cause. Of the other classes of causation, some, such as dietary deficiencies and toxins, appear unlikely on the basis of the epidemiology of the disease; for others, such as neoplasia or trauma, there is little evidence in affected individuals. Psychogenic trauma much favoured by dynamic theorists is not supported by reliable evidence of its presence and nature. Although 'expressed emotion' in relatives has been viewed as a predictor of relapse it has not been seriously advanced as an initiator. In a recent study (CRC Division of Psychiatry) of first episodes of illness, expressed emotion in relatives was a less accurate predictor of relapse than the duration of disturbance of the patient's behaviour before admission. Both may be indices of illness severity rather than its causes. Aside from the genetic component the list of classes of possible causal agent is surprisingly short: it appears restricted to infection and immunity, and autoimmune pathologies are often initiated by infections.

For these reasons genetic and infective factors in schizophrenia have received particular attention. It seems that it is amongst genes and viruses, or an interaction between them, that the aetiology of schizophrenia will be found.

THE GENETIC BACKGROUND

The greatest degree of consensus is on a genetic contribution. The evidence comes from family, twin, and adoption studies:

1. From a compilation of studies Zerbin-Rüdin (1972) estimated that morbidity risk in various categories of relatives as shown in Table 20.1. The rates are higher in first than in second degree relatives, and higher in the latter than in the general population. This is consistent with a genetic contribution although the tendency for rates to be higher in siblings than in parents (noted, for example, by Rosenthal 1970, p. 109) and in siblings than in children is unexplained.

2. Concordance rates are higher in monozygotic than in dizygotic pairs of twins. In the more recent, which may be more reliable than the earlier, studies Gottesman (1978) finds proband rates for monozygotic pairs of between 35 and 58 per cent and for dizygotic pairs between 9 and 26 per cent.

3. In adoption studies rates in individuals who are reared in separation from their relatives with schizophrenia are higher than those of comparison groups without such relatives. Thus, Heston (1966) found higher rates in the adopted-away children of schizophrenic mothers than in the adopted children of control mothers (Table 20.2).

In the converse experiment, Kety, Rosenthal, Wender, Schulsinger, and Jacobsen (1978) examined the rates of schizophrenia in the biological relatives of adopted individuals who had developed the disease and compared them with rates in the relatives of adoptees who had not (Table 20.3).

A further illuminating analysis of the literature by Karlsson (1970) compares

TABLE 20.1. *Morbidity risk in various categories of relative (Zerbin-Rüdin 1972)*

Relationship to a schizophrenic	Morbidity risk (corrected percentages)
Parents	5–10
Children	9–16
Siblings	8–14
Grandchildren	2–8
Cousins	2–6
Nieces and nephews	1–4
Uncles and aunts	2–7
Grandparents	1–2
General population	0.85

TABLE 20.2. *Rates of schizophrenic illness in adopted-away children (Heston 1966)*

	Normal mother	Schizophrenic mother
No. of offspring	50	47
Schizophrenia	0	5

$p = 0.024$

TABLE 20.3. *Rates of schizophrenic illness in relatives of adopted-away children (Kety et al. 1978)*

	n	Definite schizophrenia	Uncertain schizophrenia
Biological relatives of schizophrenic adoptees	173	11	13
Biological relatives of control adoptees	174	3	3
p =		0.026	0.009

TABLE 20.4. *Rates of schizophrenic illness in foster-reared close relatives of schizophrenic patients (Karlsson 1970)*

Relationship to index cases	No. of indivi- duals	Environmental theory		Genetic theory		Cumulative data	
		%	Cases	%	Cases	%	Cases
Monozygotic co-twins	12	0.8	0	65	8	75	9
Children of two schizophrenics	2	0.8	0	46	1	50	1
Sibs, one parent also affected	9	0.8	0	17	2	33	3
Children of one schizophrenic	100	0.8	1	11	11	11	11

the rates of illness in foster-reared close relatives of schizophrenic patients with those to be expected on an environmental theory (assuming the general population risk and that no genetic factors are operating) and the genetic theory (assuming that only genetic factors operate and that the risks are as detected in family studies by Kallman). The rates are close to the latter (Table 20.4).

Together, these studies make it difficult to avoid the conclusion that genes play at least a role in predisposing to the illness. But three cogent arguments can be advanced against the view that the genetic hypothesis is a sufficient explanation of the aetiology of the disease:

(i) concordance in monozygotic pairs of twins falls short of 100 per cent;
(ii) onset of illness is often well into adult life, and in many cases occurs after a number of years of perfectly adequate function;
(iii) the disease perists at a high prevalence in spite of the fact that biological fitness of affected individuals is diminished by a reduction in fertility (Stevens 1969).

THE ORiGINS OF THE VIRAL HYPOTHESIS

That the environmental agent in schizophrenia might be a virus appears first to have been considered following the 1918 influenza epidemic. Menninger (1926) reported a series of cases of post-influenzal psychosis and drew attention to the frequency of a 'dementia praecox-like' picture which he considered had an uncharacteristically favourable outcome. In a subsequent paper (Menninger 1928), he discussed infection as a cause of 'acute schizophrenic reactions', but in the published discussion which followed it appears that he shrank from the view that schizophrenia itself could be of similar aetiology (see Menninger 1928, p. 481). It was left to Goodall (1932) to formulate this view with precision. In the wake of the encephalitis lethargica epidemic he noted that 'there are observers who consider that there is no essential difference between psychotic disturbances connected with encephalitis (post-encephalitic) and those met with in states covered by the description schizophrenia . . .' and went on to argue that 'epidemic encephalitis, with the psychosomatic disorders which accompany it may be a virus disease and similarly caused, perhaps, are the schizophrenic states which resemble them . . .'.

Epidemic encephalitis and the influenza epidemic of 1918 may both have been due to the same virus (Ravenholt and Foege 1982), but there are other virus infections that may induce schizophrenic symptoms. Thus, Vilyuisk encephalitis, which is seen in the Yakat Republic of the USSR, is described as an episodic and often progressive condition in which the sequelae include neurological symptoms and dementia but sometimes also schizophrenic manifestations (Petrov 1970). The disease may be caused by a virus resembling the mouse encephalomyocarditis agent. In addition, there are a number of case reports in which illnesses presumed to be encephalitic and possibly viral in aetiology (sometimes on the basis of c.s.f. changes) have been accompanied by schizophrenia-like symptoms (for reviews see Torrey and Petersen 1973; Crow 1978).

Some animal viral infections are also relevant. Visna is a slowly progressive neurological disease of sheep which is seen in Iceland and is caused by a C-type retrovirus which evades the immune response (Petursson, Martin, Georgsson, Nathanson, and Palsson 1979) to induce a periventricular demyelinating process. The chronicity of the course and the location of the lesions made this model of possible interest in relation to the psychoses. The disease borna is possibly of greater relevance in that the course may be episodic rather than continuous and the agent sometimes enters a latent phase. The disease affects horses, sheep, cattle, and possibly deer, and can be transferred to rodents (Narayan, Herzog, Frese, Scheefers, and Rott 1983); it may be caused by an enveloped RNA virus. Of particular interest is the fact that it has a selectivity for the limbic system.

EPIDEMIOLOGY

(a) Seasonality

An observation which is consistent with a viral aetiology for the functional psychoses is that they show seasonal variations. There is a well-marked excess of onsets of illness in the summer months for mania and also for schizophrenia (Hare and Walter 1978), expressed in relation to admissions for other types of illness. It is not clear from the literature whether first differ from later episodes in seasonality of onset.

Even better-established with respect to schizophrenia is a season of birth effect — individuals who later develop the disease are more likely (by 4 to 8 per cent) to have been born in the months of winter and early spring than at other times of the year (Torrey, Torrey, and Petersen 1977). Similar effects are seen for mania (Hare and Walter 1978) and some relationships with seasonal temperature at or around the time of birth have been reported in the case of schizophrenia (Hare and Moran 1981).

The similarity of the two effects for affective disorder and schizophrenia raises the question of whether the two conditions are in some way related, perhaps that they share an aetiology.

(b) Temporal and geographical variations

Although it has been generally assumed that the incidence of schizophrenia has remained constant over time and is approximately similar in the various populations of the world this view has recently been challenged. Hare (1983*a*) has reviewed the evidence in the literature before the nineteenth century concerning hallucinatory states, and concludes that there is a relative lack of description of auditory hallucinations and that when noted these are seldom such as would now be regarded as characteristic of schizophrenia. Hare (1983*b*) also has presented evidence that the increase in admissions to mental hospitals which occurred in the course of the nineteenth century may not be explicable in terms of social changes, and that part at least may be attributable to a real increase in what is now described as schizophrenia.

Torrey (1980) also surveyed the historical literature with similar conclusions and assessed the question of whether there are significant geographical variations. Anomalously high rates have been reported in the north of Sweden, in Croatia, and Ireland. There are also interesting reports that the prevalence may be low in certain primitive communities before extensive contacts with western civilization have developed; for example, New Guinea (Torrey, Torrey, and Burton-Bradley 1974) and the islands of Micronesia (Dale 1981). In all these cases there are problems in estimating the prevalence of the disease in different populations with methods of assessment that are comparable, but it seems that the case that schizophrenia is a disease with a prevalence constant with respect to temporal and geographical variations has not been unequivocally established. In so far as there are significant variations, these are compatible with a role for environmental pathogens including infectious agents.

THE CONTAGION HYPOTHESIS

If schizophrenia is caused by an infectious agent, the question arises of its mode of transmission. A genetic component is not incompatible with an infectious aetiology. Twin studies of poliomyelitis and tuberculosis show monozygotic–dizygotic twin differences similar to those observed for schizophrenia (Table 20.5).

Presumably, genetic factors predispose to tuberculosis and poliomyelitis and a gene-infectious agent interaction is conceivable also for schizophrenia. Some findings of family studies are consistent with the proposition that the critical factor for a predisposed individual is proximity to someone who already has the disease (Crow 1983). For example:

(i) Concordance rates in most studies in which the appropriate comparison has been made are higher in dizygotic twins than in siblings. Dizygotic twins, of course, share genes to the same extent as do pairs of siblings, but because they are the same age they are likely to be in closer contact.

(ii) Pairs of siblings (and other first degree relatives) are more likely to be

TABLE 20.5. *Concordance rates for schizophrenia, tuberculosis, and poliomyelitis in twins*

	No. of pairs (% concordant)	
	Monozygotic	Dizygotic
Tuberculosis (Kallman and Reisner 1943)	78 (67%)	230 (23%)
Poliomyelitis (Herndon and Jennings 1951)	14 (36%)	33 (6%)
Schizophrenia (Kallman 1946)	210 (46%)	309 (14%)

concordant if they are the same than of opposite sex (Rosenthal 1962). However, this is true only for relationships (i.e. first degree) within the family, a finding consistent with the effect being environmental.

(iii) In pairs of monozygotic twins, the second twin is more likely to become ill in the first two years after illness onset in the first, but in the data of Abe (1969) this period of increased risk was confined to pairs who were together at illness onset in the first twin.

(iv) It has been claimed by Kasanetz (1979) that first episodes of illness are more likely to occur in individuals who are in contact, although unrelated to, persons who already have the disease than in those who are not so exposed.

These observations suggested that contagion could not be ruled out, although the adoption studies, and the other evidence for a genetic factor, restricts such transmission to a gene–virus interaction. Consistent with this possibility is the demonstration by Scharfetter that in cases of *folie à deux* in unrelated individuals (commonly spouses) the genetic predisposition is as great in the secondary as in the primary case.

A STUDY IN PAIRS OF SIBLINGS

The contagion hypothesis has now been subjected to a further test in pairs of siblings with the disease. According to this hypothesis, the siblings of patients with schizophrenia will include individuals at genetic risk and such individuals are also exposed to someone who already has the disease. In an analysis of five collections of such pairs on whom data are available (Crow and Done 1985 age of onset has been found strongly correlated between pairs ($r = 0.68$) and there is a shift toward earlier age of onset in the younger sibling ($X^2 = 42.45$ $p < 0.0005$).

This observation is susceptible to three explanations:

(i) age of onset is genetically determined but when the disease is seen in an elder sibling it is detected at an earlier age in a younger sibling (the 'early detection' hypothesis),

(ii) the disease is transmitted from one to the other sibling, the age shift being related to the age difference between the siblings at the time of transmission, i.e. from elder to younger or vice versa (the 'contagion' hypothesis),

(iii) age of onset is under genetic control but, because pairs are collected at the time of onset of illness in one sibling, an excess of younger siblings with earlier age of onset are included (the 'ascertainment bias' hypothesis).

A decision between these hypotheses is made possible by an analysis of the age shift (to younger age of onset in younger sibling) in relation to whether the disease occurs first in the elder or younger sibling. The 'early detection' and the 'contagion' hypotheses both predict that the age shift will be seen in the pairs of siblings in whom the illness occurs first in the elder. The selection bias hypothesis predicts the age shift will occur only in the pairs in which the younger sibling is ill first.

This latter is what is observed. Within the group of pairs in which the elder sibling is ill first, age of onset between siblings remains highly correlated but there is no tendency to earlier onset in the younger sibling.

This finding rules out the contagion hypothesis (or at least demonstrates that if contagion does occur it must be in a proportion of cases so small as not to be detectable in the series of 264 pairs of siblings available), as well as the early detection theory. It also has wider implications for the role of an environmental agent in precipitation since the apparent independence of date of onset of illness in one sibling from date of onset in the other indicates that if such an agent exists it is not defined in time and shared by the siblings. Thus, such factors as common infective illnesses of childhood and psychogenic insults (except of a kind which are unvarying with respect to the passage of time) are ruled out. Since the data on siblings are more extensive than the pairs of mono-zygotic twins examined by Abe (1969) and the first episodes of illness studied by Kasanetz (1979), and have been collected in better defined circumstances than the latter, it seems that contagion can be excluded as the usual method by which the disease is transmitted. If this had been the case, the age shift should have been observed in the pairs in which the elder sibling was ill first. The findings therefore impose significant constraints on viral hypotheses and suggest, for example, that if viruses play a role that this may occur in prenatal rather than postnatal life.

A NEW HYPOTHESIS: GENE, VIRUS, AND ONCOGENE

If both gene and virus are present at birth (and therefore that the virus persists for many years in a latent form) parsimony requires that it be considered that the two are more closely related than is suggested by the gene–virus interaction hypothesis. The two could be one and the same if the virus were integrated in the genome and passed from one generation to the next. Such a possibility, against prevailing biological opinion, was considered by Myerson (1925).

Agents now known to have the ability (by possession of the enzyme reverse transcriptase) to integrate in the host's genome are retroviruses; in the pre-implantation embryo Jaenisch (1976) has shown that the virus may become integrated into the germ line. In earlier studies retrovirus-related antigens (Payne and Chubb 1968) and tumour-inducing viruses (Bentvelzen and Daams 1969) had been found to be transmitted in chickens and mice respectively in a Men-delian fashion, and interspecies comparisons suggested that exogenously-acquired genes have in some cases become integrated in the host germ-line (Benveniste and Todaro 1974).

Thus schizophrenia (and perhaps manic-depressive psychosis) could be manifestations of infection with a retrovirus which has become integrated in the genome. The season of birth effect could be relevant to viral infection and integration occurring *in utero*; once the virus was incorporated in the germ-line the descendants of that individual would inherit susceptibility to the disease. In this case the season of birth effect would be expected in those cases in which a family history was not already present, as observed by Kinney and Jacobsen (1978). In their analysis of the Danish–American adoption study the proportion of schizophrenic patients with a low genetic risk (70 per cent) born in January to April was significantly greater than the proportion (21 per cent) of probands at a high biological risk (i.e. with a family history or history of brain damage).

This retroviral hypothesis provides explanations for some anomalies in the genetic data. It could, for example, explain the differences in rates in dizygotic twins and siblings. When disease susceptibility is inherited from a parent, concordancies will be similar in dizygotic twins and siblings, but when viral integration occurs for the first time *in utero* it may be expected that there is an increased probability that both twins will be affected. The hypothesis may also explain why morbidity risks are greater in siblings than in parents, and in children than in siblings, because there is in addition to the inherited component the possibility of *de novo* acquisition of the viral sequence.

However, the rate of discordance in monozygotic twins (generally taken as evidence for an environmental component in aetiology) is unexplained. If disease susceptibility is inherited from an affected parent it may be supposed that both twins would be affected, and this would also be expected in most of those cases in which the agent was acquired *in utero*. However, Boklage (1977) has uncovered an explanation for the discordance which is consistent with a higher degree of genetic determination than is suggested by the twin studies. Cerebral dominance is genetically determined, perhaps by a single gene for right-handedness which induces speech in the left hemisphere (Annett 1978) and which either is not present or is not systematically confined to the left hemisphere in left-handers. Pairs of monozygotic twins are not always concordant for handedness and in such pairs there is an excess of left-handers. Boklage proposes that these facts are relevant to schizophrenia in that in MZ pairs discordance for schizophrenia is related to the presence of non-righthandedness in one or other member of the pair. Thus, in an analysis of the MZ twin data of Gottesman and Shields, together with the series of Slater, he found that in 12 pairs concordant for handedness 11 (92 per cent) were concordant for schizophrenia whereas in 16 pairs in which one or both members were not unequivocally right-handed only 4 pairs (25 per cent) were concordant. These findings suggest (i) that the genetic component may be greater than has been generally assumed from recent twin studies, and (ii) that schizophrenia is in some way intimately related to the determination of cerebral dominance.

Boklage's conclusions are relevant to the modifications of the viral hypothesis advanced above. He writes that if schizophrenia 'is with rare exception (heritably) cellular in origin, the following considerations are appropriate:

1. Schizophrenic psychosis is clearly not what is inherited; that takes on the average nearly 30 years to appear, and it is not possible in the majority of cases to say that the individual 'was always more or less like that'.
2. Therefore, what is inherited or otherwise cellularly imposed before birth is some cellular *anlage*, stable for 20–60 years of growth with or without intervening development of the *anlage* itself or of identifiable behavioural deviations originating therefrom.
3. That the symptoms of schizophrenia represent lateralized pathology does not prove that the cellular *anlage* is similarly placed. However, it seems fairly safe to defy a simpler explanation . . .'.

The view that schizophrenia is a disease of the dominant hemisphere is supported by a recent post-mortem study (Brown *et al.* 1985). Brains were collected from patients dying in Runwell Hospital over a period of 26 years and groups of patients with schizophrenia and affective psychosis were selected on the basis of the Feighner criteria. After patients whose brains showed evidence of significant Alzheimer-type change or vascular disease had been excluded, and corrections for age, sex, and year of birth, had been applied the brains of the patients with schizophrenia were found to differ from those of patients with affective disorder in that (i) they were a mean 60 g lighter, (ii) the inferior horn of the lateral ventricle was approximately twice as large, and (iii) the width of the parahippocampal gyrus was reduced. For this latter change there was a significant ($p < 0.02$) diagnosis by side interaction the difference between the groups being greater on the left side. The findings offer support to views expressed on the basis of observations on the psychoses associated with temporal lobe epilepsy (e.g. Flor-Henry 1969; Taylor 1975; Lindsay, Ounsted, and Richards 1979), that schizophrenia is a disease of the dominant, whereas affective disorder disturbs the non-dominant, hemisphere.

A RELATIONSHIP BETWEEN SCHIZOPHRENIA AND MANIC-DEPRESSIVE PSYCHOSIS

This possibility is compatible with a common aetiology for the two psychoses, as suggested by the seasonality findings, the side of the disturbance (albeit under genetic control) determining the form of the psychological disturbance.

It has generally been considered that the two psychoses are independently transmitted although the existence of intermediate states ('schizo-affective psychoses') is an embarrassment to this viewpoint. A possible relationship between the conditions is that in successive generations there is a (probably small) tendency for manic-depressive psychosis to transmute into schizophrenia. Thus, Rosenthal (1970) summarized the findings concerning the incidence of schizophrenia in the relatives of patients with affective disorder and found an excess in the children (Table 20.6).

Schulz (1940) studied psychoses occurring in the children of two manic-

TABLE 20.6. *Risk of schizophrenia in relatives of manic-depressive probands*

	No. of studies	% (± S.D.)
Parents	6	0.42 ± 0.33
Siblings	9	0.79 ± 0.53
Children	5	2.30 ± 0.96

depressive parents and found 28 per cent to be affective but 12 per cent to be schizophrenic. In a case register study of parent-child pairs who had both been recorded as being given a psychotic diagnosis, Powell, Thomson, Hall, and Wilson (1973) found that amongst the children of parents with schizophrenia 9 were recorded as suffering from this disease and none from manic-depressive psychosis, whilst amongst children of parents with the latter disorder there were 10 with manic-depressive disease but 15 with schizophrenia.

Thus, the form of psychotic disorder may change in succeeding generations. Such a change implies an alteration in the gene itself, and may be relevant to the persistence of schizophrenia in the face of a decrease in fertility. For if schizophrenia originates sometimes by a modification of a gene predisposing to another condition, and that condition itself is not associated with reduced fertility, the continuation of the disease at a high and apparently constant prevalence is easier to understand, even though the mechanism of the modification remains obscure.

THE RELATIONSHIP BETWEEN DOMINANCE AND PSYCHOSIS

If schizophrenia is indeed a disease of the dominant hemisphere (or perhaps more specifically a disease of cerebral dominance) there are two possible relationships between the genetic determination of cerebral dominance and the transmission of psychosis:

(i) The genes for dominance and psychosis are separate, but have become linked, so that when the psychosis gene replicates it does so in the dominant hemisphere and the resultant psychological disturbance is manifest as schizophrenia. According to this concept, manic-depressive disease results from replication of the gene in the non-dominant hemisphere.

(ii) The gene for psychosis is but a modification of the dominance gene. This view invites attention to the evolutionary significance of dominance itself and the possible existence of balanced polymorphisms with respect to handedness.

Cerebral asymmetries (e.g. an increase in the size of the planum temporale) associated with dominance are now well established (Galaburda, Le May, Kemper, and Geschwind 1978) and presumably arise from increased growth in the dominant hemisphere during development. Growth factors are known to be acquired and transposed as 'oncogenes' by retroviruses. Thus, it seems worth considering whether dominance itself might result from the action of a retrovirus associated oncogene in one hemisphere. The capacity of retroviral mechanisms to transpose gene segments provides the possibility of further changes with adaptive gains and losses. Thus, one may speculate that whereas the activity of the oncogene on one side confers a degree of dominance (perhaps associated with the capacity for speech) and righthandedness, the presence of the oncogene on the other side as well (which might account for some cases of lefthandedness) has further advantages, e.g. ambidexterity, and increased size of the corresponding segment of the temporal lobe, as well as disadvantages, e.g. loss of dominance by one hemisphere and of the ability of the non-dominant hemisphere to develop its own specializations. Further oncogene replications (e.g. more than one in either hemisphere) could add to the occasional gains and the hazards, and might relate to the occurrence of psychosis. Thus, the functional psychoses could be the deleterious consequences of a balanced polymorphism whose evolutionary significance lies in the development of cerebral dominance and its associated benefits.

SUMMARY

The existence of a genetic component in schizophrenia is attested by the findings of adoption and twin studies although the results of the latter appear to leave room for an environmental component and the onset of the disease in adult life and persistence in the face of reduced fertility remain (on the genetic hypothesis) unexplained. Seasonality of birth and possibly of onset and some evidence of temporal and geographical variations in prevalence have been advanced as consistent with a role for a virus in aetiology. However, age of onset in pairs of siblings suggests that horizontal transmission does not occur. An alternative hypothesis is proposed:

(i) that schizophrenia (and perhaps manic-depressive psychosis) is due to a retrovirus, which occasionally is acquired *in utero* (giving rise to the season-of-birth effect in non-familial cases), that can become integrated in the genome;

(ii) that the integrated virus (the 'psychosis gene') is in some way associated with cerebral dominance being either linked with the dominance gene or constituting a modification of that gene;

(iii) that the dominance gene itself may include an oncogene responsible for the development of cerebral asymmetry;

(iv) that expression (possibly replication) of the psychosis gene (whether linked with or part of the dominance gene) outside the period of normal development results (in the dominant hemisphere) in schizophrenia and (in the non-dominant hemisphere) in affective disorder;

(v) that manic-depressive psychosis is sometimes expressed in later generations as schizophrenia; this suggests that modifications of the gene occur and that these are associated with shifts in lateralization of the psychosis gene.

REFERENCES

Abe, K. (1969). The morbidity rate and environmental influence in monozygotic co-twies of schizophrenics. *Br. J. Psychiat.* **115**, 519–31.

Annett, M. (1978). A single gene explanation of right and left handedness and brainedness. Lanchester Polytechnic, Coventry.

Bentvelzen, P. and Daams, J. H. (1969). Hereditary infections with mammary tumor viruses in mice. *J. natn Cancer Inst.* **43**, 1025–35.

Benveniste, R. E. and Todaro, G. J. (1974). Evolution of C-type viral genes: inheritance of exogenously acquired viral genes. *Nature, Lond.* **252**, 456–9.

Boklage, C. E. (1977). Schizophrenia, brain asymmetry development and twinning: cellular relationship with etiological and possibly prognostic implications. *Biol. Psychiat.* **12**, 19–35.

Brown, R., Colter, N., Corsellis, J. A. N., Crow, T. J. Frith, C. D., Jagoe, R., Johnstone, E. C., and Marsh, L. Brain weight and parahippocampal gyrus width are decreased and temporal horn area is increased in schizophrenia by comparison with affective disorder. *Arch. gen. Psychiat.* (in press).

Crow, T. J. (1978). Viral causes of psychiatric disease. *Post-grad. med. J.* **54**, 763–7.

—— (1983). Is schizophrenia an infectious disease? *Lancet* i, 173–5.

—— and Done, J. D. Age of onset of schizophrenia in siblings. *Psychiatry Research* (in press).

Dale, P. W. (1981). Prevalence of schizophrenia in the Pacific Islands of Micronesia. *J. Psychiat. Res.* **16**, 103–11.

Flor-Henry, P. (1969). Psychosis and temporal lobe epilepsy: a controlled investigation. *Epilepsia* **10**, 363–95.

Galaburda, A. M., Le May, M., Kemper, T. L., and Geschwind, N. (1978). Right–left asymmetries in the brain. *Science* **199**, 852–6.

Goodall, E. (1932). The exciting cause of certain states of disease, at present classified under 'schizophrenia' by psychiatrists, may be infection. *J. ment. Sci.* **78**, 746–55.

Gottesman, I. I. (1978). Schizophrenics and genetics: Where are we? Are you sure? In *The nature of schizophrenia* (ed. L. C. Wynne, R. L. Cromwell, and S. Matthysse), pp. 59–69. John Wiley, New York.

Hare, E. H. (1983a). Epidemiological evidence for a viral factor in the aetiology of the functional psychoses. *Adv. Biol. Psychiat.* **12**, 52–75.

—— (1983b). Was insanity on the increase? *Br. J. Psychiat.* **142**, 439–55.

—— and Walter, S. D. (1978). Seasonal variations in admissions of psychiatric patients and its relation to seasonal variations in their births. *J. epidemiol. Commun. Hlth* **32**, 47–52.

Hare, E. and Moran, P. (1981). A relation between seasonal temperature and the birth rate of schizophrenic patients. *Acta psychiat. scand.* **63**, 396–405.

Heston, L. L. (1966). Psychiatric disorders in foster home reared children of schizophrenic mothers. *Br. J. Psychiat.* 112, 819–25.

Jaenisch, R. (1976). Germ line integration and Mendeliam transmission of the exogenous Moloney leukemia virus. *Proc. natn Acad. Sci. U.S.A.* 73, 1260–4.

Karlsson, J. L. (1970). The rate of schizophrenia in foster-reared close relatives of schizophrenic index cases. *Biol. Psychiat.* 2, 285–90.

Kasanetz, E. F. (1979). Tecnica per investigare il ruolo di fattori ambientale sulla genesi della schizofrenia. *Riv. psicol. Anal.* 10, 193–202.

Kety, S. S., Rosenthal, D., Wender, P. H., Schulsinger, F., and Jacobsen, B. (1978). The biologic and adoptive families of adopted individuals who became schizophrenic: prevalance of mental illness and other characteristics. In *The nature of schizophrenia* (ed. L. C. Wynne, R. L. Cromwell, and S. Matthysse), pp. 25–37. John Wiley, New York.

Kinney, D. K. and Jacobsen, B. (1978). Environmental factors in schizophrenia: new adoption study evidence. In *The nature of schizophrenia* (ed. L. C. Wynne, R. L. Cromwell, and S. Matthysse), pp. 38–51. John Wiley, New York.

Lindsay, J., Ounsted, C., and Richards, P. (1979). Long-term outcome in children with temporal lobe seizures. III Psychiatric aspects in childhood and adult life. *Dev. med. Child Neurol.* 21, 630–6.

Menninger, K. A. (1926). Influenza and schizophrenia. An analysis of post-influenzal 'dementia praecox' as of 1918, and five years later. *Am. J. Psychiat.* 5, 469–529.

— (1928). The schizophrenic syndrome as the product of acute infectious disease. *Archs Neurol. Psychiat.* 20, 464–81.

Myerson, A. (1925). *The inheritance of mental disease.* Williams & Wilkins, Baltimore.

Narayan, O., Herzog, S., Frese, K., Sbheefers, H., and Rott, R. (1983). Behavioral disease in rats caused by immuno-pathological responses to persistent borna virus in the brain. *Science* 220, 1401–2.

Payne, L. N. and Chubb, R. C. (1968). Studies on the nature and genetic control of an antigen in normal chick embryos which reacts in the COFAL test. *J. gen. Virol.* 3, 379–91.

Petrov, P. A. (1970). Vilyuisk encephalitis in the Yakat Republic (USSR). *Am. J. trop. Med. Hyg.* 19, 146–50.

Petursson, G., Martin, J. R., Georgsson, N., Nathanson, N., and Palsson, P. A. (1979). Visna, the biology of the agent and the disease. In *Aspects of slow and persistent virus infections* (ed. D. A. J. Tyrrell), pp. 165–97. Martinus Nijhoff, The Hague.

Powell, A., Thomson, N., Hall, D. J. and Wilson, L. (1973). Parent–child concordance with respect to sex and diagnosis in schizophrenia and manic-depressive psychosis. *Br. J. Psychiat.* 123, 653–8.

Ravenholt, R. T. and Foege, W. H. (1982). 1918 influenza, encephalitis lethargica, parkinsonism. *Lancet* ii, 860–4.

Rosenthal, D. (1962). Familial concordance by sex with respect to schizophrenia. *Psychol. Bull.* 59, 401–21.

— (1970). *Genetic theory and abnormal behavior.* McGraw-Hill, New York.

Schulz, B. (1940). Erkrankungsalter schizophrenen Eltern und Kinder. *Z. Neurol. Psychiat.* 168, 709–21.

Stevens, B. C. (1969). *Marriage and fertility of women suffering from schizophrenia or affective disorders.* Oxford University Press.

Taylor, D. C. (1975). Factors influencing the occurrence of schizophrenia-like psychosis in patients with temporal lobe epilepsy. *Psychol. Med.* 5, 249–54.

Torrey, E. F. (1980). *Schizophrenia and civilization.* Jason Aronson, New York.

— and Petersen, M. R. (1973). Slow and latent viruses in schizophrenia. *Lancet* ii, 22–4.

—, Torrey, B. B., and Burton-Bradley, B. G. (1974). The epidemiology of schizophrenia in Papua-New Guinea. *Am. J. Psychiat.* 131, 567–73.

—, —, and Petersen, M. R. (1977). Seasonality of schizophrenic births in the United States. *Arch. gen. Psychiat.* 34, 1065–70.

Zerbin-Rüdin, E. (1972). Genetic research and the theory of schizophrenia. *Int. J. ment. Hlth* 1, 42–62.

PART 5
Euphoriants and stimulants

21

Opioids

MARTIN MITCHESON, RICHARD HARTNOLL AND
ROGER LEWIS

Our personal involvement with drug dependence is that of a clinical psychiatrist, and of research work investigating the effects of drug use for individuals living in the community. The first concern of a physician is with the experience of individual patients, and in reducing the harm to the individual that might result in the consumption of drugs. The second concern is with matters of public policy in relation to the control of drugs, and to the problems that may result to society as a whole from drug taking. Our expertise is not in the details of the action of drugs upon the brain; but, working within a multidisciplinary team, it is in the doctor's responsibility to be aware of pharmacological developments, particularly as they may affect the management of patients. The identification of opiate receptors and the isolation of endorphins within the brain have provided a pharmacological explanation that is consistent both with clinical experience and many literary descriptions pertaining to the effects of exogenous opioids on mental functioning, and which also underwrites the observed events occurring during withdrawal illness. Recently, these have been reviewed lucidly and comprehensively in a paper by Gold and Rea (1983). In practice, however, this exploration and explanation of brain function has not so far altered the basic problems presented by the addict to the professional person, who is attempting to assist that addict overcoming his or her addiction. We propose therefore to review the current status of the consumption of opioid drugs in the United Kingdom, and then to pose some suggestions as to how developments in pharmacology might be of value to those of us who work in drug clinics.

It is not easy to focus exclusively on one specific group of drugs. Thus, in talking about the opioids, we are almost by definition talking about multiple drug-users who have experienced a wide range of drugs prior to the opioids, and are probably, at least intermittently, consuming a continual melange concomitantly with opioids. When considering the non-medical use of any drug, apart perhaps from cannabis (and even that tends to be associated with above-average consumption of alcohol), the exclusive use of only a single drug is very much the exception to the rule of multiple drug-taking.

Generally, drug-taking conforms to the old adage of commonest things being commonest, but with consumers expanding their repertoires of drug use rather than passing on from one and leaving the other behind. Thus, there are statistical correlations with the first drug used by an individual being the commonest used by that society (Kandel and Faust 1975). In our society, that is beer, or wine, followed by distilled alcohol or nicotine, and then cannabis. For the diminishing minority of drug-takers who continue to expand their repertoire of multiple drug use, the pattern of progression is more variable. In the 1960s and early 1970s it appeared that, for working-class drug-takers, amphetamines were more likely to be used before cannabis, followed by sedatives, including barbiturates, cocaine, or LSD, and, at least commonly and usually the last to be experienced, opioids. In contrast, for middle-class drug-takers, the pattern appeared to be cannabis, then LSD, sedatives, amphetamines or cocaine, and finally opioids. In more recent years, whilst cannabis remains generally the most common initial illicit drug consumed (across all classes), the picture is more blurred regarding other drugs. Indeed, in some areas, it seems that solvents are the first drug to be used, perhaps even before alcohol.

Although firm evidence is not available, it appears, both from our own epidemiological work in north London, and from the impressions of other workers, that heroin and cocaine are being used earlier in many drug-takers' careers than was the case ten years ago. There are substantial indications that this correlates with increased prevalence of use of these two drugs.

A statistical correlation between prevalence of use of a drug, and the stage at which it is added to the repertoire of multiple drug use does not imply any necessary chemical progresssion nor any direct and inflexible causal relationship.

There have, however, been suggestions that there may be certain common pathways, involving endorphin production in the mediation of various *chemical* addictions, including alcohol, and *non-chemical* compulsive behaviours such as gambling or marathon-running.

The pattern of drug abuse since 1960 has fluctuated in response to such factors as availability, fashions in experimentation, individual susceptibility, changes in the socio-economic climate, acceptance or taboos within the individual's peer group, and the current 'image', as well as the specific effects of a particular drug. The 1960s saw an increase from 500 to nearly 3000 known cases of opioid addiction, mainly including heroin, which was prescribed to certain addicts by a limited number of independent practitioners. With the introduction of the restriction of heroin-prescribing in 1968 to specially-licensed doctors in clinics, there was a temporary peak and then a reduction in the number of new cases. The early and mid-1970s gave some hope for a stabilization of the opioid problem but saw the development of multiple drug abuse with barbiturate injection as a dangerous practice. The opioid user of that period seemed to be growing older, with a falling-off particularly of adolescent patients presenting for treatment, and a gradual ageing of what seemed to be a cohort that had been introduced to drug-taking during the 1960s.

However, since 1978/79 there has been a marked increase in heroin abuse (Fig. 21.1). At first this involved 'recruits' from the same ageing cohort. Amongst new patients who presented for treatment, the majority had had some acquain-

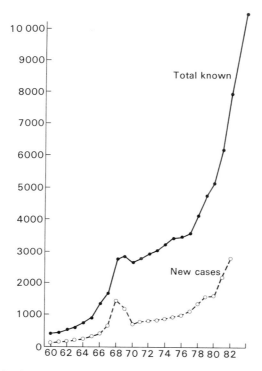

Fig. 21.1. Narcotic drug addicts known to the Home Office 1960–82. (Source: Home Office Statistical Bulletin, 13/83, 5 July 1983.)

tance with illegal drugs since their adolescence, but a dependence history of only 1–3 years. In the last two years other groups in their mid-to-late teens and early twenties have started to become involved with heroin and cocaine. These drugs seem to be readily available in groups of varied classes and cultures in any city in the UK (though not generally amongst ethnic minorities).

Epidemiological research has been undertaken in Camden and Islington, investigating several techniques and sources of information. These included multiplier formula from deaths; extrapolation from surveys of GPs; extrapolation from nominations by drug users; and capture–recapture using several combinations of sources: clinic attendances, deaths, hepatitis cases, and local court reports. See Fig. 21.2. Local trends reflect the national picture. During 1982, an estimated 2000 people (+/− 500) used opioids for non-medical reasons on a regular basis (daily/almost daily). This gives a period prevalence of about 13 per 1000 population aged 16–44. The rate at any one time (point prevalence) was lower, perhaps 7–8 per 1000. The main drug involved was (and is) illicit heroin from SW Asia.

It is not yet possible to ascertain what proportion of those not receiving treatment experience serious problems. Certainly, it is not insignificant. For

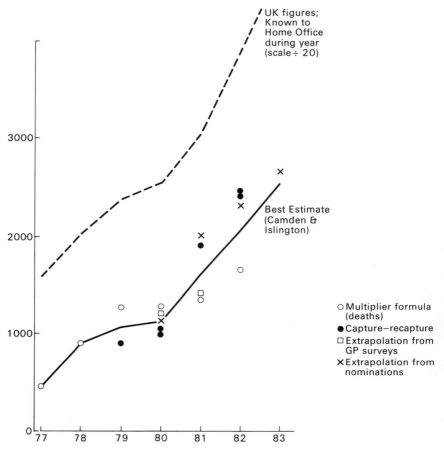

Fig. 21.2. Regular opioid use (Camden and Islington, 1977–83) 12-month period prevalence estimates.

example, out of 22 addicts in Camden and Islington who died during 1982, only two had been in contact with the clinic in the previous twelve months.

Problems associated with psychoactive drugs other than opioids are encountered at least as frequently by many agencies, and present difficulties of management which are at least as severe as cases involving opioids. Sedative/ alcohol combinations and multiple drug use involving sedatives/stimulants/ analgesics predominate. Solvent use arouses considerable anxiety, though the numbers known to most agencies are small. There are several reasons for the increase in heroin use. These include a growth in supply and availability (Fig. 21.3), together with a diminuation in price. This in turn reflects a variety of factors. One example was the Iranian revolution in 1979. Subsequent political events on the Afghanistan/Pakistan border have favoured the production of

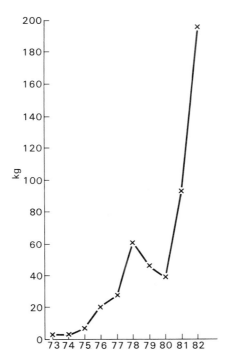

Fig. 21.3. Quantities of heroin seized (Police and H.M. Customs). (Source: Home Office Statistical Bulletin, 13/83, 5 July 1983.)

opium and its conversion to heroin in an area where no major political power has the ability to control, nor, perhaps, the will to risk alienating the local population.

Heroin, like cocaine, has become more socially acceptable amongst groups who, some years ago, would rarely have considered using heroin. The weakening of taboos surrounding heroin is in part associated with changes in methods of administration. Smoking and sniffing have become much more popular, especially amongst recent initiates. Not only do such modes of administration seem less dramatic than self-injection, but some users appear to believe that heroin is not addictive unless injected. They are, of course, mistaken. The UCH clinic sees a substantial proportion of addicted patients who have never injected drugs — they are, however, safe from syringe transmitted hepatitis or AIDS.

A further factor, which seems to be particularly relevant to the socio-economic circumstances pertaining in some connurbations, is a sense of disillusionment, associated with though not necessarily directly explained by, unemployment and urban decline.

The question that we pose, not expecting any definitive answer, but perhaps provoking some suggestions, is what developments in pharmacology might be expected to contribute to the reduction of harm to drug-takers, and to the remainder of society. In the management of addiction, a basic decision is whether the provision of a maintenance supply of a drug enables a dependent individual to lead an otherwise normal life. Leaving to one side the stimulants and sedatives, it is possible briefly to consider different styles of opioid dependence which may be characterized by the middle-aged therapeutic addict noted in the 1920s by the Rollaston Committee, in contrast to the younger heroin user addicted in the course of subcultural activities in the 1960s or 1980s. A representative sample of the younger addict receiving a heroin prescription at London clinics in 1968 was studied by Stimson and Ogborne (1976) who subdivided them into four groups according to their behaviour, described as stables, junkies, loners, and two-worlders. Of these, the stables conform most closely to the pattern of the earlier therapeutic addict with adequate social functioning and little involvement in the drug subculture. From society's point of view the maintained addict who abstains from subcultural involvement with other drug users and from criminal activity, is clearly preferable to the junky supporting a drug habit in the illegal market. From the individual's point of view the quality of that person's social and emotional life may be of paramount importance but has been little studied. An early reference in Homer's *Odyssey* (c. 800 BC) quoted by Raymond Prince (1982) in a review for psychological anthropologists, however, indicates one effect on social and emotional responsiveness: 'Into the bowl in which their wine was mixed she slipped a drug that had the power of robbing grief and anger of their sting and banishing all painful memories. No-one that swallowed this dissolved in wine could shed a single tear that day, even for the death of his mother or father, or if they put his brother or his own son to the sword and he were there to see it done.' Thus it is easy to understand the political objections to the introduction of maintenance programmes in social situations where deprivation and poverty can only be altered by drastic political and economic change.

In considering whether to offer maintenance therapy there are, therefore, factors relating to the individual patient, and factors of interest primarily to society in general, which may or may not be congruent or in conflict. Nevertheless, if a maintenance supply converts a person involved in subcultural activity and illicit drug use into a law-abiding, medically-maintained addict, then this may be regarded as advantageous by the majority of society. Research undertaken at UCH indicates that the provision of an injectable prescription does not generally achieve even this goal (Hartnoll, Mitcheson, Battersby, Brown, Ellis, Fleming, and Hedley 1980). Although the extent of criminal activity may be reduced by a prescription of heroin, the majority of such patients continue to spend a considerable proportion of their waking life in drug-related behaviour, and the majority continue to supplement a heroin prescription both with illegal opiates and with other drugs. Heroin being a relatively short-acting drug and significantly more attractive when taken by intravenous injection as opposed to by mouth, is clearly not an ideal drug to employ for stable maintenance. The synthetic opioid methadone which has a longer action and is reasonably active when taken by mouth, has been extensively employed in the United States in methadone maintenance programmes, albeit with an uncertain proportion of the addict population enrolling in such programmes. It has achieved apparent success in enabling economically deprived addicts to achieve a degree of stability and re-integration into normal society (McGlothlin and Anglin 1981).

In the United Kingdom it would appear that the majority of drug users do not find oral methadone a satisfactory substitute for the injection of heroin. A minority, however, seem to be able to utilize methadone in changing their life-style. When initially introduced by Dole, Nyswander, and Krick (1966), it was suggested that if methadone is employed in high doses of at least 100 mg daily then the patient develops fairly high tolerance to all opioid drugs. Where heroin is of poor quality, as is common in the United States, such a patient derives little pleasure from intravenous heroin use. In the UK where illegally imported heroin is retailed in London at an average purity of 45–55 per cent (Her Majesty's Government report 1982) an attempt to block the effects of heroin by cross-tolerance is unlikely to be effective. Methadone is now judged to be primarily effective as a maintenance drug by preventing the experience of significant withdrawal symptoms and drug craving. For this a dose in the region of 40/80 mg is usually sufficient, but for some patients a dose of up to 100 mg may be necessary to retain them in a programme without having recourse to other drugs (Hargreaves 1983).

A desirable drug for long-term maintenance would be one with sufficient agonist properties to obviate the occurrence of a withdrawal syndrome and drug craving, with a sufficient euphoriant action to attract the majority of drug users, *but* with sufficient antagonist properties to block the euphoriant effect of an intravenous injection of heroin. A drug such as buprenorphine may represent some advance towards such properties provided that a suitable schedule transferring patients from pure agonists could be devised (see Jasinski, Pevnick, and Griffith, 1978; Mello, Mendelson, and Kuehnle 1982). It is important to emphasize that the provision of such a drug *per se* would have little impact unless it were to be combined with a significant programme to assist patients in making structural changes in their life. The patient needs to acquire techniques of coping with personal difficulties and stress to which they have developed a habitual avoidance response of taking drugs. Because of the shortage of experienced staff prepared to work in this field and the lack of financial resources to train or employ them, an initial programme might utilize such a drug without significant external psycho-social supports. However, experience of clinics in this country indicate that a very high proportion of clients exhibit personal difficulties and are socially disadvantaged so that it is unlikely that such a programme would be effective in isolation. By combining an initial period of stabilization with social and behavioural change techniques, then a reduction programme might be initiated with a greater prospect of success and at this stage the patient's initial resolve to remain drug-free could be supported by taking an orally-active and long-acting opioid antagonist such as naltrexone (Renault 1978). A progressive programme based on such concepts was suggested by Avram Goldstein in the mid-1970s but not implemented (Goldstein 1976).

In the space available, we have not considered the pharmacology of drug-withdrawal. Clinical experience indicates that withdrawal may be relatively easily achieved where a patient is reasonably motivated and friends, relatives, or staff are able to provide substantial support. It is in no way intended to denigrate the undoubted value of both conventional techniques nor of those less common to orthodox medicine to suggest that it is the concern of the therapist and the insistence on the patient taking responsibility for achieving a healthy state that renders attempts at cure effective. That is not to say that technical services such as an incremental reduction of an agonist drug, the use of clonidine or lofexidine which suppress those withdrawal symptoms mediated by the noradrenergic system (Ginzburg 1983), electro stimulation or acupuncture which may stimulate endorphin production, do not have an important if not essential role to play in facilitating this process. Progress in the investigation of the deficiencies or disruption of the natural endorphin system certainly increase understanding of the acute and protracted withdrawal states, and may eventually yield drugs that may mitigate these symptoms and promote normal functioning. Nevertheless, there is a paradox whereby there is an ideological contradiction between the science of clinical pharmacology and an individual's cure from drug addiction. It is only, we suggest, at the point where the patient ceases to look for a magic drug to cure their addiction for them, and takes on themselves the burden and responsibility of operating a drug-free life, that the products of pharmacology are likely to be effective in enabling that individual in first achieving, and then maintaining, abstinence. The alarming increase in the incidence of heroin addiction that is affecting all social classes and all major cities in the British Isles, suggests that we need all the combined resources that pharmacology, professional psychotherapists, self-help organizations, and therapeutic communities can offer.

REFERENCES

Dole, V. P., Nyswander, M. E., and Krick, M. J. (1966). Narcotic blockade. *Arch. internal Med.* **118**, 304–9.

Ginzburg, H. M. (1983). Use of clonidine or lofexidine to detoxify from methadone maintenance or other opioid dependencies. In *Research on the treatment of narcotic addiction* (ed. J. R. Cooper). US Department of Health & Human Services, Rockville, Maryland.

Gold, M. S. and Rea, W. S. (1983). The role of endorphines in opiate addiction, opiate withdrawal and recovery. *Psychiatric clinics of North America*, Vol. 6, pp. 489–520.

Goldstein, A. (1976). New approaches to the treatment of heroin addiction: STEPS (Sequential Treatment Employing Pharmacological Supports). *Arch. gen. Psychiat.* **33**, 353–8.

Hargreaves, W. A. (1983). Methadone dose and duration for maintenance treatment. In *Research on the treatment of narcotic addiction* (ed. J. R. Cooper), pp. 19–94. US Department of Health & Human Services, Rockville, Maryland.

Hartnoll, R. L., Mitcheson, M. C., Battersby, A., Brown, G., Ellis, M. Fleming, P., and Hedley, N. (1980). Evaluation of heroin maintenance in a controlled trial. *Arch. gen. Psychiat.* **37**, 877–84.

Her Majesty's Government (1982). Report to the United Nations by Her Majesty's Government in the U.K. on the workings of the International Convention of Narcotic Drugs, p. 23.

Jasinski, D. R., Pevnick, J. S., and Griffith, J. D. (1978). Human pharmacology and abuse potential of the analgesic buprenorphine. *Arch. gen. Psychiat.* **35**, 501–16.

Kandel, D. B. and Faust, R. (1975). Sequence and stages in patterns of adolescent drug use. *Arch. gen. Psychiat.* **32**, 923–32.

McGlothlin, W. H. and Anglin, M. D. (1981). Long-term follow-up of clients of high and low-dose methadone programmes. *Arch. gen. Psychiat.* **38**, 1055–63.

Mello, N. K., Mendelson, J. H., and Kuehnle, J. C. (1982). Buprenorphine effects on heroin self-administration: an operant analysis. *J. Pharmac. exp. Ther.* **223**, 30–9.

Prince, R. (1982). The endorphines, a review for psychological anthropologists. *Ethos* **10**, 303–16.

Renault, P. F. (1978). Treatment of heroin dependent persons with antagonists, current status. *Bulletin on Narcotics* **20**, 21–9.

Stimson, G. V. and Ogborne, A. C. (1970). Survey of addicts prescribed heroin at London clinics. *Lancet* **i**, 1163.

22

Alcohol

DAVID CURSON

THE HISTORICAL PERSPECTIVE

> And Noah began to be an husbandman, and he planted a vineyard: And he drank of the wine, and was drunken; and he was uncovered within his tent.
>
> Genesis, 9:20–1.

The pharmacological activity and the behavioural effects of alcohol have been known since the dawn of civilization. Indeed, the occupational hazards of the wine trade were recognized even then!

Brewing of alcohol from dates, honey, and grapes was a common practice in the Middle East and Europe long before the rise and spread of Christianity and Islam, even though the chemistry of fermentation and distillation was ill-understood. Scholars in Persia around 800 AD believed a fine invisible powder was emitted when fermented material was boiled: the Arabic phrase for 'the powder' is *Al kohl*, hence the name alcohol (Madden 1979).

The abuse of alcohol was recognized as undesirable by Moslems, for example, though the prohibition of *Khamr* (wine) was gradual. The first Quranic revelation regarding alcohol occurred at Mecca before the Prophet Mohammed emigrated to Medina. Attention was drawn to the distinction between strong drink and good nourishment. The second Quranic revelation was a response to questions by members of Moslem communities about alcohol and gambling to Prophet Mohammed. He replied: 'They question thee about strong drink and gambling. Say: In both is great sin and some usefulness for men — but their sin is greater than their usefulness'. The third step towards complete prohibition is said to have occurred after one Imam led the prayer in Medina while he was drunk (Hammad 1983).

Since those early times there have been major technical advances in the mass production of alcoholic beverages but their use, and attempts at the prevention of abuse are clearly not new. Contemporary societies throughout the world continue to struggle with the problem while at the same time levying taxes and duties to bring in substantial, and in many instances, essential revenue to the state or nation.

THE PSYCHOPHARMACOLOGY OF ALCOHOL

The pharmacology of ethyl alcohol or ethanol is too well-known to be reiterated in detail. It has been eloquently summarized by Madden (1979). Absorption of alcohol rapidly takes place through the mucosa of the gastrointestinal tract and lungs. After drining alcohol its effects are pronounced within half an hour. Its depressant action on the central nervous system first affects the higher cerebral functions responsible for concern about personal behaviour and for self-restraint. This results in euphoria and apparent stimulation with vivacity of speech and action. As drinking progresses reaction time is slowed and muscle control impaired. Alcohol is 30 times more soluble in water than fat and is rapidly distributed throughout the body. The average rate of fall of blood alcohol concentration is about 15 mg per 100 ml per hour. Over 80 per cent of absorbed alcohol is metabolized by the liver. Tissue tolerance in the nervous system rather than metabolic tolerance occurs in regular moderate users as well as habitual heavy drinkers.

For a psychopharmacologist the response of the neurological system to varying doses and blood levels of alcohol might appear uncomplicated, but the more subtle (and sometimes not so subtle) variations of experience and actions which characterize human behaviour under the influence of alcohol are far from simple. The anticipated effect, the behavioural consequences, the tendency to repeat consumption, and the establishment of drinking patterns, are to a very large degree determined by cultural factors and the social setting in which drinking behaviour is practised and learned. MacAndrew and Egerton (1970) remind us that:

When man lifts a cup it is not only the kind of drink that is in it, the amount he is likely to take, and the circumstances under which he will do the drinking that are specified in advance for him, but also whether the contents of the cup will cheer or stupify, whether they will induce affection or aggression, guilt or unalloyed pleasure. These and many other cultural definitions attach to the drink even before it touches the lips.

Put another way, why is it that if six Glaswegian dockers and six vicars from Surrey were to drink the same amount in their separate groups at a social occasion the former would probably end up fighting and the latter giggling, telling hazardous anecdotes, and falling off their chairs?

If we are to understand alcohol, and especially its abuse, it is necessary to consider such factors. Laboratory rats may have their uses but they tell us little that is meaningful about how the drug is used by individuals and groups at different times and in different contexts. This becomes imperative for the scientific investigation of normal and abnormal drinking practices and their psychological and physical consequences. Without realistic concepts and definitions, as well as a workable classification system, the most sophisticated biochemistry will tell us nothing. Before proceeding to the abnormal, and at times harmful, use of alcohol it would be worth briefly examining at least some of the possible reasons for these intra-individual and inter-individual differences.

SOCIAL AND CULTURAL INFLUENCES ON DRINKING BEHAVIOUR

Rules and standards governing the place of drinking are well defined within single social or subcultural groups. From earliest times drinking has been integrated into social occasions, religious rituals, and various rites from the cradle to the grave. Social anthropological field studies have shown how drink-related cultural practices can range from total rejection to the most enthusiastic use. Though the form of drinking is usually explicitly stipulated, including the choice of beverage, the amount and rate of intake, the time and place of drinking, the sex and age of the drinker, and the whole range of behaviours proper to drinking, they are frequently implicit and carried informally in the culture (Robinson 1977).

In our own (late twentieth-century British) culture children acquire their knowledge by hearsay, direct observation of drinking and its consequences in their elders, and, on occasions, by experimenting themselves. Two studies in Glasgow and one in England are probably applicable to British children generally.

Jahoda and Cramond (1972) found that most children began learning about alcohol at home and had formed definite impressions before primary school. Two-fifths of six-year-olds could identify alcoholic drinks by smell, and by the age of ten three-fifths could do so. Many children tasted alcohol when quite young, they often saw it and could recognize it, and more than half of the Glasgow children attributed drunken behaviour on film to drinking. Most of those under six had encountered drunken adults. From the outset, boys were encouraged to sample drinks more than girls and there were major sex differences in later use of alcohol.

A second Glasgow study by Davies and Stacey (1972) examined alcohol use in 14- to 17-year-olds. As children grew older, home influences diminished and the teenage peer group became dominant. At 14 years, 92 per cent of boys and 85 per cent of girls had tasted alcohol. Within the next three years all but 2 per cent of the boys and 4 per cent of the girls had tried it. The extreme and negative prepubertal attitudes had changed to those in which drinkers were seen as sociable and tough, whilst abstainers were socially undesirable, weak, and unsociable. Drinking regularly occurred because their friends did it and because it was prestigious.

A more recent survey of over 7000 English children aged 13 to 18 years supported the Glasgow findings (Hawker 1978). Most children had established regular drinking habits in their early teens although the desired norm was light or moderate drinking and such approval did not extend to heavy drinking which was perceived as excessive and unsociable.

Moderate drinking parents may provide a useful model for their children, since those who go on to develop alcohol problems as adults often come from homes in which the parents were alcohol abusers or total abstainers (O'Connor 1978).

SOCIAL LEARNING AND CONDITIONING

It should be evident that drinkers are involved in some sort of learning process which involves the association of objects or events in life with specific results. Whilst many of the mechanisms are not fully understood, the law of effect suggests, as far as it goes, that if the response to a stimulus such as alcohol is pleasant or 'positive', the behaviour will be reinforced or strengthened. If drinking has beneficial results, it will tend to continue; if it is not beneficial, drinkers will be less inclined to drink (Plant 1979). For the majority, imbibing alcohol is usually pleasant. Low doses of the drug induce euphoria, relaxation, and disinhibition, in a fairly predictable and acceptable form. High dose may induce dysphoria, unacceptable social behaviour, and acute physical illness in a less predictable way. Trial and error, moulded by assimilated attitudes, permit titration of dose against anticipated and desired response. Initially, such behaviour is self-determined, until judgement is so distorted and disturbed by the drug that the achievement of anticipated response is more difficult. Modelling, social expectations, social, personal, and group reinforcement as well as the pharmacological effects on mood, perception, impulse control and behaviour all contribute to the attitudes to alcohol and the quality and frequency of drinking behaviour (Curson 1982).

Drinkers drink for differing reasons at different times and this is reflected in terms of beverage choice, place of consumption, social pressure to drink, social and financial circumstances, and social role. The reasons and antecedent cues for the first, second, third, and last drink may be quite different. Yet drinking habits are subject to change and for the majority of young alcohol abusers, for example, this change is frequently facilitated by the development of enduring personal relationships or a change in occupational status which serves to disengage them from a heavy-drinking peer group (Cahalan, Cissin, and Crosslev 1969). When someone drinks heavily it is usually for social and personal reasons, but it may be linked to type of job, availability of alcohol, and financial resources. For many male heavy drinkers in our own culture drinking is their main social activity. The 'local pub' and the 'club', be it working mens' or golf, are familiar centres for such pursuits.

Superimposed upon the social context of drinking, and irrespective of culture, are the specific and personal effects that alcohol may have on anxiety, depression, boredom, loneliness, premenstrual tension, and many other states of mind or circumstances. When seen against a background of constitutional factors such as trait anxiety, temperament, predisposition to hangover effect, impulse control, and perhaps inherited characteristics which determine amount consumed (*British Medical Journal*, 1980); each drinker develops values and behaviours which originate from multiple sources and experiences and each may have a different degree of impact at different times.

DEPENDENCE AND ABUSE

Even this briefest of reviews of some social and cultural aspects of drinking behaviour should alert the unwary to the problems ahead in defining and classifying alcohol abuse and dependence.

The World Health Organization (1974) attempted to define psychological dependence as a condition in which a drug not only promotes a feeling of satisfaction but also a drive to repeat the consumption of that drug in order to induce pleasure or avoid discomfort. However, it is not a clearly-defined state and not necessarily abnormal in its own right (Davies 1976). If some type of activity were substituted for 'drug' the same then could apply to golf, football, hang-gliding, gambling, crosswords, skiing, financial dealing on the stockmarket, and even sex. There may be something more than the intrinsic pharmacological properties of a chemical in the concept of dependence or addiction.

The more severe degrees of alcohol dependence may be identified reliably and accurately and some homogeneity emerges. The alcohol dependence syndrome (Edwards and Gross 1976) is characterized by a number of features varying in degree of intensity. These are: the narrowing of drinking repertoires, the salience of drink seeking behaviour, increased tolerance, physical withdrawal symptoms, subjective awareness of a compulsion to drink, drinking to relieve and allay withdrawal symptoms, and the reinstatement of the syndrome after a period of abstinence. The utility of the concept was explored by Hodgson, Stockwell, Rankin, and Edwards (1978) and Stockwell, Hodgson, Edwards, and Rankin (1979), and its predictive value in terms of drinking outcome was described in a follow-up study (Hodgson 1980). The syndrome (ADS) does not imply an illness state in its own right but is a psychobiological state with significant social and cultural components.

The psychopharmacologist may now sense some uniformity and the hope of measurable indices of disorder or dysfunction. Alas, it is a false dawn. Although such phenomena are measurable and have predictive value under certain circumstances they are generally relevant only when the person is actively drinking or returning to drinking. An alcohol-dependent person is just like anyone else when not drinking.

We are now in the field of alcoholism and rather than getting easier the terrain gets more difficult. While similarities emerge as total alcohol consumption rises, often to quite heroic levels, the differences increase once drinking ceases. The notion of the typical 'alcoholic personality' can be dismissed. No such evidence exists for the overwhelming majority of problem drinkers (Kessel and Walton 1969; Kammeier, Hoffman, and Loper 1973) and as Lederman (1956) observed as per capita alcohol consumption increases in a society, more 'normal' people develop drinking problems. The principle cause of alcoholism appears to be alcohol (Royal College of Psychiatrists 1979).

To add to the semantic confusion (alcoholism, alcohol dependence, alcohol-related disability, alcohol addict, problem drinker, etc.) there is a continuing dispute over alcoholism as a 'disease' entity. The complex philosophical and nosological issues have been well-reviewed by Madden (1979), and Heather and Robertson (1981). The rediscovery of a disease model over 40 years ago, in which Alcoholics Anonymous and its medical sympathizers played a major part, was motivated by practical rather than theoretical issues. In the words of Room (1972):

the promulgation of disease concepts of alcoholism has been brought about essentially as a means of getting a better deal for the 'alcoholic' rather than as a logical consequence of scholarly work and scientific discoveries.

In effect, the disease model removes the alcoholic's behaviour from the realm of choice and moral obligation, and absolves him (or her) from responsibility for his deviant actions in law.

The scientific basis of the disease model was seriously flawed from the outset. Litman (1982) observed that E. M. Jellinek rightly deserves tribute as one of the great pioneers of research into alcoholism. What is not so widely recognized is that many of his statements about alcoholism as a disease and the phenomena of 'loss of control' were actually obtained from a questionnaire designed by members of Alcoholics Anonymous and circulated through their official organ. Based on only 98 responses received, Jellinek concluded:

Loss of control means that as soon as a small quantity of alcohol enters the organism a demand for more alcohol is set up which is felt as a physical demand by the drinker. The drinker has lost the ability to control the quantity once he has started (Jellinek 1952).

That such myths have been perpetuated and virtually unchallenged during the next three decades is not the fault of Jellinek.

One principle characteristic of severe alcohol-dependence is that it tends to be a chronic, relapsing condition (Litman 1982). Yet remarkably little research into relapse has been conducted until recently. There would appear to be a variety of reasons for the lack of interest in relapse and some of these might be attributed to the disease model. If a return to drinking is caused by 'craving' and the continuation of drinking is due to 'loss of control', what further enquiry is necessary? The residues of the moralistic model of alcoholism may have also contributed, since the explanations given by the drinker for a return to drinking were dismissed as excuses or alibis. Research into process rather than outcome reveals that the natural history of the condition is for people to move into and out of phases of problem drinking and dependence, and so-called spontaneous remission further complicates the measurement of efficacy of treatment (Polich, Armor, and Braiker 1979; Cahalan *et al.* 1969; Yates and Norris 1981). The nature of relapse precipitants has been studied only relatively recently, though relapse itself has been the concern of clinicians for decades (Litman, Eiser, Rawson and Oppenheim 1977). For the majority of alcoholics studied in this way such precipitants (and the reciprocal coping strategies) appear to be cognitively based (Marlatt and Gordon 1980; Litman, Stapleton, Oppenheim, and Peleg 1983). Alcohol-induced brain damage, whether reversible or irreversible, is one of the potentially catastrophic complications of prolonged heavy drinking. If the reliable self-evaluation of drinking behaviour and the appropriate coping strategies are cognitively-mediated, the research on CT scans and neuropsychological impairment (Ron 1983) has major repercussions for the continuation of such a habit, the initiation of help-seeking, and the response to treatment or help offered.

THE ROLE OF DRUGS IN ALCOHOLISM TREATMENT

So what has psychopharmacology got to offer in the way of aetiological explanation, prevention, and even treatment of alcohol dependence and problem drinking, which are reaching epidemic proportions in the Western world? At our present state of knowledge, the answer has to be: very little for the vast majority of uncomplicated cases. Indeed, untimely and inappropriate pharmacological intervention with drugs such as the benzodiazepines (Petursson and Lader 1981) almost certainly complicates and often exacerbates the existing problem. Benzodiazepines and Chlormethiazole are useful in very short courses during detoxification. Anticonvulsants, vitamin B preparations, and phenothiazines may prevent some of the more serious neuropsychiatric complications of alcohol withdrawal. Disulfiram and calcium carbamide are an important and effective adjunct to treatment for motivated problem drinkers who wish to pursue a goal of total abstention (Costello 1975). It should be noted, however, that they work psychologically and not chemically as a deterrent. The decision to use them is the drinker's.

Any clinician who has been involved in trying to help those with drinking problems knows that dependence may develop as a result of or in association with psychiatric disorders such as affective illnesses and phobic anxiety states. Yet the psychiatric assessment of people who consume large quantities of a depressant substance which leads to depressing consequences is extremely difficult. Whilst the prevalence of phobic states in alcoholics may be found in about a third of those admitted to a treatment unit (Mullaney and Trippett 1979), it is unclear how much phobic anxiety may contribute to the development and perpetuation of abnormal drinking. There is some evidence that excessive alcohol consumption may worsen existing phobic anxiety states and even cause them (Smail, Stockwell, Canter, and Hodgson 1984; Stockwell *et al.* 1984).

The effective treatment of affective illness and phobic anxiety which are not artefacts of heavy drinking will invariably improve the prognosis provided that simultaneous treatment is offered for the drinking problem. This approach to treatment is no more than the induction of change in relapse precipitants or antecedent drinking cues and is not a direct influence on drinking behaviour or dependence (Murray and Murphy 1978).

CONCLUSION

A realistic appreciation of the complexity of drinking behaviour and the current concepts of drinking problems, alcohol dependence, and alcoholism would seem to be essential if valid comparison is to be made between samples of drinkers with the aim of establishing biochemical and pharmacological correlates and associations. The old, simplistic classification must be abandoned but, as yet, no new system of classification has emerged. This is one of the great challenges of contemporary behavioural science.

Psychopharmacology may have something to offer on a long-term basis. Littleton (1984) has suggested that the most profitable areas for continuing research would include the identification of the individual at risk of specific alcohol-related physical disease, intervention to reduce the positively reinforcing effects of alcohol ingestion as well as the negatively reinforcing properties of abstinence, and prevention of alcohol-induced harm.

Sitting in an armchair at the end of a long day and nursing a gin and tonic, it is tempting to speculate about the future. It is theoretically possible to combine advances in immunology with developments in the pharmacokinetics of alcohol metabolism (Kidger 1984). Isoenzymes of alcohol dehydrogenase probably operate differentially at high and low levels of alcohol concentration — high Km and low Km (Von Wartburg 1984). Monoclonal antibodies might be developed to knock out either. This would offer two types of 'vaccination': one for controlled drinkers, who would experience the equivalent of a disulfiram reaction after more than a couple of drinks, and one for total abstainers, who would experience the same reaction at very low levels of alcohol consumption. Attractive as this idea may sound, the ethical considerations make those of psychosurgery pale into insignificance.

REFERENCES

British Medical Journal (1980). Alcoholism: an inherited disease? **281**, 1301–2.

Cahalan, D., Cissin, I. H., and Crossley, H. M. (1969). *American drinking practices: a national study of drinking behavior and attitudes*. Monograph No. 6. Rutgers Centre for Alcohol Studies, New Brunswick.

Costello, R. M. (1975). Alcoholism treatment and evaluations: In search of Methods II Collation of Two year follow-up studies. *Int. J. Addict.* **10** (5), 857–67.

Curson, D. A. (1982). Alcoholics, drinkers, and drunks. In *Personal Meanings* (ed. E. Shepherd and J. P. Watson). John Wiley, Chichester.

Davies, D. L. (1976). Definitional issues in alcoholism. In *Alcoholism: interdisciplinary approaches to an enduring problem*. Addison-Wesley, Mass.

Davies, J. and Stacey, B. (1972). *Teenagers and alcohol: A developmental study in Glasgow*, Vol. 1. HMSO, London.

Edwards, G. and Gross, M. M. (1976). Alcohol dependence: provisional description of a clinical syndrome. *Br. med. J.* **1**, 1058–61.

Hammad, G. (1983). Alcoholism: a new danger in the Islamic World. First International Medical Seminar, Tehran (unpublished manuscript).

Hawker, A. (1978). *Adolescents and alcohol*. Edsall, London.

Heather, N. and Robertson, I. (1981). *Controlled drinking*. Methuen, London.

Hodgson, R., Stockwell, T., Rankin, H., and Edwards, G. (1978). Alcohol dependence: the concept, its utility and measurement. *Br. J. Addict.* **73**, 339–42.

Hodgson, R. J. (1980). Treatment strategies for early problem drinkers. In *Alcoholism treatment in transition* (ed. G. Edwards and M. Grant). Croom-Helm, London.

Jahoda, G. and Cramond, J. (1972). *Children and alcohol: A developmental study in Glasgow*, Vol. 1. HMSO, London.

Jellinek, E. M. (1952). The phases of alcohol addiction. *Q. J. Stud. Alcohol* **13**, 673–84.

Kammeier, M. L., Hoffman, H., and Loper, R. G. (1973). Personality of alcoholics as college freshmen and at the time of treatment. *Q. J. Stud. Alcohol* **34**, 390–9.

Kessel, N. and Walton, H. (1969). *Alcoholism*. Penguin, London.

Kidger, T. (1984). Personal communication.

Lederman, S. (1956). *Alcool, alcoolisme, alcoolisation*. Institut National d'Etudes Demographiques Cahiers No. 29, Presses Universitaires de France, Paris.

Litman, G. K. (1982). Personal meanings and alcoholism survival: translating subjective experience into empirical data. In *Personal meanings* (ed. E. Shepherd and J. P. Watson). John Wiley, Chichester.

—, Eiser, J. R., Rawson, N. S. B., and Oppenheim, A. N. (1977). Towards a typology of relapse: a preliminary report. *Drug & Alcohol Depend.* **2**, 157–62.

—, Stapleton, J., Oppenheim, A. N., and Peleg, M. (1983). An instrument for measuring coping behaviours in hospitalized alcoholics: implications for relapse prevention treatment. *Br. J. Addict.* **78**, 269–76.

Littleton, J. M. (1984). The future could be bright. In *Pharmacological treatments for alcoholism* (ed. G. Edwards and J. M. Littleton). Croom-Helm, London & Sydney; and Methuen, New York.

Madden, J. S. (1979). *Alcohol and drug dependence*. John Wright, Bristol.

MacAndrew, C. and Egerton, R. B. (1970). *Drunken comportment; a social explanation*. Nelson, London.

Marlatt, G. A. and Gordon, J. R. (1980). Determinants of relapse: Implications for the maintenance of behaviour change. *Behavioural medicine: changing health life styles* (ed. P. O. Davidson and S. M. Davidson). Brunner Mazel, New York.

Mullaney, J. A. and Trippett, C. J. (1979). Alcohol dependence and phobias: clinical description and relevance. *Br. J. Psychiat.* **135**, 656–73.

Murray, R. M. and Murphy, D. N. (1978). Drug response and psychiatric nosology. *Psychol. Med.* **8**, 667–81.

O'Connor, J. (1978). *The young drinkers*. Tavistock, London.

Petursson, H. and Lader, M. H. (1981). Benzodiazepine dependence. *Br. J. Addict.* **76** (2), 133–46.

Plant, M. A. (1979). Learning to drink. In *Alcoholism in perspective* (ed. M. Grant). Croom-Helm, London.

Polich, J. M., Armor, D. J., and Braiker, H. B. (1979). *The course of alcoholism: four years after treatment.* The Rand Corp., Santa Monica.

Robinson, D. (1977). Factors of influencing alcohol consumption. In *Alcoholism: new knowledge and new responses* (ed. G. Edwards and M. Grant). Croom-Helm, London.

Ron, M. A. (1983). *The alcoholic brain: CT scan and psychological findings. Psychol. Med.* Monogr. Suppl. 3.

Room, R. (1972). Comments on Robinson D. 'The alcohologists addiction'. *Q. J. Stud. Alcohol* **33**, 1049-59.

Royal College of Psychiatrists (1979). *Alcohol and alcoholism:* The report of a Special Committee of The Royal College of Psychiatrists (Chairman: G. Edwards). Tavistock, London.

Smail, P., Stockwell, T., Canter, S., and Hodgson, R. (1984). Alcohol dependence and phobic anxiety states I A prevalence study. *Br. J. psychiat.* **144**, 53-7.

Stockwell, T., Hodgson, R., Edwards, G., and Rankin, H. (1979). The development of a questionnaire to measure severity of alcohol dependence. *Br. J. Addict.* **74**, 79-87.

——, Smail, P., Hodgson, R., and Canter, S. (1984). Alcohol dependence and phobic anxiety states II A retrospective study. *Br. J. Psychiat.* **144**, 58-63.

Von Wartburg, J. P. (1984). Pharmacokinetics of alcohol in the normal and alcoholic subject. In *Pharmacological treatments for alcoholism* (ed. G. Edwards and J. M. Littleton). Croom-Helm, London & Sydney; and Methuen, New York.

World Health Organization (1974). *Expert committee on drug dependence: Twentieth report.* WHO Tech. Rep. Ser. No. 55.

Yates, F. E. and Norris, H. (1981). The use made of treatment: an alternative approach to the evaluation of alcoholism services. *Behav. Psychother.* **9** (4), 291-309.

23

Central nervous system stimulants

L. G. BROOKES

INTRODUCTION

A large number of natural and synthetic substances are capable of effecting stimulation of the central nervous system (CNS) in man and other animals, but few have a legitimate role in therapeutics today. This chapter will address those compounds commonly referred to as the 'amphetamines' and will not include the analeptics or convulsants such as strychnine, picrotoxin, or pentylenetetrazol since these latter drugs are now mostly only of toxicological interest.

The amphetamines are sympathomimetic amines that differ from the catecholamines primarily in that they are effective when given orally, and most have comparatively long biological half-lives. Chemically, the amphetamines, like the biogenic amines adrenaline and noradrenaline, can be represented as derivatives of phenylethylamine. Amphetamine, methylamphetamine, ephedrine, and methylphenidate, probably the best known members of this group of compounds, and well recognized for their psychomotor stimulant properties, were all widely prescribed for a variety of conditions for many years. Newer molecules subsequently introduced for the more selective treatment of the conditions indicated but without the attendant CNS stimulant effects of amphetamine, have now almost completely replaced that drug in therapeutic practice, although its uncontrolled, illicit use has increased significantly. Amphetamine has a very limited application in medicine today, but it is of key importance in psychopharmacology, being relevant to the mechanisms of action of both antipsychotic and antidepressant drugs, catecholamine physiology and pharmacology, and also to the psychoses produced.

In this chapter, information is presented on the pharmacological and psychopharmacological effect of the amphetamines and their mode of action, together with a review of their current use and abuse, attendant side-effects and toxicity and methods for treating drug overdose, dependence, and psychosis.

ABSORPTION, DISTRIBUTION, METABOLISM, AND EXCRETION

The intensity of psychomotor stimulant action depends on the specific activity of the stimulant and on its concentration at the site of action, i.e. the neurones in certain areas of the brain. The concentration of drug in the brain in turn depends on the drug plasma concentration, but this relationship has not yet been well defined in respect to the amphetamines.

Following oral administration, the amphetamines are readily absorbed, predominantly from the small intestine, and attain a peak plasma concentration within 1–2 h following administration. Absorption is essentially complete in 2.5–4 h and is accelerated rather than impeded by ingestion of a simple meal. All amphetamines are rapidly distributed extravascularly and are readily absorbed into the brain and the cerebrospinal fluid. By comparison, the catecholamines pass the blood–brain barrier only with difficulty.

The metabolism of the amphetamines has been the subject of many investigations in man and other animal species for several years (see Caldwell 1980, and references cited therein). There are well-defined species differences in the metabolism of these compounds, which must be considered when animal species are being chosen for experiments purporting to have relevance to the human situation. Metabolism of amphetamine in the dog and monkey most closely resembles its biotransformation in man. As Caldwell has pointed out, a knowledge of the metabolism of the amphetamines is essential in the area of drug abuse since it has important pharmacological and forensic implications.

Many of the metabolites of the amphetamines retain pharmacological activity and may be responsible for or contribute to certain effects of these drugs. In particular, certain hydroxylated metabolites (see later) resemble noradrenaline so closely in structure as to be able to be stored in noradrenergic neurones and replace noradrenaline and to undergo release and reuptake in the same way as the neurotransmitters (Brodie, Cho, and Gessa 1970). Such metabolites are termed 'false neurotransmitters' and have been causally related to the development of tolerance to certain actions of amphetamine.

All the amphetamines are partially excreted via the kidney unchanged. In addition to glomerular filtration, there is tubular secretion. Tubular reabsorption of the amphetamines is substantial and is related to their structures and physical properties, the most significant of which is their lipid solubility.

PHARMACOLOGY AND MODE OF ACTION

It is not possible to identify the exact mode of action of amphetamine and the observed effects are thought to be due to a number of contributory mechanisms. Four possible mechanisms of action of the drug are currently considered as of importance; (a) inhibition of monoamine oxidase activity, (b) release of catecholamines from neuronal binding sites, (c) inhibition of neuronal reuptake of catecholamines and serotonin, and, (d) direct action on the catecholamine and serotonin receptors. These four theories all appear to contribute towards the net effect of amphetamine, but the release of catechoamines appears to be the most important of the actions listed. Amphetamine is also capable of promoting the release *in vivo* of extragranular stores of serotonin from the serotonergic nerve terminals of the corpus striatum and high doses of amphetamine have been shown to enhance the release of acetylcholine from the cerebral cortex.

In the striatum, but not elsewhere, amphetamine decreases dopamine synthesis. The drug activates the diffuse projection systems both upwards to the cerebral cortex through ascending reticular pathways and downwards to the brain stem and spinal cord.

The behavioural effects of amphetamine comprise enhanced locomotor activity, alertness, facilitation of conditioned reflexes, self stimulation and an elevation of mood — all of which are probably mainly related to noradrenergic pathways. It is this powerful CNS stimulant activity which gives the amphetamines their high abuse potential. Amphetamine is a potent anorectic and elevates both plasma free fatty acids and body temperature. The peripheral effects are all of the sympathomimetic type; a constriction of blood vessels, an increase in blood pressure and heart rate, dilatation of the pupils and bronchioles and relaxation of the smooth muscle of the gastrointestinal tract. In higher doses, excessive pupillary dilatation, hypertension, and tachycardia prevail. The various psychomotor stimulant drugs differ greatly in their relative potencies of central stimulant and peripheral sympathomimetic effects and some observers have noted a mixed heterogeneous response in humans; some become drowsy, with reduced electrical brain activity in the first hours of drug administration, whereas others show increased alertness with increased electrical brain activity (Cole 1967).

Noradrenaline and dopamine are now generally considered to be neurotransmitters in the brain and these compounds have received considerable attention with respect to their contributions to the action of amphetamine.

Reserpine, which causes 80–90 per cent depletion of neuronal noradrenaline, has little effect on the locomotor activity or stereotyped behaviours elicited by amphetamine. Inhibition of the ongoing biosynthesis of catecholamines with α-methyltyrosine, however, abolishes these effects of amphetamine. Both effects can be restored by levodopa. On this evidence, it has been suggested that some of the central actions of amphetamine, particularly stereotyped behaviour, depend upon release of dopamine. Amphetamine is able to facilitate self-stimulation in rats implanted with electrodes in reward areas of the hypothalamus and in midbrain areas. This effect can be blocked by dopamine-β-hydroxylase inhibitors, and is reversed by intraventricular administration of noradrenaline but not dopamine. This also suggests that noradrenaline plays an important role in certain aspects of amphetamine's central action (Caldwell and Sever 1974). The role of 5-hydroxytryptamine in the mediation of amphetamine-induced CNS stimulation is at present a matter for speculation. It has been shown that in rats the development of tolerance to the effects of amphetamine upon operant behaviour is accompanied by release of brain 5-HT, in contrast to the drug naïve state, in which noradrenaline only was released. Treatments which inhibit the degradation of catecholamines, such as monoamine oxidase inhibitors, enhance the behavioural effects of amphetamine.

There is normally a surge in prolactin secretion associated with sleep, throughout the night. Shaywitz, Hunt, and Jatlow (1982) have provided evidence to show that a clinical response to methylphenidate is related to a significant reduction in plasma prolactin concentration and an increase in growth hormone levels. Plasma levels of methylphenidate correlated well with percentage improvement in the clinical response. This endocrine change has also been noted by other workers using amphetamine in chronic therapy for hyperkinetic children. Within one month of treatment with amphetamine the prolactin surge was markedly diminished even though sleep patterns remained as normal. Since prolactin secretion is inhibited by dopamine it is considered that its suppression was due to amphetamine's dopaminergic action. Although growth hormone was secreted as normal, every child treated also displayed a reduced growth velocity during this period. Since prolactin is a growth factor it is possible that its suppression accounted for this side-effect of amphetamine therapy.

Groves and Rebec (1976) have made an excellent review of the correlates of long-term amphetamine administration in which they demonstrate the significant contribution of the hydroxylated metabolites of amphetamine to its apparent pharmacological actions. The metabolite primarily responsible is *p*-hydroxynorephedrine, a secondary metabolite produced by the action of dopamine-β-hydroxylase on the primary metabolite *p*-hydroxyamphetamine. The half-life of *p*-hydroxynorephedrine in the brain is considerably longer than that of either amphetamine or its *para*-hydroxylated metabolite, suggesting that this compound could be responsible, at least in part, for the sustained reduction in levels of noradrenaline during chronic amphetamine intoxication. Indeed, there seems to be a stoichiometric relationship between the persistence of noradrenaline depletion and the tissue concentration of *p*-hydroxynorephedrine. Both hydroxylated metabolites of amphetamine, however, are capable of promoting the release and blocking the reuptake of catecholamines almost as efficiently as the parent compound. They are also capable of producing locomotor and stereotyped behaviours following intraventricular injection in rats. The ability of these hydroxylated metabolites to alter brain dopamine levels, however, is transient and not so pronounced.

AMPHETAMINE PSYCHOSIS

The most frequent and serious toxic manifestation associated with the consumption of (any of) the amphetamines is the 'amphetamine psychosis', a clinical syndrome in which the drug elicits a peculiar series of motor behaviours and thought disturbances. This psychotic reaction closely resembles paranoid schizophrenia. The psychosis generally (though not necessarily always) follows chronic drug administration, with an increased incidence in persons consuming large doses. However, there have been isolated instances where a single dose of 55 mg free base equivalent or more has produced the same effect, particularly when administered intravenously. The amphetamines generally are capable of precipitating a psychotic reaction in patients with an underlying schizophrenic tendency and (especially with methylphenidate) in this context have been used to diagnose the condition. Once an amphetamine psychosis has occurred it is generally more likely that a relapse may be precipitated with only a large single dose. This aspect of amphetamine toxicity was first comprehensively reviewed by Connell in 1958, and subsequently by several other authors including Kalant (1973), and Davis and Schlemmer (1981). Interestingly, the occurrence of an amphetamine psychosis is an extremely rare event during the treatment of hyperkinetic children with amphetamine.

Kokkinidis and Anisman (1980) have presented a comprehensive review of amphetamine models of paranoid schizophrenia in which they evaluate the neurochemical and behavioural changes induced by acute and chronic amphetamine administration, particularly as they pertain to drug-induced psychosis and paranoid schizophrenia.

Patients presenting with an amphetamine psychosis may display any or all of the following characteristics; delusions of persecution (most cases), anxiety, fear and terror, agitation, hyperactivity, hostility, depression, and auditory, visual, tactile and/or olfactory illusions or hallucinations, paranoid ideation, stereotyped, compulsive behaviour, social withdrawal, autistic behaviour, and hypervigilance. However, virtually all patients remain orientated, although they are easily distracted and have poor powers of attention and concentration. The clinical condition is indistinguishable from paranoid schizophrenia and, since the physical signs of amphetamine intoxication are not always present, the diagnosis of amphetamine psychosis has been based on the fact that the symptoms disappear in a matter of days or weeks following drug withdrawal. Connell recommended that chemical tests for detecting amphetamines in urine should also be applied rather than rely solely on the disappearance of the symptoms of the psychosis. Two dissimilarities between the characteristics of amphetamine psychosis and schizophrenia are: (a) more visual hallucinations are seen during amphetamine psychosis than are seen with schizophrenia, and (b) the amphetamine psychosis is almost uniformly a paranoid psychosis, while schizophrenia need not be.

The principal effects noted by the drug users themselves included increased energy, cheerfulness, talkativeness, anorexia, thirst, dry mouth, tremors (particularly of the hands), insomnia and depression on withdrawal, and an inclination to suicide. Libido is not consistently affected. These signs are not considered to be of diagnostic significance however because they could also have resulted from extreme anxiety.

Stereotyped behaviour, or stereotypy, is of particular interest because it is also readily observed in animals (in the form of licking, biting, gnawing, and sniffing), especially rats and mice treated with amphetamine. Rats treated with amphetamine sufficient to produce this stereotypy also tend to demonstrate social withdrawal, to remain hypervigilant and to display many of the other characteristics also seen in man when amphetamine psychosis is present. The occurrence of locomotor activity and stereotyped behaviours following amphetamine administration is dose-dependent and sequentially patterned. Although the stereotypy seen in animals is less complex than that seen in man, the study of amphetamine psychosis in animals is of particular value as a model in the study of paranoid schizophrenia or other endogenous psychoses in man. Monkeys are the best animal model for man.

McMillen (1983) has discussed how the CNS behavioural stimulants can be subdivided into two classes of drugs, depending on whether or not the induced stereotypies and locomotor activities are inhibited by reserpine. Amphetamine, methylamphetamine, and phenmetrazine are not inhibited by reserpine-induced depletion of catecholamines whereas methylphenidate (and cocaine and pipradol) are potently inhibited by reserpine pretreatment. In contrast, if α-methyl-p-tyrosine is used to inhibit catecholamine synthesis, only amphetamine, methylamphetamine and phenmetrazine are inhibited. These results clearly demonstrate two mechanisms of action for producing CNS stimulation. Results from several laboratories have more recently implicated the release of dopamine rather than noradrenaline, by both classes of drugs in the rat brain, as the cause of stereotyped behaviour. Thus, there must be two different mechanisms for enhancing the release of dopamine.

The magnitude of the withdrawal syndrome seen following cessation of dosing with amphetamine, correlates well with the dose(s) used and the chronicity of use, although the lapsed time period between cessation of treatment and the onset of delirium can be of several days. Fatigue and depression are the most common symptoms experienced, together with confusion, sleepiness, and occasionally an enhanced appetite. However, most if not all the psychological and physiological effects of amphetamine are reversible over a period of time. The most obvious symptoms disappear within a few days although some, e.g. confusion, loss of memory, and delusional ideas, may persist for weeks or months. In rare instances a psychosis may persist indefinitely after drug withdrawal, if not treated.

EFFECT OF AMPHETAMINES ON HUMAN PERFORMANCE AND MOOD

The illicit use of amphetamines is almost invariably prompted by the desire to benefit from their effects on performance and/or mood. The review by Weiss and Laties (1962) is probably the most comprehensive of its kind on this subject and they concluded that amphetamine actually does produce a superior performance in a multiplicity of tasks and does not merely restore to a normal level performance degraded by fatigue, boredom or other influences. Both (a) in laboratory studies, when volunteers performed various tasks requiring a high rate of energy input, such as on a bicycle or hand ergometer, and (b) in military field studies, when military personnel performed a wide variety of tasks such as long hikes or marches (with full pack), driving tanks, performing sentry duty, or flying on bombing missions, amphetamines have been shown to be able to

improve performance, increase endurance and reduce fatigue. Athletic performance in such events as putting the shot, swimming, and running has also
been shown to benefit from the administration of these drugs, reaction time
in both normal and fatigued personnel has been reduced, steadiness has increased
and coordination, particularly with more complex tasks, improved. At least in
the short term, amphetamine has been shown to reduce learning time for new
tasks but does not lead to improved intellectual performance except, perhaps,
when normal performance has been degraded by fatigue or boredom. Generally, there was less of an improvement in performance in highly-motivated
individuals.

There are many conflicting reports on the effects of amphetamines on judgement and many have not been adequately controlled studies, but the general
indication is that the amphetamines cause a mild time-distortion which translates
into impaired judgement. In a review of various experimental treatments that
affect memory processes in animals, Lipton, diMascio, and Killam (1978)
describe some studies involving amphetamine and other sympathomimetic
agents. Behaviourally, amphetamine has been shown to disrupt performance of
previously well-learned responses, particularly those requiring timing functions
or active inhibition of behaviour. There is substantial evidence to show that
amphetamine can alter acquisition of a variety of behaviours. For example,
active-avoidance learning is facilitated by amphetamine administered prior to
acquisition. It was concluded that both serotonin and catecholamines were
involved in performance changes induced by amphetamine.

The literature is replete with reports of studies on the effects of the amphetamines on mood. Again, one sees distinct differences from one individual to
another and from drug to drug but the 'positive' effects experienced by subjects
taking these drugs generally include: a feeling that it is relatively easy to perform
a task, coupled with a considerable increase in the desire for work, euphoria,
exhilaration, a feeling of general well-being and an increase in energy, good
humour, talkativeness, restlessness and excitement. Subjects have also reported
feeling less fatigued from the day's work, an increase in mental activity and
efficiency, a more business-like attitude, and feeling clearheaded, efficient,
and ambitious. 'Negative' effects also seen in subjects taking amphetamines
include: anxiety, slowness in reasoning, vertigo, difficulty in concentrating,
exhaustion and tremor, indifference, inward tension, nervousness, irrespons-
ible behaviour, dreaming or drunk feelings, quarrelsomeness, impulsive and
inappropriate activity, irritability and restlessness, and suicidal inclinations.
Mood responses to stimulants are generally thought to be due to actions leading
to stimulations of central catecholamine receptors and Silverstone, Wells, and
Trenchard (1983) have shown the effect of amphetamine on mood to be dose-
related.

TOLERANCE AND DEPENDENCE

Tolerance to many of the effects of the amphetamines develops rapidly and there are several well documented accounts of the regular use of doses of as high as one gram per day, compared to the normal therapeutic dose of 10 mg to 30 mg. This cannot be explained on the basis of increased metabolism or rate of excretion. Chronic administration of amphetamine leads to the persistent depletion of noradrenaline in both central and peripheral sympathetic nervous systems, this being brought about by *p*-hydroxynorephedrine. In animals, tolerance does not develop to the stereotyped behaviour observed with amphetamine nor apparently to the increased locomotor activity. Thus, it appears that the false transmitter hypothesis, which may account for the acquisition of tolerance to noradrenergically mediated effects of amphetamine, cannot account for tolerance developed to other effects of amphetamine, which may be initiated through alternative neuronal mechanisms.

All of these theories as to the development of tolerance to amphetamines are currently speculative but it is undoubtedly the case that several mechanisms are involved.

It is considered that the amphetamines cause drug-dependence, and dependent persons are prone to accidents and psychotic episodes, and display aggressive, antisocial behaviour. While dependence of the amphetamine type does not generally lead to physical dependence, withdrawal is followed by mental and physical depression. Kalant (1973) has presented a comprehensive review of the differences in medical opinion on whether or not these amphetamines are considered habituating or addictive. There is no clear answer to this question since the amphetamines do not fully meet all the requirements of either description.

THERAPEUTIC USE

Prinzmetal and Bloomberg (1935) were the first to use amphetamine in a clinical situation and this was in the treatment of narcolepsy. Other conditions for which amphetamine and certain related compounds were subsequently used included depression, anxiety and agitation, enuresis, post-encephalitic Parkinsonism and hyperkinesis (in children). These drugs were also used to alleviate fatigue and increase endurance in combat troops in World War II. Amphetamine-barbiturate mixtures were used for the treatment of depression but, because of the rapid development of tolerance, neither these drug combinations nor the amphetamines alone were of any permanent value in such situations and were replaced by the tricyclic antidepressants as soon as they became available. The treatment of narcolepsy is now the only unequivocal indication for psychomotor stimulant drug use (Editorial 1968), although even for that use it is now being replaced by tricyclic antidepressants such as clomipramine.

It is their cortical arousal actions which underlie the usefulness of the amphetamines in the management of narcolepsy and this action may also contribute to their well demonstrated usefulness in the childhood syndrome known as 'hyperactivity', hyperkinesis or 'minimal brain dysfunction'. So-called hyperactive or hyperkinetic children have abnormal ECGs, are typically restless, quarrelsome, irritable, and inattentive. Amphetamines act by increasing the attention span and lessening antisocial behaviour. The mechanism whereby the amphetamines affect hyperactive children is not fully understood and, unfortunately, improvement may not persist despite continued treatment. The amphetamines should not be used with psychotic, autistic or brain-damaged children, as increased excitement, agitation or paranoid reactions may develop. Amphetamine is, however, considered to be more effective than chlordiazepoxide in reducing the manifestations of the hyperkinetic syndrome in children.

As indicated earlier, the amphetamines can precipitate a psychotic reaction in patients with an underlying schizophrenia tendency and have been used as a diagnostic agent in this situation.

A second diagnostic use for amphetamine and methylphenidate which has been investigated more recently is in the prediction of response to antidepressants (Sabelli, Fawcett, Javaid, and Bagri 1983). Some studies in psychiatric patients with major depressive disorders indicated that some responded to imipramine or desipramine but not to amitriptyline or nortripytline and vice versa, although plasma levels of the tricyclic antidepressants were within therapeutic ranges. Mood elevation by amphetamine and methylphenidate predicted marked improvement from treatment with imipramine or desipramine but not with amitriptyline or nortriptyline. When amphetamine or methylphenidate failed to improve mood, patients responded favourably to amitriptyline and nortriptyline but not to desipramine. Acute behavioural changes following 20 mg amphetamine i.v. have also been shown to predict the antipsychotic and antidepressant effects of lithium treatment in schizophrenic patients (van Kammen, Docherty, Marder, and Bunney 1981) — the greater the increases in the amphetamine-induced changes in the thought disorder cluster, the greater the antipsychotic effects of lithium. It has also been noted that patients who show a positive mood response to amphetamine and are more responsive to imipramine have a low level of 3-methoxy-4-hydroxyphenylglycol (MHPG), a metabolite of noradrenaline. Patients responsive to amitriptyline have much higher levels of MHPG. Amphetamine has been seen to worsen mood in such patients. In patients with tardive dyskinesias, the intravenous administration of amphetamine has been shown to increase dyskinetic movements, and it has been considered as a diagnostic technique in patients with very minimal symptoms and in those where there is a sound reason to suspect the possibility of such a disorder.

In certain instances, several of the amphetamines have been used beneficially in the treatment of aggression and the suppression of emotional reactions to anger-provoking situations. Occasionally, depressed patients (and especially those with pain) and those with apathy, who have been refractory to treatment with all other antidepressants, have responded positively to amphetamines.

Amphetamines have also been used as anorectic agents in obese patients and Silverstone *et al.* (1983) have presented date to show that the appetite-suppressant effect of amphetamine is independent of its stimulant effects.

ILLICIT USE

In the 1960s an explosive increase in the non-medical use of amphetamines occurred as part of the general increase in the consumption of a variety of psychoactive drugs. Consumption of these drugs occurred predominantly in North America and in some parts of Europe. Surveys showed that the extent of use of amphetamines in North America, particularly by late teenagers and young adults was exceeded only by that of alcohol, tobacco and marihuana. In Sweden and Czechoslovakia and some other countries, phenmetrazine was the drug of choice, while in the UK, a short-lived epidemic of intravenous use of methyl-amphetamine occurred in 1968. From the time of this increase in the 1960s, the pattern of amphetamine use developed from mainly oral to more predominantly parenteral administration with the specific additional complication of the rapidity and intensity of the onset of drug effect, and hence the rate and strength of development of psychological dependence. However, the basic problems associated with amphetamine abuse are common to both methods of intake. Essentially, where there is dependence on amphetamines, behavioural and psychiatric complications develop in a comparable manner, regardless of the mode of intake and of the age, social status or life-style of the user (see Kalant 1973, and references cited therein).

Since the introduction of stricter legislation, which has significantly curbed the prescribing of amphetamines, there has been a marked increase in the use of phenylpropanolamine (norephedrine). This drug substance is currently available in a plethora of over-the-counter preparations (in slimming aids and nasal decongestants) which, in Australia and the USA in particular, have been heavily promoted on television, in magazines, and in the press. Unfortunately, phenylpropanolamine is also a sympathomimetic compound with actions very similar to amphetamine and ephedrine, and it has the potential for producing exactly the same side-effects, many of which have already been sustained (Blum 1981). More recently, there have been an increasing number of reports of the illicit use (primarily in Australia) of a new hallucinogen, 2,5-dimethoxy-4-bromoamphetamine, commonly known as 'Bromo DMA'. This drug is now considered to be taking over in popularity from LSD and will doubtless feature increasingly in future reports on drugs of abuse (Buhrich, Morris, and Cook 1983).

TOXICITY

The toxicity of the amphetamines varies considerably, depending on the specific amphetamine in question, the magnitude of dose and duration of treatment, etc. There is also substantial variation in the patient-to-patient response. Kalant (1973) has presented an excellent review of the acute and subacute toxicity of the amphetamines, together with a report on over seventy case histories. In general, the toxic effects experienced following administration of amphetamines, as for any other psychomotor stimulants, are primarily the response to over-stimulation of the central or peripheral sympathetic nervous system. Toxic symptoms include those 'negative' effects cited earlier (p. 270) and also dysphoria, somnolence, confusion and delirium. There may also be profuse sweating, mydriasis, rapid breathing, headache, pallor, paresthesia, palpitation, tachycardia, hypertension and cardiac arrythmias or circulatory collapse. High doses of amphetamines for prolonged periods have been known to cause muscular joint pain, severe tremors, severe chest pains and increase in diastolic and systolic blood pressure. Changes in libido may occur and there may be skin rashes. Continuous central stimulation usually gives way to fatigue and mental depression, which may be followed by convulsions and coma. There have been many reports of intracranial haemorrhages and necrotising angiitis (Citron, Halpern, McCarron, Lundberg, McCormick, Pincus, Tatter, and Haverback 1970; Margolis and Newton 1971) occurring following the administration of large doses of amphetamines, especially when given intravenously. Cardiomyopathy has also been diagnosed in a number of amphetamine takers and eosinophilia has been observed in some patients following i.v. administration of methylphenidate. In children, amphetamine and methylphenidate in particular have been shown to cause a depression of growth in weight or height — an effect which can lead to a rebound gain in weight on cessation of treatment (see also p. 267). Finally, a somewhat bizarre toxic effect increasingly seen in patients who administer extracts of tablets or capsule formulations of the amphetamines, and particularly methylphenidate, is disc and peripheral retinal neovascularization, caused by deposits of talc and corn starch. Low doses of amphetamine, even when used for prolonged periods of time rarely cause any permanent changes or damage to the personality. High doses may lead to permanent changes and to a variety of chronic personality disorders. The implication here is that high doses may damage the nervous system and limit its adaptive capacities.

TREATMENT OF DEPENDENCE

There has been relatively little research on methods of treatment of amphetamine-dependence — the only sure method currently available is to remove the subject from the source of the drug and to relocate outside the drug subculture. In general, relapse is the rule and prognosis is at least as bad as in opiate-dependence. However, phenelzine has been used successfully as a prophylactic in the prevention of amphetamine-type drug abuse and desipramine has been shown to be effective in treating amphetamine dependency and (probably does so by selectively blocking noradrenaline uptake). (This method of treatment does carry some risks, however — see Maletzky 1977).

TREATMENT OF OVERDOSE

The general treatment for casual or spontaneous overdose with all CNS stimulants involves supportive and symptomatic therapy. In severe overdose the stomach should be emptied by aspiration and lavage and diazepam may be given to control CNS stimulation and convulsions. In cases of marked excitement or when the patient is hallucinating, chlorpromazine may be administered — its α-adrenoceptor blocking properties may be useful for the management of hypertension. In cases of more severe hypertension, phentolamine or a comparable drug may be required, and propranolol or a more cardioselective β-adrenoceptor blocking agent may be required to control cardiac arrythmias.

Lithium carbonate has also been used to advantage in a large number of patients suffering from overdose of amphetamines by modifying the mood and behavioural alterations. Specifically, lithium significantly reduces the level of arousal–activation, euphoria–grandiosity and the total score of manic-state ratings following a (methylphenidate) challenge. Also, lithium carbonate appears to be capable of modifying the general hormone response to methylphenidate. Barbiturates are of limited value because of the uncertainty of response by the patient.

The neuroleptic drugs such as chlorpromazine, thioridazine, droperidol, and haloperidol have all been shown to be beneficial in the treatment of amphetamine overdose and appear to be specific antagonists to this drug (Espelin and Done 1968). Haloperidol has also been highly successful in the treatment of overdose with Bromo-DMA (Buhrich *et al.* 1983). Reserpine pretreatment prevents the peripheral effects of the amphetamines but some central effects such as the stereotypies are resistant. Older measures include the intramuscular administration of paraldehyde and hypertonic magnesium sulphate. Hydration is also important in helping the patient recover.

In earlier studies, the lethal dose of amphetamine was shown to be much lower when administered to groups of animals, as opposed to animals housed singly (Chance 1947). It is important to treat human patients under conditions of as much sensory deprivation as possible — this has been shown to be of practical value in at least one case of amphetamine toxicity in a child (Patuck 1956). Also, mice have been shown to salivate profusely and convulse following the parenteral administration of ephedrine and amphetamine at room temperature whereas animals transferred to an environment of 4 °C were protected from death. This observation would also be well worth considering the care of patients suffering from overdose.

TREATMENT OF PSYCHOSIS

As described previously, the symptoms of amphetamine psychosis fade quite rapidly following drug withdrawal and so symptomatic and supportive treatment is called for. Attention should also be focused on the underlying disability that led the patient to abuse the drugs in the first place. Obviously, where an amphetamine either precipitates or exacebates schizophrenia, the treatment should be that which is currently in use for that condition. Acidification of the urine (with, e.g., ammonium chloride) will ensure the most rapid elimination of drug from the body and, unless contraindicated, may be of value in treating amphetamine psychosis. Following a psychotic reaction induced by amphetamine the patient generally experiences depression, exhaustion, apathy and fatigue. The feelings of depression and exhaustion can last for many weeks but may be ameliorated by the tricyclic antidepressants. The mood elevating and stimulating effects of the amphetamines can be blocked by lithium, which is also known to be able to increase monoamine oxidase activity in both brain and platelets. Antidepressant drugs may also be of similar value.

CONCLUSION

In conclusion, the group of drugs collectively known as the 'amphetamines' have a very limited application in medicine today. Methylphenidate and amphetamine *per se* continue to be prescribed in only a few cases, as appropriate, for the treatment of narcolepsy and hyperkinesis in children. However, there has been a significant increase in their use for illicit purposes. The amphetamines are now considered 'old' drugs but from the research carried out on these compounds over the years it has been possible to develop newer molecules with more selective modes of action, which have now largely replaced the parent compounds. Interestingly, amphetamine and its congeners have begun to enjoy a new lease of life in recognition of their importance in psychopharmacology as tools for a better understanding of the mechanisms of action of both antipsychotic and antidepressant drugs.

REFERENCES

Blum, A. (1981). Phenylpropanolamine: an over-the-counter amphetamine? *J. Am. med. Assoc.* 245, 1346–7.

Brodie, B. B., Cho, A. K., and Gessa, G. L. (1970). Possible role of p-hydroxynorephedrine in the depletion of norepinephrine induced by d-amphetamine and in tolerance to this drug. In *Amphetamines and related compounds* (ed. E. Costa and S. Garattini), pp. 217–30. Raven Press, New York.

Buhrich, N., Morris, G., and Cook, G. (1983). Bromo-DMA: the Australasian hallucinogen. *Aust. N.Z. J. Psychiat.* 17, 275–9.

Caldwell, J. (1980). The metabolism of amphetamines and related stimulants in animals and man. In *Amphetamines and related stimulants: chemical, biological, clinical, and sociological aspects*. (ed. J. Caldwell) pp. 29–46. CRC Press, London.

— and Sever, P. S. (1974). The biochemical pharmacology of abused drugs. *Clin. Pharmac. & Ther.* 16 (4), 625–38.

Chance, M. R. A. (1947). Factors influencing the toxicity of sympathomimetic amines to solitary mice. *J. Pharmac. exp. Ther.* 89, 289–96.

Citron, B. P., Halpern, M., McCarron, M., Lundberg, G. D., McCormick, R., Pincus, I. J., Tatter, D., and Haverback, B. J. (1970). Necrotising angiitis associated with drug abuse. *New Engl. J. Med.* **283**, 1003-11.

Connell, P. H. (1958). In *Amphetamine psychosis*. Chapman & Hall, London.

Cole. S. O. (1967). Experimental effects of amphetamine: A review. *Psychol. Bull.* **68**, 81-90.

Davis, J. M. and Schlemmer, R. F. (1981). The amphetamine psychosis. In *Amphetamines and related stimulants: chemical, biological, clinical and sociological aspects* (ed. J. Caldwell), pp. 161-73. CRC Press, London.

Editorial (1968). *Drug Ther. Bull.* **6**, 33-4.

Espelin, D. E. and Done, A. K. (1968). Amphetamine poisoning. Effectiveness of chlorpromazine. *New Engl. J. Med.* **278**, 1361-6.

Groves, P. M. and Rebec, G. V. (1976). Biochemistry and behaviour: some central actions of amphetamine and antipsychotic drugs. *A. Rev. Psychol.* **27**, 91-121.

Kalant, O. J. (1973). In *The amphetamines: toxicity and addiction*. Univ. of Toronto Press, Toronto.

Kokkinidis, L. and Anisman, H. (1980). Amphetamine models of paranoid schizophrenia: an overview and elaboration of animal experimentation. *Psychol. Bull.* **88** (3), 551-79.

Lipton, M. A., di Mascio, A., and Killam, K. F. (1978). *Psychopharmacology. A generation of progress*. Raven Press, New York.

Maletzky, B. M. (1977). Phenelzine as a stimulant drug antagonist: a preliminary report. *Int. J. Addict.* **12**, 651-5.

Margolis, M. T. and Newton, T. H. (1971). Methamphetamine ('speed') arteritis. *Neuroradiology* **2**, 179-82.

McMillen, B. A. (1983). CNS stimulants: two distinct mechanisms of action for amphetamine-like drugs. *Trends in Pharmacological Sci.* **4**, 429-32.

Patuck, D. (1956). Acute dexamphetamine sulphate poisoning in a child. *Brit. med. J.* (i), 670-1.

Prinzmetal, M. and Bloomberg, W. (1935). The use of benzedrine for the treatment of narcolepsy. *J. Am. med. Assoc.* **105**, 2051-4.

Sabelli, H. C., Fawcett, J., Javaid, J. I., and Bagri, S. (1983). The methylphenidate test for differentiating desipramine-responsive depression. *Am. J. Psychiat.* **140**, 212-14.

Shaywitz, S. E., Hunt, R. D., and Jatlow, P. (1982). Psychopharmacology of attention deficit disorder. Pharmacokinetic, neuroendocrine and behavioural measures following acute and chronic treatment with methylphenidate. *Paediatrics* **69**, 688-94.

Silverstone, T., Wells, B., and Trenchard, E. (1983). Differential dose-response effects of dexamphetamine sulphate on hunger, arousal and mood in human volunteers. *Psychopharmacology* **79**, 242-5.

Van Kammen, D. P., Docherty, J. P., Marder, S. R., and Bunney, W. E. (1981). Acute amphetamine response predicts antidepressant and antipsychotic responses to lithium carbonate in schizophrenic patients. *Psychiatry Res.* **4**, 313-25.

Weiss, B. and Laties, V. G. (1962). Enhancement of human performance by caffeine and the amphetamines. *Pharmac. Rev.* **14**, 1-36.

24

Central effects of caffeine in man

M. KENNY AND A. DARRAGH

INTRODUCTION

The three most commonly used psychoactive drugs are alcohol, nicotine, and caffeine. In clinical situations, a great deal of attention is given to alcohol and nicotine, while caffeine is often overlooked, although it is the only one to which we may be continually exposed throughout life from infancy.

Caffeine can exert pharmacological effects on the central nervous system in doses from 85–200 mg, resulting in a reduction in drowsiness and fatigue, an elevation in mood, improved alertness and productivity, increased capacity for sustained intellectual effort and a rapid and clearer flow of thought (Rall 1980). At these doses caffeine may also produce diuresis, relax smooth muscle, activate gastric acid secretion and can affect heart rate, blood pressure and blood vessel diameter. Doses of caffeine in excess of 250 mg are generally considered to be high and may cause headaches, irritability, and nervousness. The Diagnostic and Statistical Manual of Mental Disorders (DSM-III, 1980) describes caffeine intoxication at doses exceeding 250 mg. Dependency and withdrawal reactions may occur following daily doses of 600 mg.

The amount of caffeine present in tea and coffee beverages varies considerably depending on the method of brewing. Caffeine is also present in significant amounts in cocoa, chocolate, soft drinks and many over-the-counter preparations, including analgesics, common cold remedies, diuretics and patent stimulants (Table 24.1), and pharmacologically-active doses may inadvertently be attained. In small children, significant doses could easily be consumed in the form of soft drinks, cocoa, and chocolate.

Caffeine is readily absorbed from the gastrointestinal tract and is rapidly distributed throughout all tissues and organs. Peak blood levels are reached within 15–45 min after oral administration in man, although the type of drink may affect the absorption rate (caffeine is absorbed more slowly from coca cola than from tea or coffee (Marks and Kelly 1973)). Caffeine crosses the placenta and is secreted in maternal milk.

The half-life in plasma shows considerable inter-individual variation with values ranging from 3.0–10 h. It is significantly shorter in smokers than in non-smokers while the use of oral contraceptives may double the half-life. It is also prolonged in pregnancy, particularly in the last trimester, when it can

TABLE 24.1. *Sources of caffeine*

Source	Concentration
Beverages	
Brewed coffee*	100–150 mg/180 ml
Instant coffee*	60–80 mg/180 ml
Decaffeinated coffee*	3–5 mg/180 ml
Brewed tea*	40–100 mg/180 ml
Pepsi cola†	16 mg/240 ml
Coca cola†	26 mg/240 ml
Lucozade†	43 mg/240 ml
Food	
Milk chocolate‡	6 mg/ounce
Cooking chocolate‡	35 mg/ounce
Over-the-counter medications*	
Cojene	105 mg/tablet
Aqua Ban	100 mg/tablet
Hedex Seltzer	60 mg/sachet
Phensic	50 mg/tablet
Beechams hot lemon	50 mg/sachet
Codural	50 mg/tablet
Pro-Plus	50 mg/tablet
Anadin maxi strength	32 mg/capsule
Solpadeine	30 mg/tablet

Obtained from *Martindale 1982; †Darragh, Lambe, Hallinan, and O'Kelly 1981; ‡Scientific Status Summary 1983.

reach 20 h. Newborn babies do not have the enzymes necessary to metabolize caffeine until several days after birth, and the half-life has been reported as approximately 82 h. This gradually decreases to reach 2–3 h after about six months (see Curatolo and Robertson 1983, for review).

Coffee consumption has been associated with a variety of disorders including hypertension, myocardial infarction, peptic ulcer, and cancers of the gastro-intestinal and urinary tracts, but this chapter will be confined to the effects on the central nervous system.

EFFECTS OF CAFFEINE ON PERFORMANCE AND SLEEP

The effects of caffeine on performance in a variety of mental and motor tests have been investigated in healthy volunteers. In tasks analogous to night-driving, there were significantly fewer attention lapses after 200–400 mg caffeine (Baker and Theologus 1972). However, when the effects begin to wear off a rebound drowsiness may occur. In this situation car accidents are more likely to occur if the plasma caffeine level cannot be maintained.

Caffeine is said to counteract the decrement in various kinds of performance tasks that is caused by fatigue or boredom (Goldstein, Kaiser, and Warren 1965a), but there is no convincing evidence that it is capable of enhancing performance above control levels. The first study reported in the literature, which was sponsored by the Coca-Cola company in 1912, found that 65–130 mg caffeine resulted in beneficial motor and mental efforts, while doses of 390 mg produced tremor, poor motor performance, and insomnia. (Hollingsworth 1912, in Stephenson 1977). The results of more recent studies investigating the effects of caffeine on mental tasks are equivocal. Some investigators have confirmed Hollingsworth's observations, but others have failed to find evidence that caffeine is capable of altering numerical reasoning, verbal fluency, short-term memory, or skill on the digit symbol substitution test. The effects of caffeine on performance may be dependent on personality, a marked difference in response being observed between extraverts and introverts. When subjects were further subdivided according to impulsiveness, the effects of caffeine were dependent on the time of day. Another variable in such studies, which is not always taken into account, may be the individual's normal pattern of caffeine consumption. Differences between low and high users in the effects of caffeine on performance have also been observed (for review, see Sawyer, Julia, and Turin 1982).

Clearly there is plenty of scope for definitive studies in this area. While the exact nature of the effects of caffeine on psychomotor behaviour remain to be defined, it is apparent that in healthy volunteers caffeine can significantly alter the results of performance tests and should be routinely excluded from the diet in clinical investigations of psychoactive drugs. However, care should be taken in the selection of subjects, to avoid heavy caffeine-users who could be susceptible to withdrawal symptoms, see below.

There is little doubt that caffeine taken before going to bed may interfere with both the quality and quantity of normal sleep; such sleep disturbances resemble those reported by insomniacs. A 150 mg dose of caffeine administered 30 min before retiring had a marked effect including an increase in sleep latency, a reduction in total sleep time and sleep efficiency, and a decrease in the number of REM periods (Okuma, Matsuoka, Matsue, and Toyomura 1982). Heavy caffeine users reported sounder sleep than usual on caffeine-free nights, suggesting that they suffer chronically from some degree of sleep impairment (Goldstein, Warren, and Kaiser 1965b). While large inter-individual differences are encountered, it has been demonstrated that coffee has a disturbing effect on sleep EEG patterns in addition to subjective evaluation of sleep characteristics (Karacan, Thornby, Anch, Booth, Williams, and Salis 1975). These effects appear to be more pronounced in light users of caffeine. In a study on the effects of caffeine on sleep in late middle-age, Brezinova (1974) observed that 300 mg caffeine taken before retiring resulted in an average decrease in total sleep time of approximately two hours. In addition, the sleep cycle was altered, in that REM sleep shifted to the earlier part of the night and stages III and IV shifted to the later part.

Caffeine can also influence the effects of hypnotics. Forrest, Belville, and Brown (1972) examined the interaction between caffeine and pentobarbital on the sleeping patterns in a number of medical and surgical patients. As expected, caffeine adversely affected sleep while pentobarbital facilitated sleep. When administered together, the effects of the individual drugs were cancelled and no difference in sleep pattern was found between the combination and placebo.

CAFFEINE, A HIDDEN COMPLICATION IN DIAGNOSIS

Adverse physiological and psychiatric reactions to large doses of caffeine have been described in the literature since 1892. When coffee was first introduced into Great Britain in the seventeenth century there was great resistance to its entry because of the behavioural changes known to be associated with its use. High doses of caffeine can produce symptoms which are indistinguishable from those of anxiety neurosis, and both conditions may exist simultaneously. Caffeinism has been defined as a pharmacological state of acute or chronic toxicity that results from ingestion of high doses of caffeine. It is characterized by anxiety and affective symptoms, sleep disruption, psychophysiological complaints, and withdrawal manifestations. Symptoms may include restlessness, irritability, nervousness, dizziness, tremulousness, sensory disturbances, periods of agitation and depression, diuresis, gastrointestinal complaints, headache, insomnia, palpitations, flushing, and arrythmias (Greden 1974).

The latest edition of the *Diagnostic and Statistical Manual of Mental Disorders* describes caffeine intoxication as a condition simulating an anxiety attack in which the patient may experience nausea, insomnia, restlessness, and jitteriness. In general, 600 mg/day appears to be the cut-off point between euphoric and dysphoric effects although individual sensitivities vary considerably. An intake in excess of 600 mg/day greatly increases the risk of developing clinical signs of caffeinism.

Greden (1974), in his paper entitled 'Anxiety or caffeinism: a diagnostic dilemma', illustrates very clearly the need for routine enquiry about a patient's normal caffeine consumption. He described three patients with a variety of symptoms which were initially attributed to anxiety neurosis. Subsequent inquiry revealed that they had been consuming more than 1000 mg caffeine/day. The symptoms resolved following cessation of caffeine and reappeared when 'challenged' with caffeine after a period of abstinence. Shortly afterwards, Molde (1975) described a patient with severe anxiety symptoms that were unrelieved by high doses of minor tranquillizers or by other psychoactive drugs.

It was then disclosed that he was consuming approximately fifty cups of coffee per day. A marked improvement in symptoms occurred within a few days when his total coffee consumption was reduced by 60 per cent.

Psychiatric patients may drink large quantities of caffeine-containing beverages to relieve the thirst produced by the anticholinergic effects of some psychoactive drugs, or to combat the sedative effects of many of these drugs. In a group of severely retarded aggressive psychiatric in-patients, who had a high caffeine-intake, the benefits observed following substitution of decaffeinated coffee (without the knowledge of patients or staff) led to the permanent exclusion of caffeine from the hospital diet (Podboy and Mallory 1977). Similarly, in a group of schizophrenic in-patients, a significant improvement was observed when caffeine intake was reduced, suggesting that 'chronic caffeine use created clinically significant levels of anxiety and tension that could be reversed by decreasing caffeine intake'; this improvement was reversed when regular coffee was reintroduced (de Freitas and Schwartz 1979).

Caffeinism may also complicate the diagnosis of affective disorders. Self-medication with caffeine may either be the cause or the result of an affective episode, and may totally alter the clinical presentation of the illness. In one study, the caffeine intake of patients with anergic, hypersomnic unipolar depression was markedly higher than in patients with uncomplicated unipolar depression (1250 vs. 280 mg). Many of these patients had been initially mis-diagnosed because of symptoms of agitation and hyposomnia, which disappeared when caffeine intake was limited. They had all consciously increased their caffeine intake substantially above their usual amount following the onset of an episode of anergic hypersomnic depression, in an attempt to combat decrements in performance and diminished energy-levels. They reported transient improvement in concentration and performance and decreased fatigue, but this was invariably followed by an increase in nervousness, irritability, sleep disturbance, and dysphoric mood (Neil, Himmelhoch, A. G. Mallinger, J. Mallinger, and Hanin 1978).

A number of studies have been carried out recently both in healthy volunteers and in psychiatric patients in which low, and high caffeine users have been found to differ markedly in several respects. High consumers (750 mg/day or more) scored significantly greater on the State–Trait Anxiety Index and the Beck Depression Scale than did moderate and low consumers (Gilliland and Andress 1981; Greden, Fontaine, Lubetsky, and Chamberlin 1978). High consumers described significantly more clinical symptoms, felt that their physical health was not as good, and reported greater use of minor tranquillizers and sedative hypnotics. They also used more tobacco and alcohol than did low consumers, while there was no significant difference between the two groups in the use of neuroleptics, antidepressants, lithium, or stimulants. Similar patterns were found in both psychiatric and non-psychiatric patients (Greden, Proctor, and Victor 1981).

Marked variation in response to caffeine is also observed between low and high users. Low users reported that caffeine makes them jittery and nervous, while heavy users reported stimulant and euphoric effects and experienced irritability, headache, and restlessness in its absence (Goldstein and Kaiser 1969). Differences between the two groups in the degree of sleep impairment and in the effects on performance tasks have already been mentioned above. In the past, such effects have been attributed to a difference in sensitivity at the site of action. However, a recent report on caffeine metabolism shows that the plasma half-life in subjects with a history of caffeine-induced insomnia is significantly longer than in those subjects not affected by caffeine (mean half-life 7.4 vs. 4.2 h, Levy and Zylber-Katz 1983). In this study, only non-smokers were used because the half-life of caffeine in smokers is significantly shorter than in non-smokers, an effect attributed to induction of hepatic enzymes by tobacco. Animal studies have shown that caffeine is also capable of hepatic enzyme-induction, and it remains to be seen whether such an effect could be responsible for the observed differences in half-life between light and heavy users, or whether an inherent sensitivity to caffeine in light users is responsible for their limited consumption. Heavy users of caffeine may develop a dependence on it and exhibit classical withdrawal symptoms following abstinence, which may include severe headache, rhinorrhea, nervousness, irritability, drowsiness and lethargy, and an inability to work effectively. These symptoms are relieved by caffeine (Goldstein, Kaiser, and Whitby 1969). In the Jewish community, one of the most common complaints encountered during 24-hour fasts is headache and this has been attributed to the abrupt withdrawal of caffeine in moderate to heavy users (Shorofsky and Lamm 1977). Withdrawal headaches have been produced experimentally, the symptoms of which were quite constant (Dreisbach and Pfeiffer 1943). The subjects experienced lethargy in the morning of the day of withdrawal. A diffuse throbbing headache usually began early in the afternoon, reaching a peak approximately 16 h after the last intake. Nausea and vomiting occurred in some subjects. Mental depression, drowsiness, yawning, and disinclination to work were also noted. The most effective treatment was caffeine. Caffeine-withdrawal headaches, the criteria for which include regular consumption of at least 600 mg caffeine per day, the development of tolerance, and the sudden discontinuation, often occur during weekends when patterns of caffeine ingestion may be markedly reduced (Greden, Victor, Fontaine, and Lubetsky 1980). Patients with frequent headaches often take caffeine-containing analgesics which relieve the headaches temporarily but which can start a vicious circle of recurring headaches.

   Caffeinism should be suspected as a complicating factor in all patients presenting with anxiety, sleep disturbance, psychophysiological problems and atypical anxious depression. It should also be suspected in patients who do not seem to respond to minor tranquillizers or night-time hypnotics and in patients with recurrent headache, who routinely use caffeine-containing analgesics. Diagnosis can be confirmed by caffeine challenge following a period of withdrawal. Children who complain of tachycardia, or insomnia, but who are otherwise healthy, may be drinking excessive amounts of cola drinks.

Identification of caffeine abuse in psychiatric patients is of the utmost importance both for accurate diagnosis and for design of effective treatment. The most frequently encountered situations are summarized in the following points:

1. Caffeinism may be mis-diagnosed as anxiety neurosis, resulting in additional psychoactive drugs being prescribed rather than reduction of caffeine.

2. Caffeine can modify the clinical manifestations of affective disorders resulting in an inappropriate therapeutic regimen.

3. Caffeine has been reported to precipitate or exacerbate psychosis and to increase agitation in psychiatric in-patients.

4. Caffeinism may be a complicating factor in anorexia.

5. Caffeine may interact with other psychoactive drugs.

Since caffeine is a convulsant at high doses and it antagonizes the anticonvulsant efforts of diazepam in animals (Marangos, Martino, Paul, and Skolnick 1981), its use to counteract the sedative effects of anticonvulsants such as phenytoin would be inadvisable.

INTERACTION WITH ALCOHOL AND THE BENZODIAZEPINES

Because of the extensive consumption of caffeine in the general population, its ingestion in combination with ethanol and with the benzodiazepines must also be widespread. As mentioned above, high caffeine users are also more likely to take minor tranquillizers and alcohol than moderate or light users. Interactions with alcohol have been reported since 1911, but there is still considerable doubt whether caffeine actually antagonizes ethanol. Studies of the effects of caffeine on ethanol-induced deterioration in human performance show no conclusive evidence of antagonism. In fact, some authors found a further deterioration by caffeine (Curatolo and Robertson 1983). No evidence for a possible restorative effect of coffee during alcohol-intoxication has been reported and the net effect of administering coffee after an excessive amount of alcohol may simply be a difficult-to-handle 'wide-awake drunk'.

Interactions between caffeine and the benzodiazepines have been investigated at both the behavioural and receptor levels. In a series of electrophysiological and behavioural tests, which are sensitive to the benzodiazepines, caffeine was consistently found to antagonize various effects of diazepam but not those of phenobarbitone. Fairly large doses of caffeine were required to prevent the anticonvulsant effects of diazepam, while low doses counteracted its anticonflict and muscle relaxing action (Polc, Bonetti, Pieri, Cumin, Angioi,

Mohler, and Haefely 1981). Caffeine-induced insomnia in man can be eliminated by the administration of temazepam (Okuma *et al.* 1982), and in psychometric studies, caffeine reduced the lorazepam-induced impairment on some tests (File, Bond, and Lister 1982). At higher doses (500 mg), it also counteracted the anti-anxiety effects of lorazepam. Similar effects were reported by Mattila, Palva, and Savolainen (1982), who observed that the diazepam-induced impairment in performance was antagonized by 250 mg caffeine, while 500 mg was found to counteract the calming effect of 10 mg diazepam during stress. The observation that caffeine competitively inhibits ^{3}H-diazepam binding to brain synaptosome membranes (Marangos, Paul, Goodwin, Syapin, and Skolnick 1979), led to the suggestion that some of the central effects of caffeine may be due to an interaction with benzodiazepine receptors. However, since large doses of caffeine did not affect binding of ^{3}H-flunitrazepam *in vivo* (Polc *et al.* 1981), the competition would appear to be selective and could not be responsible for the observed behavioural interactions between benzodiazepines and caffeine.

MECHANISM OF ACTION OF CAFFEINE

The molecular basis for the central effects of caffeine still remains to be defined. Caffeine affects calcium disposition and catecholamine turnover but only at very high concentrations. For many years it was generally accepted that inhibition of cyclic nucleotide phosphodiesterases by caffeine provided a reasonable basis for its central and peripheral actions, but more recent studies show that the concentration of caffeine in brain tissue never reaches that required to inhibit these enzymes (see Daly, Butts-Lamb and Padgett 1983, for review).

Adenosine plays a physiological role as a regulator in several cells and tissues. There is now an impressive amount of evidence to indicate that the central actions of adenosine are mediated through specific adenosine receptors. It has marked sedative and anticonvulsant activity which can be potentiated by the benzodiazepines and antagonized by caffeine (Daly, Bruns, and Synder 1981). In fact, some authors have suggested that the behavioural interactions between caffeine and the benzodiazepines might be explained in part by an interaction at adenosine receptors. In human brain, caffeine was found to be a more potent inhibitor of adenosine receptors than of benzodiazepine receptors (Boulenger, Patel, and Marangos 1982).

The stimulant effects of caffeine have been shown to be correlated with its potency as an inhibitor of binding of adenosine receptor ligands (Snyder, Katims, Annau, Bruns, and Daly 1981), and more recent studies give further support to the hypothesis that caffeine exerts its stimulant effects by blocking central adenosine receptors (Katims, Annau, and Snyder 1983). However, at least two major classes of adenosine receptors which are sensitive to caffeine have been described (Daly *et al.* 1981, 1983). A high-affinity A1 receptor functions to inhibit adenylate cyclase and a low-affinity stimulatory A2 receptor activates cyclic AMP systems. Furthermore, another A2 receptor has been identified in striatal and limbic regions which differs from the A2 receptors found in the rest of the brain in its affinity for adenosine. Caffeine exhibits a similar affinity for all three receptor populations *in vitro*. However, Daly *et al.* (1983), postulate that the susceptibility of these receptor types to competitive inhibition by caffeine *in vivo* may depend on their relative affinities for adenosine.

These recent studies open a whole new area in the investigation of the mechanism of action of caffeine. Using more selective antagonists it may be possible to identify sub-populations of receptors which are implicated in specific effects of caffeine.

ACKNOWLEDGEMENTS

The authors are grateful to Professor B. E. Leonard for his helpful comments, and to V. Brennan and P. McCann who typed the manuscript.

REFERENCES

Baker, W. J. and Theologus, G. C. (1972). Effects of caffeine on visual monitoring. *J. appl. Psychol.* **56**, 422–7.

Boulenger, J.-P., Patel, J., and Marangos, P. J. (1982). Effects of caffeine and theophylline on adenosine and benzodiazepine receptors in human brain. *Neurosci. Lett.* **30**, 161–6.

Brezinova, V. (1974). Effect of caffeine on sleep: EEG study in late middle age. *Br. J. clin. Pharmac.* **1**, 203–8.

Curatolo, P. W. and Robertson, D. (1983). The health consequences of caffeine. *Ann. int. Med.* **98**, 641–53.

Daly, J. W., Bruns, R. F., and Snyder, S. H. (1981). Adenosine receptors in the central nervous system: relationship to the central actions of methylxanthines. *Life Sci.* **28**, 2083–97.

——, Butts-Lamb, P., and Padgett, W. (1983). Subclasses of adenosine receptors in the central nervous system: interaction with caffeine and related methylxanthines. *Cell mol. Neurobiol.* **3**, 69–80.

Darragh, A., Lambe, R. F., Hallinan, D., and O'Kelly, D. A. (1979). Caffeine in soft drinks. *Lancet* i, 1196.

De Freitas, B. and Schwartz, G. (1979). Effects of caffeine in chronic psychiatric patients. *Am. J. Psychiat.* **136**, 1337–8.

Diagnostic and statistical manual of mental disorders (1980), 3rd edn, pp. 160–1. American Psychiatric Association, Washington.

Dreisbach, R. H. and Pfeiffer, C. (1943). Caffeine withdrawal headache. *J. lab. clin. Med.* **28**, 1212–19.

File, S. E., Bond, A. J., and Lister, R. G. (1982). Interaction between effects of caffeine and Lorazepam in performance tests and self-ratings. *J. clin. Psychopharmac.* **2**, 102–6.

Forrest, W. H., Bellville, J. W., and Brown, B. W. (1972). The interaction of caffeine with pentobarbital as a nighttime hypnotic. *Anaesthesiology* **36**, 37–41.

Gilliland, K. and Andress, D. (1981). Ad lib caffeine consumption, symptoms of caffeinism, and academic performance. *Am. J. Psychiat.* **138**, 512–14.

Goldstein, A. and Kaiser, S. (1969). Psychotropic effects of caffeine in man. III. A questionnaire survey of coffee drinking and its effects on a group of housewives. *Clin. Pharmac. Ther.* **10**, 477–88.

—, —, and Warren, R. (1965*a*). Psychotropic effects of caffeine in man. II. Alertness psychomotor coordination and mood. *J. Pharmac. exp. Ther.* **150**, 146–51.

—, —, and Whitby, O. (1969). Psychotropic effects of caffeine in man. IV. Quantitative and qualitative differences associated with habituation to coffee. *Clin. Pharmac. Ther.* **10**, 489–97.

—, Warren, R., and Kaiser, S. (1965*b*). Psychotropic effects of caffeine in man. I. Individual differences in sensitivity to caffeine induced wakefulness. *J. Pharmac. exp. Ther.* **149**, 156–9.

Greden, J. F. (1974). Anxiety or caffeinism: a diagnostic dilemma. *Am. J. Psychiat.* **131**, 1089–92.

—, Procter, A., and Victor, B. (1981). Caffeinism associated with greater use of other psychotropic agents. *Comp. Psychiat.* **22**, 565–71.

—, Fontaine, P., Lubetsky, M., and Chamberlin, K. (1978). Anxiety and depression associated with caffeinism among psychiatric inmates. *Am. J. Psychiat.* **13**, 963–6.

—, Victor, B., Fontaine, P., and Lubetsky, M. (1980). Caffeine-withdrawal headache: a clinical profile. *Psychosomatics* **21**, 411–18.

Karacan, I., Thornby, J A., Anch, M., Booth, G. H., Williams, R. L., and Salis, P. J. (1975). Dose related sleep disturbances induced by coffee and caffeine. *Clin. Pharmac. Ther.* **20**, 682–9.

Katims, J. J., Annau, Z., and Snyder, S. H. (1983). Interactions in the behavioural effects of methylxanthines and adenosine derivatives. *J. Pharmac. exp. Ther.* **227**, 167–73.

Levy, M. and Zylber-Katz, E. (1983). Caffeine metabolism and coffee-attributed sleep disturbances. *Clin. Pharmac. Ther.* **33**, 770–5.

Martindale (1982). *The extra pharmacopoeia*, 28th edn, Caffeine and other xanthines, p. 340. Pharmaceutical Press, London.

Marangos, P. J., Martino, A. M., Paul, S. M., and Skolnick, P. (1981). The benzodiazepines and inosine antagonise caffeine-induced seizures. *Psychopharmacology* **72**, 269–73.

—, Paul, S. M., Goodwin, F. K., Syapin, P., and Skolnick, P. (1979). Purinergic inhibition of diazepam binding to rat brain (*in vitro*). *Life Sci.* **24**, 851–8.

Marks, V. and Kelly, J. F. (1973). Absorption of caffeine from tea, coffee and coca cola. *Lancet* i, 827.

Mattila, M. J., Palva, E., and Savolainen, K. (1982). Caffeine antagonises diazepam effects in man. *Med. Biol.* **60**, 121–3.

Molde, D. A.. (1975). Diagnosing caffeinism. *Am. J. Psychiat.* **132**, 202.

Neil, J. F., Himmelhoch, J. M., Mallinger, A. G., Mallinger, J., and Hanin, I. (1978). Caffeinism complicating hypersomnic depressive episodes. *Comp. Psychiat.* **19**, 377–85.

Okuma, T., Matsuoka, H., Matsue, Y., and Toyomura, K. (1982). Model insomnia by methylphenidate and caffeine and use in the evaluation of temazepam. *Psychopharmacology* **76**, 201–8.

Podboy, J. W. and Mallory, W. A. (1977). Caffeine reduction and behaviour change in the severely retarded. *Ment. Retard.* **15**, 40.

Polc, P., Bonetti, E. P., Pieri, L., Cumin, R., Angioi, R. M., Mohler, H., and

Haefely, W. E. (1981). Caffeine antagonises several central effects of diazepam. *Life Sci.* **28**, 2265–75.

Rall, T. W. (1980). Central nervous system stimulants: the xanthines. In *The pharmacological basis of therapeutics* (ed. A. G. Gilman, L. S. Goodman, and A. Gilman), 6th edn, pp. 597–607. Macmillan, New York.

Sawyer, D. A., Julia, H. L., and Turin, A. C. (1982). Caffeine and human behaviour: arousal, anxiety, and performance effects. *J. behav. Med.* **5**, 415–39.

Scientific Status Summary (1983). Caffeine. *Food Technol.*, 87–91.

Shorofsky, M. A. and Lamm, N. (1977). Caffeine withdrawal headache and fasting. *New York State J. Med.* **77**, 217–18.

Snyder, S. H., Katims, J. J., Annau, Z., Bruns, R. F., and Daly, J. W. (1981). Adenosine receptors and behavioural interactions of methylxanthines. *Proc. natn Acad. Sci. U.S.A.* **78**, 3260–4.

Stephenson, P. E. (1977). Physiological and psychiatric effects of caffeine on man. *J. Am. diet. Assoc.* **71**, 240–7.

25

Aphrodisiacs

ROBERT B. GREENBLATT, JASWANT S. CHADDHA,
ANA ZULLY TERAN, AND CEANA H. NEZHAT

> In Xanadu did Kubla Khan
> A stately pleasure-dome decree:
>
> . . . . . .
>
> For he on honey-dew hath fed,
> And drunk the milk of Paradise.
>   COLERIDGE

It has been alleged that power is the greatest aphrodisiac. Yet so powerful a conqueror as Kubla Khan sought out such presumed aphrodisiacal agents as honey-dew and the milk of Paradise. Perhaps power was not enough.

In the Bible, the second book of Samuel unfolds a scenario of sexual dysfunction in all its ramifications: first, the introduction of voyeurism as a stimulus to lust unrestrained; then, the insinuation of psychogenic forces, abetted by advancing age resulted in the loss of sexual prowess; and finally, the employment of an age-old aphrodisiacal device to test potentia.

King David, standing on the balcony of his palace, lustfully watched a nude woman bathing on the roof of her house. The woman, Bathsheba, was the wife of a captain serving in the King's army at the battlefront. Sexually aroused, David summoned her to his rooms and seduced her. Soon Bathsheba was with child. When the prophet Nathan admonished the God-fearing David, 'Thou art the man', conscience took reason prisoner; the King's remorse deepened with the years. In time, rumours of his impotence became current, and the Israelites, who equated leadership with virility, applied the test. A young and beautiful Shunamite maiden was chosen to lie with the king, but 'he gat no heat' – 'love's labours' lost. David failed the test and was forced to abdicate in favour of his son Solomon, he of the thousand wives (Greenblatt 1977).

THE ROLE OF THE PSYCHE AND THE NERVOUS SYSTEM IN SEXUAL PERFORMANCE

The eminent British surgeon, John Hunter (1728–93) predated today's physicians when he pointed out that a relationship existed between emotional stress and psychogenic impotence. The mind is subject to many a caprice that affects sexual performance. Thus, in order to overcome sexual inadequacy, men and women have sought means to stimulate sexual ardour by resorting to foodstuffs, plants, herbs, spices, philtres, love potions, alcoholic beverages, imagery, the body beautiful, and even sacrifices and prayers to the gods. In recent years, pharmacologic agents and hormones have been employed as aphrodisiacs to provoke libidinous drive, enhance or maintain penile erection, and stimulate vaginal lubrication and hyperaemia.

Sexual arousal depends on the five senses in hormonally-prepared individuals, but organic response is dependent on an intact autonomic nervous system conditioned by the state of the mind. Penile erection, however, is not necessarily hormone-dependent, for this phenomenon has been observed in the foetus-in-utero, in boys during early childhood, and in men castrated after adolescence. Parasympathetic nervous system activation dominates the initial phase of sexual excitement while progressive cholinergic impulses are involved in orgasm and ejaculation (Wiedenking, Ziegler, and Lake 1979). In the male frog (*Rana pipiens*), both gonadotropins and adrenergic agents stimulate the sympathetic ganglia to release sperm; a response which adrenolytic drugs can abolish (Greenblatt, Clark, and West 1950) (Fig. 25.1).

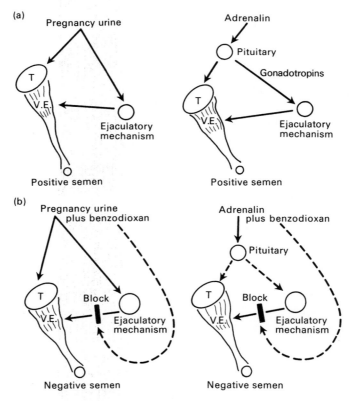

Fig. 25.1. Both pregnancy urine and adrenalin stimulate the ejaculatory mechanism in the *Rana pipiens*. Adrenolytic agents abolish the response. (From Greenblatt 1979).

ASPECTS OF THE NEUROPHYSIOLOGY OF SEXUAL BEHAVIOUR

Sexual behaviour and potency have been associated with alterations in levels of brain serotonin and dopamine. The depletion of serotonin has an invigorating effect on sexually sluggish rats, but no effect on rats whose baseline activity is normal. Hormonal interactions with serotonin and other neurotransmitters may be instrumental in the modification of sexual behaviour (Zitrin, Dement, Barchas *et al.* 1973). In the female rat, castration (*ovariectomization*) results in a rise, oestrogens in a fall of brain noradrenaline. Testosterone administered to one-day-old male rats prevent the usual twelfth-day rise in serotonin (Fig. 25.2). When new-born female rats are injected with testosterone, the hypothalamus is masculinized, preventing the initiation of cyclic oestrus (Barraclough and Gorsi 1968). There is a wealth of material defining the role of a variety of pharmacologic agents which influence the neurotransmitters of the brain of experimental animals, but thus far, application of this knowledge to human sexual behaviour has not proved promising (Tucker and File 1983). In the last resort, human reactions can only be studied in man.

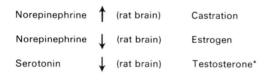

Norepinephrine	↑	(rat brain)	Castration
Norepinephrine	↓	(rat brain)	Estrogen
Serotonin	↓	(rat brain)	Testosterone*

*Blocks 12th day rise if injected on day 1.

Fig. 25.2. Oestrogens and androgens influence brain content of neurohormones of the brain.

TEMPORAL ASPECTS OF SEXUAL AROUSAL IN MEN AND WOMEN

Women are subject to episodic changes in hormone levels throughout the menstrual cycle. Dramatic surges of oestradiol (E_2) and luteinizing hormone (LH) initiate ovulation; soon thereafter, progesterone levels rise then fall precipitously to trigger the menstrual process. Testosterone and prolactin levels also show cyclic shifts. Hormonal status may influence sexuality; some women experience their greatest sexual urge at the time of ovulation, others during the luteal or premenstrual phase, and not a few during menstruation. Males, on the other hand, are not subjected to such hormonal swings. Like stags in rutting season, most men remain in a continuous state of readiness. Perhaps Henry Higgins' query in *My Fair Lady*, 'Why can't a woman be more like a man?' referred to the inconstancy of her moods and behaviour — a reflection of the gyrations in hormonal tides.

THE ROLE OF GONADAL STEROIDS IN SEXUAL BEHAVIOUR

Nottebohn (1983), puzzled by the fact that only male canaries sing, injected adult females with testosterone. Within ten days, the female canaries burst into song. He and his associates found an area in the forebrain that increases in volume following testosterone administration. Perhaps women, too, who bemoan their loss of sexual drive can be made 'to sing' following the judicious use of this hormone. The danger of drawing facile parallels is apparent, but the canary experience serves to emphasize that the brain is a target organ.

The metabolic fate of testosterone involves conversion into E_2 and 5α-dihydrotestosterone (DHT); one of the enzymes in the pathway of biosynthesis has aromatase activity. The intracerebral administration of an aromatase blocker (andros-1,4,6-triene-3,17-dione) will inhibit masculine sex behaviour in spite of the systematic presence of testosterone (Baum and Starr 1980). It appears that E_2 and DHT are essential for expression of these behaviours, rather than the parent steroid testosterone (Christensen and Clemens 1975) (Fig. 25.3).

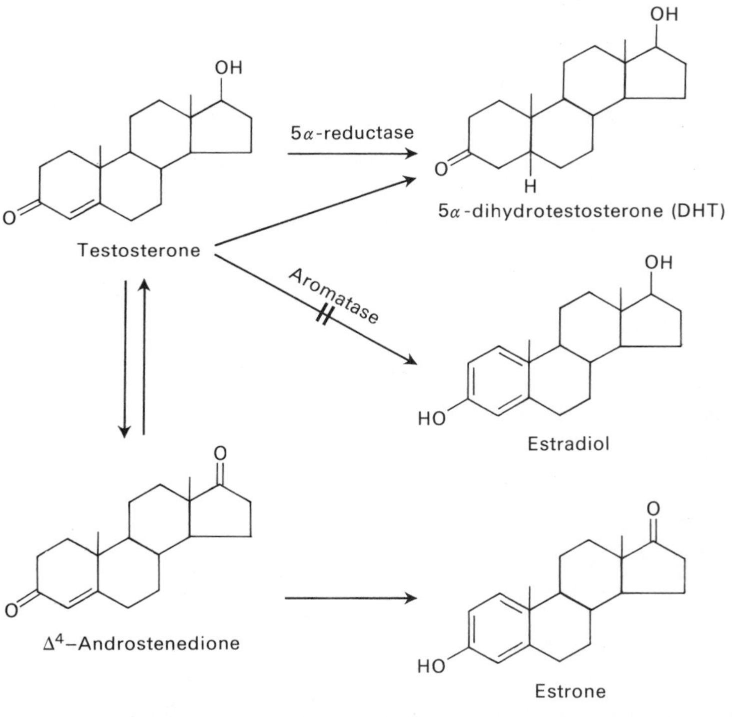

Fig. 25.3. A blockade of aromatase activity will inhibit sexual behaviour in spite of the systemic presence of testosterone. E_2 and DHT are essential for expression of sexual behaviour. (After Christensen and Clemens (1975) *Endocrinology* **97**, 1545–51).

Newman and Northup (1983) report that about thirty years ago an experiment was performed in which an adult woman received an intravenous injection of testosterone (then available for experimental use). Within a few minutes there was intense vulvar flushing, vaginal hyperaemia, a rise in uterine temperature accompanied by a distinct increase in libido. Masters and Johnson (1977), in their clinical studies, observed similar changes in females during sexual excitement.

Men and women with hypopituitarism due to an hypothalamic lesion resulting in anosmia and secondary hypopituitarism (Kallmann's syndrome), or those with primary hypopituitarism (idiopathic or caused by a tumour) exhibit all the signs of sexual infantilism, absence of sexual hair, and libidinous drives. In females, the results of hormone replacement therapy are striking. Cyclic oestrogen and progestin therapy will induce regular withdrawal uterine bleeding periods and breast development, but sexual arousal remains poor, and pubic hair fails to appear. When androgen is added to the oestrogen-progestin regimen, sexual hair grows and sex drive becomes very positive (Fig. 25.4). When a placebo is substituted for the androgen, then both sexual hair and libido regress completely (Greenblatt 1945). This human experiment helps delineate the role of gonadal steroids in sexual drive.

APHRODISIACAL EFFECT OF OESTROGEN-TESTOSTERONE ADMINISTRATION FOR SEXUAL DYSFUNCTION IN WOMEN

Despite the scepticism of the medical establishment concerning the value of hormones in the treatment of sexual dysfunction in women, the many positive reports cannot be ignored (Salmon 1941; Greenblatt, Mortara, and Torpin 1942; Dempsey, Hertz, and Young 1935; Studd 1978). There is no doubt that oestrogens will relieve dyspareunia when due to atrophic vaginitis; and that oestrogens and testosterone properly administered will increase sexual dreams and appetites and will promote orgasmic responses in many women. Oral oestrogens and androgens in the usually recommended doses often prove inadequate because hormones taken orally enter the enterohepatic system where the liver conjugates, detoxifies, and neutralizes, while parenteral hormones avoid the first pass through the liver and, hence, are more effective (Campbell and Whitehead 1977). Our most recent study of 136 depressed menopausal women involves the subcutaneous implantation of one or two pellets of 17β-oestradiol (E_2) (25 mg each) or a combination of one or two E_2 pellets with one or two pellets of testosterone (75 mg each). Almost every woman in this series complained of loss of sexual desire. The hormone therapy resulted in an increase in free and total tryptophan (Alyward 1973) (Table 25.1). We are not certain whether the improvement in emotional status or the changes in tryptophan metabolism were responsible for the increased sexual responsiveness, but what emerged from this study is that gonadal steroids not only exert an anti-

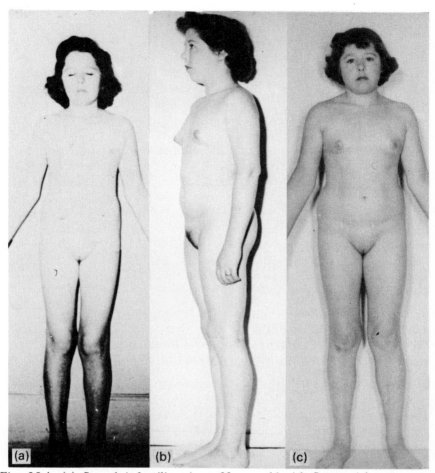

Fig. 25.4. (a) Sexual infantilism in a 23-year-old girl. Sequential oestrogen-progestin therapy-induced breast development and withdrawal uterine bleeding periods, but neither pubic hair nor libido. (b) The addition of an oral androgen resulted in sexual-hair growth and stimulated libido. (c) The replacement of the androgen with a placebo caused complete regression of the hair growth, with loss of sexual desire. (From Greenblatt (1945) *West. J. Surg.* **53**, 222–6).

depressant effect (Herrmann and Beach 1976), but that such therapy is associated with a return of sexual drives.

The question will be asked, What about untoward reactions and possible risks of cancer? The answer is that only a few women on such a regimen develop hairiness, mild acne, and more rarely, voice changes or slight enlargement of the clitoris. Reversal of the untoward signs usually takes place if further androgen therapy is discontinued. Many women, however, do not wish to eliminate

TABLE 25.1. *Tryptophan† in depressed menopausal women with loss of libido*

Serum free and total tryptophan increased to almost normal values on hormone replacement therapy in depressed menopausal women. The more frequent sexual response to the oestrogen-testosterone regimen over that of oestrogens alone suggests that the role of androgen is more important than the simple increase in free tryptophan.

Free		Total		Libido	Depression
Before	After	Before	After	25–100% Improvement	
3.76 ± 0.09	4.41* ± 0.19	34.66 ± 0.89	35.51 ± 1.28	50% on E_2	70% on E_2
				90% on E_2 + T	70% on E_2 + T
$n = 136$	$n = 90$	$n = 136$	$n = 90$		

*p = <0.05 E_2 = Estradiol pellets T = Testosterone.

	Free	Total
†Non-depressed menopausal patients	5.12 ± 0.34 $n = 20$	44.8 ± 2.87 $n = 20$

androgen medication because, for them, the benefits far outweigh the undesirable reactions. The risk of endometrial cancer on prolonged oestrogen therapy can be reduced to less than the normally expected incidence by the administration of an oral progestin for seven to ten days each month (Gambrell 1980; Greenblatt and Gambrell 1980). As to breast cancer, we feel that there is no hard evidence to support the allegation of an association. Horwitz and Stewart (1984) reviewed eleven of the most recent studies dealing with the subject. Their verdict was that with the removal of bias factors, there appears to be no increased risk.

THE USE OF PARENTERAL TESTOSTERONE (IMPLANTS OR INJECTIONS) IN NORMAL MEN WITH SEXUAL DYSFUNCTION

The male, complaining of loss of libido and/or erectile capacity, may have low or normal serum testosterone values. Normal values do not necessarily reflect the interaction between the hormone and the target cells, nor the receptivity of testosterone receptors. We have previously reported on a double-blind study in which less than 50 per cent of men experienced mild to moderate response to oral androgens (Greenblatt, Oettinger, and Bohler 1976; Greenblatt, Nezhat, Roesel, and Natrajan 1979). However, parenteral androgen therapy (implants of 75 mg pellets, one per 10–15 lb of body weight at six month intervals or injections of 100–200 mg of a long-acting testosterone, enanthate or cypionate, preparation (every 7–14 days) is far more effective than oral therapy. In our experience improvement in sexual drive and/or erections may be expected in about two-thirds of the patients (Greenblatt and Karpas 1983), (Figures 25.6 and 25.7). Men on drugs (antiphypertensives, α-β-blockers, tranquillizers), alcoholics, and diabetics, usually fail to benefit.

Untoward reactions are few, and these are prostatic enlargement and physiologic polycythemia. In the former, medication is discontinued, and in the latter, old-fashioned phlebotomy may be practised (donation of a pint of blood to a blood bank at six week intervals) to reduce haemoglobin concentration and elevated hematocrit. Occasionally, nipple tenderness is experienced. A decided increase in low and very low density lipoproteins and a decrease in high-density lipoproteins has been found to occur following oral synthetic androgens (Solym 1971), but we have not seen any significant changes after implantation of pure testosterone (Fig. 25.8).

Although the role of suggestion may be strong, the proof that implants do not act as placebos, is the fact that as the pellets are absorbed in four to five months there is, in most cases, an abrupt loss of libido and/or erectile capacity corresponding to a fall in serum testosterone levels (Fig. 25.5(a)), and a concommitant rise in serum FSH and LH levels (Fig. 25.5(b)).

IS THERE A TRUE APHRODISIAC?

The view generally held is that one expressed by Benkert (1980): 'No pharmacotherapy is known that has been experimentally substantiated. The therapeutic results obtained in controlled studies were no better than placebos.' For more than forty years we have evaluated various endocrine preparations, i.e. oestrogens, progestogens, androgens, corticoids, gonadotrophins, etc. Many of our studies were double-blind and only one effective regimen consistently has stood the test of time, and that is a preparation that contained an androgen (Albeaux-Fernet, Bohler, and Karpas 1978; Greenblatt, Barfield, and Garner *et al.* 1950) (Table 25.2).

No one will deny that testosterone administration to the hypogonadal male will result in sexual drive and erection, but what is debatable is its usefulness in the treatment of sexual dysfunction in men with normal or even subnormal serum testosterone values, and in women. It is futile to offer a course of oral therapy for a few weeks and come to a conclusion, as Bancroft (1983) did, that there were no 'significant differences between androstenedione and placebo'. Androstenedione is a very weak androgen and quite inappropriate for such a study. The key to success, it appears, is persistent therapy with potent hor-

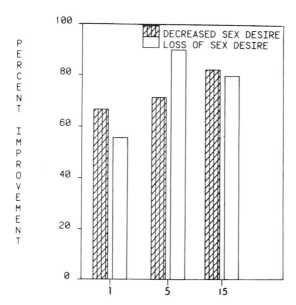

Fig. 25.6. One hundred men received testosterone pellet implants every six months. Note degree of improvement of libido after first, fifth, and fifteenth implantation.

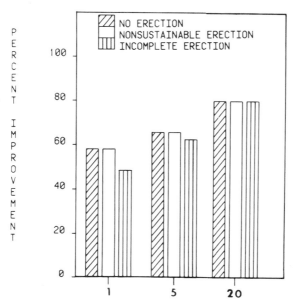

Fig. 25.7. Note degree of improvement in erectile capacity after first, fifth, and twentieth implantation.

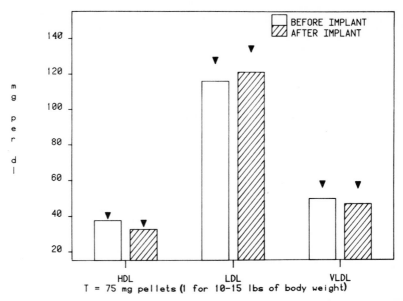

Fig. 25.8. No significant changes in high (HDL), low (LDL), and very-low-density lipoproteins (VLDL) were observed after testosterone pellet implantation.

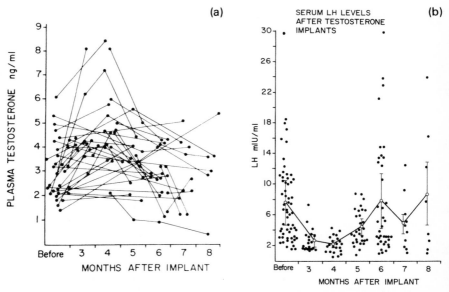

Fig. 25.5. (a) Serum testosterone levels fall after the fourth month of implantation, usually accompanied by a loss of libido and/or erectile capacity. (b) LH levels fall after testosterone pellet implantation and begin to rise coincident with loss of libido and/or erectile capacity.

TABLE 25.2.

In a double-blind study using an oestrogen (AE1), an oestrogen-androgen (AE2). an androgen (AE3), and a placebo (AE4) in the treatment of menopausal hot flushes, 12.3 per cent of the patients volunteered the information that the oestrogen increased libidinous drives, 65.5 per cent after androgens, and only 1.8 per cent on the placebo. (From Greenblatt *et al.* 1950.)

Mrs J.S., w.f. 52. Menopause. Hot flushes and formication. (Hysterectomy)

AE	1	2	3	4	
July	X				Complete relief. Slight increase in libido.
Aug.					Symptoms returned 3 wks. after stopping AE-1.
Sept.		X			90% relief. Increased libido, nervousness.
Oct.					
Nov.			X		Better than AE-2 or AE-1.
Dec.					Recurrence of symptoms.
Jan.				X	No relief. Smear 2-3 plus.
Feb.			X		80% relief. Occasional hot flushes. Smear 3 plus.
Mar.			X		Not as good as AE-1 now.
Apr.				X	No relief. Complete return of symptoms.

mones, preferably by the parenteral route. Specific agents can restore sexual function in individuals with certain disorders, such as thyroxin in the hypothyroid; and propylthiouracil in the hyperthyroid; bromocriptine in individuals with hyperprolactinaemia and acromegaly; and L-DOPA in Parkinson's disease (Calne and Sandler 1977; Spark, White, and Connolly 1980; Thorner and Besser 1976). These very agents proved of little value in normal individuals with sexual dysfunction (Ambrosi, Bara, and Fagler 1977). Although oestrogens may increase a woman's sexual ardour, and progestins may do so for others, it is our experience that women who once have known libido but lost it respond almost universally to oestrogen–androgen therapy.

CONCLUSIONS

Psychodelic drugs, serotonin-antagonists, pharmacologic drugs with vasodilator action, adrenergic blocking agents, nephrogenital irritants, plants and herbs, foodstuffs, alcoholic beverages, and organic material that have some semblance to male genitalia — Paracelsus's doctrine of signatures (i.e. tubers, rhinoceros horn) — are believed to be sexual stimulants. For some, they indeed are, but only temporarily. Suggestion is a powerful ally and, in this regard, pornography does actually stimulate sexual arousal and fantasies.

The psychophysiological complexity of the normal sexual response involves central, spinal, vascular, sympathetic, and parasympathetic elements. Oestrogens and androgens modulate the neurotransmitters of the brain and indirectly influence the autonomic nervous system. In the female, androgens are powerful stimulants of sexual dreams and fantasies, while improving vaginal hyperaemia and lubrication, often increasing clitoral sensitivity and turgescence and orgasmic experience. In the male, testosterone in large doses, preferably administered parenterally, over a sufficient length of time, has proved in our hands capable of overcoming sexual dysfunction in about two-thirds of normal men with low or normal testosterone levels. Gonadal hormones are psychotrophic drugs, participating in both physiological and psychological components of sexual behaviour.

REFERENCES

Albeaux-Fernet, M., Bohler, C. S.-S., and Karpas, A. E. (1978). Testicular function in the ageing male. In *Geriatric endocrinology* (ed. R. B. Greenblatt), pp. 201–16. Raven Press, New York.

Alyward, M. (1973). Plasma tryptophan levels and mental depression in postmenopausal subjects. Effect of oral piperazine oestrone sulfate. *Med. Sci.* 1, 30.

Ambrosi, B., Bara, R., and Fagler, G. (1977). Bromocriptine in impotence. *Lancet* 2, 987.

Bancroft, J. (1983). The role of androgens in female sexuality. In *Medical sexology* (ed. F. Romano and W. Pasini), p. 210. PGS Publishing, Littleton, Mass.

Barraclough, C. A. and Gorsi, R. A. (1968). Evidence that the hypothalamus is responsible for androgen induced sterility in the female rat. *Endocrinology* 68, 61.

Baum, M. J. and Starr, M. S. (1980). Inhibition of sexual behaviour by dopamine antagonist or serotonin agonist drugs in castrated male rats given estradiol or dihydrotestosterone. *Pharmac. Biochem.* 1 (3), 47–67.

Benkert, O. (1980). Pharmacology of sexual impotence in the male. *Mod. Probl. Pharmacopsychiat.* 15, 158–73.

Calne, D. B. and Sandler, M. (1977). L-dopa and Parkinsonism. *Nature, Lond.* 226, 21–4.

Campbell, S. and Whitehead, M. (1977). Oestrogen therapy and the menopausal syndrome. In *Clinics in obstetrics and gynaecology* (ed. R. B. Greenblatt and J. W. W. Studd), p. 30. W. B. Saunders, Philadelphia and London.

Christensen, L. W. and Clemens, L. G. (1975). Blockade of testosterone-induced mounting behaviour in the male rat with intracranial application of the aromatization inhibitor andros-1,4,6-triene-3,17-dione. *Endocrinology* 97, 1545–51.

Dempsey, E. W., Hertz, R., and Young, W. C. (1935). Experimental induction of oestrus (sexual receptivity in normal and ovariectomized guiney pigs). *Am. J. Physiol.* 116, 201.

Gambrell, R. D. Jr. (1980). Role of estrogens and progestogens in the etiology of breast and endometrial neoplasia. In *The menopause and postmenopause* (ed. N. Pasetto, R. Paeletti, and J. L. Ambrus), pp. 389–404. MTP Press, Lancester, England.

Greenblatt, R. B. (1945). Sexual infantilism in the female. *West. J. Surg.* **53**, 222–6.

— (1977). *Search the scriptures: modern medicine and biblical personages.* Lippincott, Philadelphia.

— (1979). Les mechanismes hypothalamo-hypophysaires. In *Pathiologie génitale de la femme au troisième age*, pp. 65–78. Masson, Paris.

— and Gambrell, R. D. Jr. (1980). Endometrial changes in the infertile woman with particular reference to atypism and its management. In *The endometrium* (ed. F. A. Kimball), pp. 57–81. Spectrum Publications, New York.

— and Karpas, A. E. (1983). Hormone therapy for sexual dysfunction. *Postgrad. Med.* **74**, 78–89.

—, Barfield, W. E., and Garner, J. F. (1950). Evaluation of an estrogen, androgen, estrogen-androgen combination and a placebo in the treatment of the menopause. *J. clin. Endocrinol.* **10**, 1547–58.

—, Clark, S. L., and West, R. M. (1950). Hormonal factors producing the gametokinetic response in the male frog (rana pipiens). *J. clin. Endocrinol.* **10**, 265–9.

—, Mortara, R., and Torpin, R. (1942). Sexual libido in the female. *Am. J. Obstet. Gynecol.* **44**, 658–63.

—, Oettinger, M., and Bohler, C. S.-S. (1976). Estrogen-androgen levels in aging men and women: therapeutic considerations. *J. Am. Geriatr. Soc.* **24**, 173–8.

—, Nezhat, C., Roesel, R. A., and Natrajan, P. K. (1979). Update on the male and female climacteric. *J. Am. Geriatr. Soc.* **27**, 481–90.

Hermann, W. M. and Beach, R. C. (1976). Psychotropic effects of androgens: A review of clinical observations and new human experimental findings. *Pharmakopsychiatr. Neuropsychopharmakol.* **9**, 205–19.

Horwitz, R. I. and Stewart, K. R. (1984). Effect of clinical features on the association of estrogens and breast cancer. *Am. J. Med.* **76**, 192–8.

Masters, W. H. and Johnson, V. E. (1977). *Human sexual response.* Little Brown, Boston.

Newman, H. F. and Northup, J. D. (1983). Problems in male organic sexual physiology. *Urology* **31**, 443–9.

Nottebohn, F. (1983). 1983 lecture on series on 'Brains' at the Rockefeller University's Field Research Center for Ecology and Ethology.

Salmon, U. J. (1941). Rationale for androgen therapy in gynecology. *J. clin. Endocrinol.* **1**, 162.

Solym, A. (1971). Effects of androgens on serum lipids and lipoprotein. *Lipids* **7**, 100–5.

Spark, R., White, R., and Connolly, P. (1980). Impotence is not always psychogenic. *J. Am. med. Assoc.* **243**, 705–5.

Studd, J. W. W. (1978). The climacteric syndrome. In *Female and male climacteric* (ed. P. A. van Keep, D. M. Serr, and R. B. Greenblatt), pp. 23–33. MTP Press, Lancaster, England.

Thorner, M. and Besser, G. (1976). Hyperprolactinemia and gonadal function: Results of bromocriptine treatment. In *Serono symposia on prolactin and human reproduction* (ed. P. Crosignani and C. Robyn). Academic Press, New York.

Tucker, J. C. and File, S. E. (1983). Serotonin and sexual behaviour. In *Psychopharmacology and sexual disorders* (ed. D. Wheatley), pp. 22–49. Oxford University Press.

Wiedenking, C., Ziegler, M. G., and Lake, C. R. (1979). Plasma noradrenaline and dopamine-beta-hydroxylase during human sexual activity. *J. Psychiat. Res.* **15**, 139–45.

Zitrin, A., Dement, W. C., Barchas, J. D. *et al.* (1973). Brain serotonin and male sexual behavior. In *Contemporary sexual behavior* (ed. J. Zubin and J. Money), pp. 321–36. Johns Hopkins University Press, Baltimore.

26

Nicotine pharmacology and smoking dependence

R. J. WEST AND M. A. H. RUSSELL

INTRODUCTION

Cigarette smoking induces dependence. Most smokers say they would like to give up, but when they try they usually fail. Although it has long been recognized that nicotine may be the cause of smoking dependence, it is principally in the last ten years or so that evidence has emerged to substantiate such a view. Progress has occurred on a number of fronts: it has been shown that nicotine can act as a primary reinforcer; that nicotine has actions which correspond with smokers' expressed motives for smoking; that smokers may regulate their nicotine intake; and that temporary nicotine replacement following smoking cessation can alleviate withdrawal effects and help smokers to remain abstinent. In this chapter an attempt is made to draw the various threads together and to consider how far we have come in understanding the pharmacology of smoking dependence.

NICOTINE AS A PRIMARY REINFORCER

If a drug is dependence-inducing, it should act as a primary reinforcer. That is, animals (including humans) should respond to obtain it for its own sake, as, for example, with morphine, amphetamines, cocaine, barbiturates, and alcohol. Such a demonstration has proved more difficult in the case of nicotine. In early studies of nicotine self-injection in animals, rates of responding were low compared with other drugs such as cocaine (Yanagita 1977). However, in most of these studies nicotine was given after each response or every few responses, and the frequency of dosage depended on the rate of responding. As response rates increased, the doses occurred in more rapid succession resulting in high cumulative doses which may have been aversive.

More recent studies in squirrel monkeys and beagle dogs have shown that when the schedule of nicotine delivery is arranged to avoid the problem of high cumulative dosage, high rates of responding may be obtained (e.g. Spealman and Goldberg 1982; Risner and Goldberg 1983). Spealman and Goldberg used a 'second order' schedule in which every tenth response produced a brief light, and the first component of 10 lever press responses which was completed after a given interval (e.g. 5 min) produced both light and nicotine. Under this schedule very high rates of responding were obtained ranging from 0.8 to 1.6 per second. These response rates were only slightly lower than those obtained with cocaine reinforcement under a similar schedule.

It is interesting to note that self-administration was completely abolished by pretreatment with the central cholinergic blocker, mecamylamine. This ties in with recent studies suggesting that the central actions of nicotine are mediated by its occupation of nicotinic–cholinergic receptor sites in the brain (Romano and Goldstein 1980). The reinforcing actions of nicotine may also involve non-specific reward systems in the brain. For example, it has been shown that nicotine stimulates firing of dopaminergic neurones arising from the substantia nigra (Lichensteiner, Hefti, Felix, Huwlyer, Melamed, and Schlumpf 1982), an area of the brain in which electrical stimulation acts as a potent reinforcer. Smoking also stimulates β-endorphin release and this, too, might underlie its reinforcing potential (Pomerleau, Fertig, Seyler, and Jaffe 1983).

Henningfield, Goldberg, Miyasato, Spealman, and Jasinski (1982) have studied whether intravenous nicotine will reinforce lever-press responding in humans. They found that smokers responded at a higher rate for nicotine than for saline, whereas the opposite was true for non-smokers. While these results are consistent with the view that nicotine is a primary reinforcer in some people, it leaves open the possibility that its reinforcing properties are acquired by association with some other aspect of smoking.

NICOTINE AND EXPRESSED MOTIVES FOR SMOKING

A number of studies have used questionnaires to try to identify the main factors in smoking motivation (Russell, Peto, and Patel 1974). From these studies smoking appears to serve several functions. The three most important are: providing a source of pleasure; modifying arousal levels (i.e. stimulating or sedating); and relieving withdrawal symptoms. An additional motivating factor for some smokers may be the effects of smoking in reducing hunger and weight. This section will consider each of these motives except for relief of withdrawal which will be dealt with separately.

Nicotine and smoking for pleasure

There may be many sources for the pleasure which people derive from smoking tobacco. One potential source is the slight subjective 'drug' effect produced, particularly after the first cigarette of the day. A similar effect is produced by a droplet of nicotine placed in the nose (Russell, Jarvis, Feyerabend, and Ferno 1983). In a series of double-blind studies, Henningfield *et al.* (1983) showed that intravenous nicotine produced a clearly identifiable 'drug' effect whereas there was no effect from saline. The intensity of this effect increased with increasing dosage and was rated as somewhat similar to that of cocaine and amphetamines. Smokers rated it as pleasurable, and their degree of liking for it increased with increasing dosage. On the other hand, non-smokers did not seem to enjoy the nicotine injections, possibly because they had not become tolerant to adverse effects such as nausea.

As already noted, the subjective drug-effect produced by smoking tends to occur only with the first cigarette of the day, suggesting that it is subject to acute (though not necessarily chronic) tolerance. Jones, Farrell, and Herning (1978) found some support for this view. When intravenous nicotine was given repeatedly at 60-min intervals to a group of smokers, the subjective effect decreased with successive doses.

Nicotine and the control of arousal

Arousal is a term which is used loosely to refer to a variety of physiological, subjective and behavioural dimensions. For example, EEG desynchronization, anxiety, raised plasma adrenaline concentrations, and increased behavioural activity, are usually considered to reflect heightened arousal; whereas synchronized low-frequency EEG, calmness, and decreased activity, are often taken to indicate lowered arousal. The effects of nicotine on the various dimensions associated with arousal are complex and not fully understood. Nevertheless, there is evidence that nicotine can have both stimulant and sedative actions analogous to those which smokers report.

Stimulant effects

The stimulant effects of nicotine have been demonstrated at both the behavioural and physiological level. At the behavioural level, it has been shown that after an initial depressant action, nicotine increases locomotor activity in rats (Clarke and Kumar 1983). Tolerance is soon acquired to the depressant effect leaving an unequivocal dose-dependent stimulant action. Tolerance to the initial depressant effect persists after a period of at least 90 days without nicotine (Stolerman, Fink, and Jarvik 1973). Both the stimulant and depressant effects are blocked by mecamylamine, but not by the peripheral cholinergic blocker hexamethonium, indicating that they are centrally mediated.

In humans, nicotine and smoking enhance performance in vigilance tasks, suggesting an increase in alertness. They do this primarily by counteracting the normal tendency to lose concentration as the task progresses. For example, Wesnes and Warburton (1983) report that nicotine tablets which were crushed and held in the mouth to enable buccal absorption (swallowed nicotine is rapidly metabolized by the liver) improved vigilance performance in a combined group of smokers and non-smokers. Smoking may also improve reaction time and memory consolidation, possibly reflecting a stimulant action (e.g. Andersson 1975).

At the physiological level, it has long been known that smoking and nicotine have stimulating actions both centrally and peripherally. The main central effect is desynchronization of the EEG. More recently it has been shown that smoking decreases both alpha and theta power (Herning, Jones, and Bachman 1983), and increases the dominant α-frequency (Knott and Venables 1977). These effects, like overall desynchronization, have been taken to represent increased arousal. Studies in animals have shown that nicotine infusions can have analogous effects. For example, Armitage, Hall, and Sellers (1969) found that low doses of nicotine caused desynchronization of the EEG accompanied by an increase in the release of cortical acetylcholine.

Well-known peripheral actions of smoking and nicotine include increased heart rate, blood pressure and skin conductance, and, through vasoconstrictive action, decreased distal skin temperature. More recently, it has been found that smoking and nicotine increase plasma adrenaline and noradrenaline concentrations (Cryer, Haymond, Santiago, and Shah 1976), as well as causing release of other stress-related hormones such as cortisol and growth hormone (Pomerleau *et al.* 1983; Wilkins, Carlson, van Vunakis, Nill, Gritz, and Jarvik 1983). The effect of nicotine on release of cortisol is of particular interest because it does not seem to be mediated by increased circulating levels of adrenocorticotrophic hormone (Pomerleau *et al.* 1983). It may therefore occur as a result of direct action at the adrenal cortex.

Sedative effects

The sedative effects of nicotine are complex and probably do not constitute a unitary phenomenon. Many of them appear to depend on dose, the individual and the situation.

At the behavioural level, it has already been noted that nicotine has an initial depressant effect on locomotor activity in rats. Nicotine also decreases predatory behaviour and shock induced aggression in cats and squirrel monkeys (Hutchinson and Emley 1973; Bernston, Beattie, and Walker 1976). Hall and Morrison (1973) found that nicotine facilitated the performance of rats during an unsignalled shock-avoidance task (which is very stressful) but not during signalled shock-avoidance (which is less stressful). This finding was taken to imply that over-arousal of the animals in the stressful task impaired performance and that in this situation nicotine sedated the animals sufficiently to enable more effective avoidance responding.

Other evidence related to a possible sedative action of nicotine comes from studies by Nelsen (1978) who found that nicotine counteracted the disruptive effect of electrical stimulation of the reticular formation on selective attention. Nelsen suggested that this was because nicotine alleviated the hyperstimulated, anxious state created by excess reticular activity. However, it is also possible that her results arose because of a direct effect of nicotine on selective attention. Smokers appear to pay less attention to incidental stimuli when smoking than when abstinent (Andersson and Hockey 1977), and Wesnes and Warburton (1983) report that nicotine tablets improve performance on the 'Stroop' colour-naming task. In this task, subjects are presented with a list of words written in different colours. They are required to name the colours as fast as possible.

When the words are themselves colour names (not corresponding to the colours in which they are written), speed of colour-naming is considerably slowed. This appears to be because of interference from semantic information automatically extracted from the words. It seems that nicotine helps to block out this intrusive information.

Demonstrations of the sedative effects of nicotine on physiological responses have focused on the EEG. Golding and Mangan (1982) found that, while smoking had a stimulant effect on the EEG during periods of under-stimulation, it had a de-arousing effect under stress conditions. Sham smoking had similar but smaller effects suggesting that the effect of smoking was attributable to nicotine. Armitage *et al.* (1969) had previously shown that nicotine tended to have a stimulant effect on the EEG in small doses, but a mixed stimulant and depressant effect when the doses were given in larger boli. Thus it may be that the findings of Golding and Mangan (1982) reflected a dose response relation, with smokers inhaling more in the stress condition.

Ashton, Marsh, Millman, Rawlins, Telford, and Thompson (1978), using a measure of arousal based on EEG recordings, also reported dose-related stimulant and depressant effects of smoking and intravenous nicotine. They looked at a phenomenon known as 'contingent negative variation' (CNV). This consists of a small surface negative potential which builds up during a period between a warning stimulus and a signal requiring action from the subject (e.g. pressing a button). It has been assumed that the larger this potential the higher the level of arousal. Thus, Ashton *et al.* were able to show that caffeine increased the amplitude of the CNV, while nitrazepam decreased it. The results with smoking were complex. In some subjects there was a consistent increase in arousal and in others there was a decrease. Subjects who showed an increase in arousal tended to take in nicotine at a slower rate than subjects who showed a decrease, and a later study confirmed that high doses of intravenous nicotine produced a depressant effect on CNV while small doses had a stimulant effect.

We mentioned earlier that nicotine may improve behavioural responses under stress by a sedative action. An analogous finding has been reported with physiological data. Friedman, Horvath, and Meares (1974) showed that smoking increased the rate of habituation of the EEG response to loud noise and suggested that smoking might act as a 'stimulus barrier' by attenuating sensory input and thereby lowering arousal. The sedative effects of nicotine may also be associated with, or mediated by, a decrease in muscle tension, although this decrease seems to be limited to certain muscle groups such as the masseter (Hutchinson and Emley 1973).

In summary, nicotine can have actions which a smoker may interpret as both stimulating and sedating. It can increase alertness during vigilance tasks, and produce physiological arousal as measured by EEG, cardiovascular responses, and release of stress related hormones. It can also improve selective attention and enhance coping responses in stressful situations. At least in higher doses it can lead to de-arousing effects on some physiological variables.

Nicotine, hunger, and weight

The role of weight and hunger in maintaining smoking has not received much attention in the past, despite the fact that for many smokers it may be of great importance.

Smokers as a group weigh less than non-smokers and it seems that this effect is attributable to nicotine. In a recent study, young rats given chronic nicotine administration gained less weight than did controls given saline (Grunberg 1982). The rats given nicotine consumed fewer calories due to a decrease in consumption of a sugar solution. However, it is not clear how much the difference in weight between smokers and non-smokers is attributable to differences in caloric intake. The caloric intake of smokers and non-smokers have been found to be similar in some studies but not in others.

Any effect of nicotine in decreasing caloric intake could be related to its action of raising blood glucose levels (Spohr, Hofman, Steck, Harenberg, Walter, Hengen, Augustin, Morl, Koch, Horsch, and Weber 1979) since it is known that there are glucoreceptors in the hypothalamus which are involved in hunger regulation, and that small doses of glucose can decrease food intake (Martin, Geiselman, and Novin 1982).

NICOTINE REGULATION IN SMOKING

If smokers were simply smoking out of habit or for reasons related to the *activity* of smoking, the nicotine content of the cigarettes should not make much difference to how many they smoke, or how they smoke them. Yet smokers of low-yielding cigarettes compensate for their reduced deliveries, mainly by increased puffing and inhalation (e.g. Russell, Jarvis, Iyer, and Feyerabend 1980). These cigarettes have reduced tar as well as nicotine deliveries, and it has not been clearly established whether the compensation is directed at the 'scratch' of the smoke in the throat, its taste, or the amount of nicotine delivered. Some studies have sought to vary nicotine and tar deliveries independently, but the problem with these is that the perceived strength or taste of the smoke may not simply be a function of the *amount* of tar delivered. For example, the process of curing the tobacco and its effect on the pH of the smoke may also play a role.

Information on whether smokers tend to regulate their nicotine intake can also be obtained in other ways. Schachter (1978) has reported that smokers smoke at a higher rate when nicotine excretion is increased by acidification of the urine, although whether it is the increased rate of nicotine excretion which is important, or some other consequence of the acidification procedure, is not clear. Some studies have shown that giving nicotine by another route decreases smoking (e.g. Lucchesi, Schuster, and Emley 1967), although others have failed to find this effect (Kumar, Cooke, Lader, and Russell 1977).

In general, there is some evidence that smokers regulate their nicotine intake, but the degree to which they do so, and the influence of situational factors on this process are as yet unclear.

NICOTINE, CIGARETTE WITHDRAWAL EFFECTS, AND SMOKING CESSATION

When smokers abstain, many of them experience unpleasant withdrawal symptoms. The most commonly reported abstinence effects are irritability, depression, inability to concentrate, restlessness, hunger, and craving (Shiffman 1979). These are accompanied by physiological and performance changes including decreased vigilance, a decrease in dominant α-frequency and an increase in α-abundance in the resting EEG, a drop in excreted levels of adrenaline and noradrenaline, a drop in heart-rate and a rise in skin-temperature.

These changes are by and large mirror images of the effects of smoking and nicotine which we considered earlier. There are two issues which need to be addressed: whether or not a given abstinence effect is caused by loss of nicotine; and, if it is, whether it represents an abnormal physiological state (or 'rebound') resulting from long-term adaptation to the effects of nicotine rather than simple absence of those effects.

It is only very recently that an answer has been forthcoming to the first of these questions. Several recent studies have shown that nicotine replacement by means of nicotine chewing gum reduces a number of withdrawal symptoms by comparison with a placebo (cf. West 1984). On the other hand, in the only study that measured it, nicotine gum failed to alleviate a drop in urinary adrenaline concentration. Moreover, there appeared to be little or no effect on craving. The nicotine gum produced blood nicotine levels of only a third to a half of those obtained from smoking and it is possible that more complete nicotine replacement would produce more complete alleviation of withdrawal. Indirect evidence that nicotine is implicated at least partially in craving comes from the finding that the higher the pre-abstinence plasma nicotine concentration, the more severe the craving (West 1984), whereas craving does not appear to correlate with the usual daily cigarette consumption.

The issue of whether withdrawal effects represent more than a return to the non-smoking state (i.e. contain a rebound element) is less clear-cut. A rebound element in a particular withdrawal effect could be identified in two ways: by demonstrating a return over time to a new baseline different from that prevailing in the acute phase of withdrawal; or by demonstrating that smokers after withdrawal are different from non-smokers. This latter approach entails the assumption that smokers would have been similar to non-smokers if they had never smoked.

Self-reports of subjective effects of withdrawal such as irritability appear to show an amelioration over time. However, this could be because people simply become accustomed to the change. As regards the behavioural changes, Wesnes and Warburton (1983) found that abstaining smokers were no less alert than non-smokers. On the other hand, Heimstra, Bancroft, and DeKock (1967) had previously shown that the performance of deprived smokers in a simulated driving task was worse than that of non-smokers. In a rather different vein, rats who had been given nicotine during unsignalled shock avoidance, performed less well after deprivation than rats who had never received nicotine (Hall and Morrison 1973). With physiological changes during withdrawal, Knott and Venables (1977) found that deprived smokers showed slower dominant alpha rhythms than non-smokers, suggesting a 'rebound' state.

The weight-gain during cigarette abstinence is of particular interest. A recent study by Carney and Goldberg (1984) showed that smokers have elevated levels of lipoprotein lipase which appears to be a counter-regulatory response to the weight decreasing properties of smoking. The levels of this enzyme prior to abstinence correlated highly with the amount of weight gain experienced during abstinence. This raises the possibility that at least part of the weight-gain experienced on smoking cessation is due to a rebound arising from the body's attempt to counteract the effects of smoking.

Thus while there is now good evidence that loss of nicotine underlies many of the changes which take place during smoking withdrawal, it is not clear to what extent these changes involve a rebound element. However, from the smoker's point of view it is probably not important whether or not cigarette withdrawal effects are due to physiological adaptation. What he or she notices is a change for the worse when not smoking and a change for the better when smoking. It is these changes which underlie the smoker's difficulty in giving up smoking. It is now apparent that temporary nicotine replacement by use of nicotine chewing gum following smoking cessation can increase the chances of long term abstinence (e.g. Jarvis, Raw, Russell, and Feyerabend 1982). Success with the gum does appear to depend, however, on additional psychological support to ensure that patients persevere with its use despite its initially unpleasant taste.

NICOTINE AND SMOKING DEPENDENCE: CONCLUSIONS

In the preceding sections we have looked at a wide range of behavioural, physiological, and pharmacological data which all point towards a substantial role for nicotine in smoking motivation and smoking dependence. Perhaps the most impressive feature is that although the data arise from such disparate sources, they all seem to point in the same direction. The evidence really falls into two classes: data showing that nicotine is important in smoking without necessarily indicating in what way, and data showing *how* the actions of nicotine might make it an important feature of smoking motivation. The first type of evidence comes from studies showing that nicotine is a primary reinforcer, that smokers may regulate their nicotine intake, and that nicotine replacement following smoking cessation can improve the chances of maintaining abstinence. The second type of evidence comes from studies showing that nicotine has actions which appear to be analogous to smokers' expressed reasons for smoking, including relief of withdrawal effects.

There are, however, important gaps in our knowledge which remain to be filled. Of most concern is the fact that dependence on smoking involves more than simply wanting to obtain certain effects or avoid withdrawal symptoms. It involves an overwhelming *need* to smoke despite having made a decision not to. The hunger, mood changes, and somatic symptoms attending smoking abstinence can be distressing and may plausibly provide the basis for a need to return to smoking. However, it seems to be the craving for cigarettes *per se* which is the most important factor in precipitating relapse. It is hard to understand such craving in terms of the various actions of nicotine which we have considered. The euphoriant effect is slight and intermittent, and craving is by no means limited to situations of understimulation or stress. The evidence so far that nicotine is implicated in craving is largely circumstantial. Therefore, it is possible that craving arises out of behavioural aspects of smoking, or an interaction between nicotine and those behavioural aspects. For example, the fact that the effects of smoking doses of nicotine are relatively slight and such as to enhance rather than impair performance, may indirectly lead to dependence. They enable the smoker to continue to function normally in every-day tasks, and therefore make it possible for the smoker to self-administer nicotine almost continuously throughout the day. The intermittent pairing of the behaviour of smoking with the subjective effects of nicotine could establish the behaviour of smoking as a potent secondary reinforcer to which craving might become directed.

This explanation is only one of a number of possibilities. If we are to understand smoking dependence, as opposed to smoking motivation, there is a considerable amount of work to be done in identifying the basis of craving. The fact that craving for a cigarette and relapse to smoking may occur long after the point of giving up suggests that a full understanding of the pharmacology of smoking dependence will also require a full understanding of the psychology of smoking dependence.

ACKNOWLEDGEMENTS

We are grateful to Ian Stolerman, Malcolm Lader and Heather Ashton for providing us with helpful comments, and to the Medical Research Council for providing funding.

REFERENCES

Andersson, K. (1975). Effects of cigarette smoking on learning and retention. *Psychopharmacologia* **41**, 1-5.
— and Hockey, G. R. J. (1977). Effects of cigarette smoking on incidental memory. *Psychopharmacology* **52**, 223-6.

Armitage, A. K., Hall, G. H., and Sellers, C. M. (1969). Effects of nicotine on electrocortical activity and acetylcholine release from the cat cerebral cortex. *Br. J. Pharmac.* **35**, 152–60.

Ashton, H., Marsh, V. R., Millman, J. E., Rawlins, M. D. Telford, R., and Thompson, J. W. (1978). The use of event-related slow potentials of the brain as a means to analyse the effects of cigarette smoking and nicotine in humans. In *Smoking behaviour: physiological and psychological influences* (ed. R. Thornton), pp. 54–69. Churchill-Livingstone, London.

Bernston, G. C., Beattie, M. S., and Walker, J. M. (1976). Effects of nicotinic and muscarinic compounds on biting attack in the cat. *Pharmac. Biochem. & Behav.* **5**, 235–9.

Carney, R. M. and Goldberg, A. P. (1984). Weight gain after cessation of cigarette smoking: a possible role for adipose-tissue lipoprotein lipase. *New Engl. J. Med.* **310**, 614–16.

Clarke, P. B. S. and Kumar, R. (1983). The effects of nicotine on locomotor activity in non-tolerant and tolerant rats. *Br. J. Pharmac.* **78**, 329–37.

Cryer, P. E., Haymond, M. W., Santiago, J. V., and Shah, S. D. (1976). Norepinephrine and epinephrine release and adrenergic mediation of smoking-associated hemodynamic and metabolic events. *New Engl. J. Med.* **295**, 573–7.

Friedman, J., Horvath, T., and Meares, R. (1974). Tobacco smoking and a stimulus barrier. *Nature, Lond.* **248**, 455–6.

Golding, J. and Mangan, G. L. (1982). Arousing and de-arousing effects of cigarette smoking under conditions of stress and mild sensory isolation *Psychopharmacology* **19**, 449–56.

Grunberg, N. E. (1982). The effects of nicotine and cigarette smoking on food consumption and taste preferences. *Addict. Behav.* **7**, 317–31.

Hall, G. H. and Morrison, C. F. (1973). New evidence for a relationship between tobacco smoking, nicotine dependence and stress. *Nature, Lond.* **243**, 199–201.

Heimstra, N. W., Bancroft, N. R., and DeKock, A. R. (1967). Effects of smoking upon sustained performance in a stimulated driving task. *Ann. N.Y. Acad. Sci.* **142**, 295–307.

Henningfield, J. E., Goldberg, S. R., Miyasato, K., Spealman, R. D., and Jasinski, D. R. (1982). Functional properties of nicotine in monkeys and humans. *Fed. Proc. Fedn Am. Socs exp. Biol.* **41**, 7406.

—, Miyasato, K., Johnson, R. E., and Jasinski, D. R. (1983). Rapid physiologic effects of nicotine in humans and selective blockade of behavioral effects by mecamylamine. In *Problems of drug dependence* (ed. L. S. Harris), pp. 259–63. NIDA Research Monograph 43, US Department and Human Services.

Herning, R. I., Jones, R. T., and Bachman, J. (1983). EEG changes during tobacco withdrawal. *Psychophysiology* **20**, 507–12.

Hutchinson, R. R., and Emley, G. S. (1973). Effects of nicotine on avoidance, conditioned suppression and aggression response measures in animals and man. In *Smoking Behaviour: Motives and Incentives* (ed. W. L. Dunn), pp. 179–96. Winston, Washington, DC.

Jarvis, M. J., Raw, M., Russell, M. A. H., and Feyerabend, C. (1982). Randomized controlled trial of nicotine chewing-gum. *Br. med. J.* **285**, 537–40.

Jones, R. T., Farrell, T. R., and Herning, R. I. (1978). Tobacco smoking and nicotine tolerance. In *Self-administration of abused substances: methods for study* (ed. N. A. Krasnegor), pp. 202–8. NIDA Research Monograph 20, Department of Health, Education and Welfare.

Knott, V. J. and Venables, P. H. (1977). EEG alpha correlates of non-smokers, smokers, smoking and smoking deprivation. *Psychopharmacology* **14**, 150–5.

Kumar, R., Cooke, E. C., Lader, M. H., and Russell, M. A. H. (1977). Is nicotine important in tobacco smoking? *Clin. Pharmac. & Ther.* **21**, 520–9.

Lichensteiger, W., Hefti, F., Flexi, D., Huwlyer, T., Melamed, E., and Schlumpf, M. (1982). Stimulation of nigrostriatal dopamine neurones by nicotine. *Neuropharmacology* **21**, 963–8.

Lucchesi, B. R., Shuster, C. R., and Emley, G. S. (1967). The role of nicotine as a determinant of cigarette smoking frequency in man with observations of certain cardiovascular effects associated with the tobacco alkaloid. *Clin. Pharmac. & Ther.* **8**, 789–96.

Martin, J. R., Geiselman, P. J., and Novin, D. (1982). Feeding pattern of rabbits following intraduodenal glucose infusion as a function of caloric load, fasting interval, and vagal denervation. *Physiol. Psychol.* **10**, 273–9.

Nelsen, J. M. (1978). Psychological consequences of chronic nicotinisation: a focus on arousal. In *Behavioural effects of nicotine* (ed. K. Battig), pp. 1–17. S. Karger, Basel.

Pomerleau, O. F., Fertig, J. B., Seyler, L. E., and Jaffe, J. H. (1983). Neuro-endocrine reactivity to nicotine in smokers. *Psychopharmacology* **81**, 61–7.

Risner, M. E. and Goldberg, S. R. (1983). A comparison of nicotine and cocaine self-administration in the dog: fixed-ratio and progressive-ratio schedules of intravenous drug infusion. *J. Pharmac. exp. Ther.* **224**, 319–26.

Romano, C. and Goldstein, A. (1980). Stereo specific nicotine receptors on rat brain membranes. *Science* **210**, 647–9.

Russell, M. A. H., Jarvis, M. J., Feyerabend, C., and Ferno, O. (1983). Nasal nicotine solution: a potential aid to giving up smoking. *Br. med. J.* **286**, 683–4.

—, Jarvis, M. J., Iyer, R., and Feyerabend, C. (1980). Relation of nicotine yield of cigarettes to blood nicotine concentrations in smokers. *Br. med. J.* **280**, 972–6.

—, Peto, J., and Patel, U. A. (1974). The classification of smoking by factorial structure of motives. *J. R. Statist. Soc.,* **A 137**, 313–46.

Schachter, S. (1978). Pharmacological and psychological determinants of smoking. *Ann. int. Med.* **88**, 104–14.

Shiffman, S. M. (1979). The tobacco withdrawal syndrome. In *Cigarette smoking as a dependence process* (ed. N. Krasnegor), pp. 158–85. NIDA Research Monograph 23, US Department of Health, Education and Welfare.

Spealman, R. D. and Goldberg, S. R. (1982). Maintenance of schedule-controlled behavior by intravenous injections of nicotine in squirrel monkeys. *J. Pharmac. exp. Ther.* **223**, 402–8.

Spohr, U., Hofmann, K., Steck, J., Harenberg, J., Walter, E., Hengen, N., Augustin, J., Morl, H., Koch, A., Horsch, A., and Weber, E. (1979). Evaluation of smoking-induced effects on sympathetic, hemodynamic and metabolic variables with respect to plasma nicotine and COHb levels. *Atherosclerosis* **33**, 271–83.

Stolerman, I. P., Fink, R., and Jarvik, M. E. (1973). Acute and chronic tolerance to nicotine measured by activity in rats. *Psychopharmacologia* **30**, 329–42.

Wesnes, K. and Warburton, D. M. (1983). Smoking, nicotine and human performance. *Pharmac. & Ther.* **21**, 189–208.

West, R. J. (1984). Psychology and pharmacology in cigarette withdrawal. *J. psychosom. Res.* **28**, 379–86.

Wilkins, J. N., Carlson, H. E., Van Vunakis, H., Nill, M. A., Gritz, E., and Jarvik,

M. E. (1982). Nicotine from cigarette smoking increases circulating levels of cortisol, growth hormone and prolactin in male chronic smokers. *Psychopharmacology* **78**, 305–8.

Yanagita, T. (1977). Brief review on the use of self-administration techniques for predicting abuse potential. In *Predicting dependence liability of stimulant and depressant drugs* (ed. T. Thompson and K. Unna), pp. 409–12. University Park Press, Baltimore.

27

How amphetamine works

TREVOR SILVERSTONE AND ELIZABETH GOODALL

INTRODUCTION

Shortly after amphetamine came into clinical use some fifty years ago as a nasal decongestant and bronchodilator its central stimulant and anorexiant properties became apparent (Davidoff and Riefenstein 1937). And it was this combination of properties which led the drug to be considered as particularly effective for the treatment of obesity: '. . . on the one hand it decreases the appetite, and on the other so increases the sense of well being and of energy that physical activity is spontaneously increased.' (Lesses and Myerson 1938). Its popularity as a slimming drug rapidly increased and it came to be widely prescribed for this purpose all over the world. Unfortunately, those very characteristics which had earlier seemed so beneficial, that is, its stimulant and euphoriant effects, began to cause problems.

Amphetamine was being increasingly employed as a drug of abuse, not so much by the overweight patients for whom it was prescribed but by otherwise healthy adolescents and young adults seeking a 'high'. As a result the therapeutic application of amphetamine fell into disfavour and its use became strictly curtailed, with its current therapeutic indications being limited to narcolepsy and the hyperkinetic syndrome in children. Nevertheless, however limited its therapeutic role may be, amphetamine's combination of stimulant, euphoriant, and anorexiant actions has an obvious potential interest for psychiatrists interested in the pathogenesis of affective disorders.

An appreciation of how amphetamine causes its effects on arousal, mood, and appetite in human subjects could well lead to a greater understanding of how the disturbances of arousal, mood, and appetite which are seen in patients suffering from major affective disorders might arise. And such an understanding will undoubtedly hasten the development of more effective treatments.

In normal subjects, amphetamine produces a dose-related elevation of mood and an increase in the subjective sense of arousal as evaluated by visual analogue scales, with 20 mg producing a much greater effect than 10 mg (Silverstone, Wells, and Trenchard 1983), Figs 27.1 and 27.2.

Although amphetamine also causes a dose-related reduction in hunger (Silverstone and Stunkard 1968) the dose-relationship for hunger suppression is not

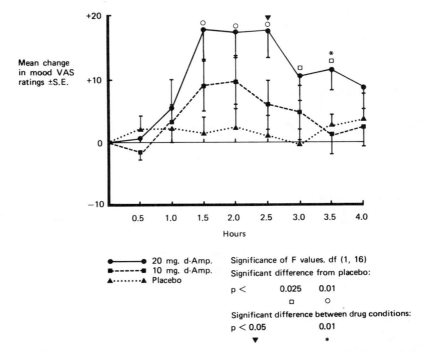

Fig. 27.1. The effect of 10 and 20 mg d-amph and placebo on subjective ratings of mood in nine male subjects.

the same as for its stimulant actions; 20 mg producing no greater anorexia than 10 mg (Silverstone *et al.* 1983), Fig. 27.3.

Such a difference in dose-response relationships between the stimulant and euphoriant action of amphetamine on the one hand and its anorectic action on the other could well reflect an underlying difference in neuropharmacological activity. In laboratory animals, amphetamine acts in the brain largely by releasing preformed noradrenaline (NA) and dopamine (DA) from presynaptic terminals and inhibiting their reuptake (Carlsson 1970).

Could it be, therefore, that the anorectic action of amphetamine results more from release of one of these two neurotransmitters while its stimulant and euphoriant actions comes from release of the other?

In a series of studies involving normal human subjects we have attempted to answer this question by examining the interaction of amphetamine with a number of relatively specific receptor blocking compounds, using both subjective and objective measures to evaluate the effects of such interactions. For ratings of subjective changes we used visual analogue scales (VAS); for objective measure of arousal we used skin conductance (Lader 1975) and for objective measurement of food intake we used an automated solid food dispenser (Silverstone, Fincham, and Brydon 1980).

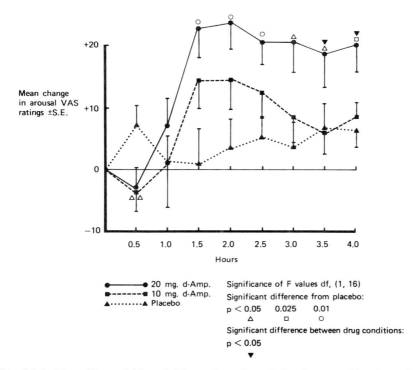

Fig. 27.2. The effect of 10 and 20 mg d-amph and placebo on subjective ratings of arousal in nine male subjects.

DOPAMINE RECEPTOR BLOCKADE

In order to determine the effect of DA receptor blockade on the stimulant and anorectic action of amphetamine (amph) we have used the selective DA receptor-blocking drug pimozide (PMZ) (Anden, Butcher, Corrodi, Fuxe, and Ungestedt 1970).

In our first experiment using PMZ we administered a single oral dose of 2 mg PMZ or matching placebo, two hours before giving a single oral dose of 10 mg dextroamphetamine (d-amph) or a second matching placebo to eight healthy female subjects. The subjects completed VAS ratings for arousal, mood, and hunger before receiving the first tablet and at hourly intervals thereafter for the next six hours.

Unfortunately, we were unable to determine the effects of PMZ in d-amph-induced euphoria, as the dose of d-amph used did not produce a significant elevation of mood. However, Jonsson (1972), using a much higher dose of d-amph had reported that PMZ inhibits the euphoriant effect of d-amph in previously addicted subjects. Thus, what evidence there is supports the view that the euphoriant action of d-amph is likely to be DA-indicated.

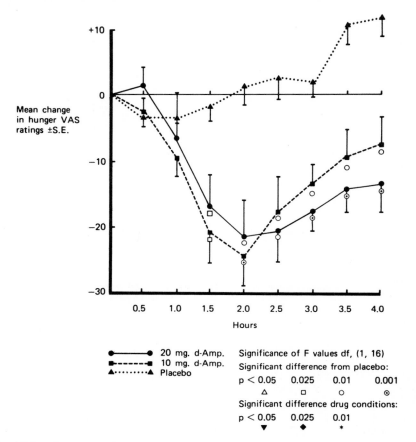

Fig. 27.3. The effect of 10 and 20 mg d-amph and placebo on subjective ratings of hunger in nine male subjects.

As far as subjective arousal was concerned we did observe a significant affect of d-amph; and this effect was significantly attenuated by pretreatment with 2 mg PMZ, Fig. 27.4. This finding suggests that d-amph-arousal is also DA-mediated.

In contrast, hunger VAS ratings, which were markedly reduced by d-amph remained unaffected by PMZ, Fig. 27.5, indicating that d-amph-anorexia, unlike d-amph arousal and euphoria, is not mediated primarily through DA pathways.

In a second study involving PMZ we measured the response to d-amph objectively by recording skin conductance before and after a single oral dose of 20 mg d-amph, with and without pretreatment with 2 or 4 mg PMZ (Jacobs and Silverstone, in preparation). As before, matching placebos were used to maintain strict double-blind conditions, d-Amph increased both the basal level of skin conductance and the number of spontaneous fluctuations in skin con-

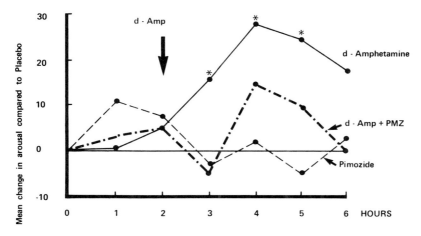

Fig. 27.4. The changes in arousal ratings following d-amph alone, PMZ alone and d-amph preceded by PMZ less the changes observed in each subject following placebo; the means of these differences are presented. Statistically significant differences ($T < 3, p < 0.05$) between drugs and placebo are marked*.

ductance. PMZ reversed these changes in a dose-related manner, a result in keeping with d-amph arousal being DA-mediated.

NORADRENALINE RECEPTOR BLOCKADE

(a) Alpha-1 receptors

Thymoxamine (TMX) is considered to have a relatively specific action on alpha-NA-receptors (Besser, Butler, Ratcliffe, Rees, and Young 1968), and has been shown to be active centrally. In order to assess the effects of NA blockade on d-amph arousal and anorexia we administered 80 and 160 mg TMX, or matching placebo one hour before giving a single oral dose of 20 mg d-amph to twelve healthy male volunteers. As far as subjective mood ratings were concerned TMX, if anything, *increased* d-amph-induced euphoria and irritability. A similar pattern was seen in the VAS arousal ratings, with TMX enhancing the effect of d-amph. Changes in skin conductance measurements were consistent with those observed in the subjective ratings.

In sharp contrast to what was observed with d-amph-induced arousal, d-amph-anorexia was partially *attenuated* by the higher dose of TMX, Fig. 27.6. This finding suggests that d-amph anorexia may well be NA-mediated, a view consistent with some of the animal data (Ahlskog 1974). However, in a second study involving healthy female subjects in which we measured food intake directly, in addition to assessing subjective hunger, we failed to replicate our previous finding that TMX attenuates d-amph anorexia (Silverstone, Trenchard,

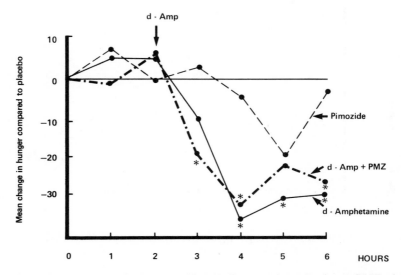

Fig. 27.5. The changes in hunger ratings following d-amph alone, PMZ alone and d-amph preceded by PMZ less the changes observed in each subject following placebo; the means of these differences are presented. Statistically significant differences ($T < 3$, $p < 0.05$) between drugs and placebo are marked*.

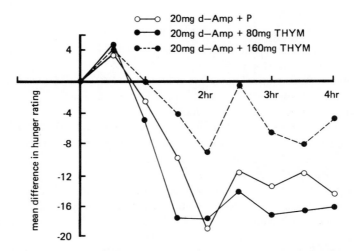

Fig. 27.6. Attentuation by the NA receptor-blocking drug thymoxamine (THYM) of the anorectic activity of 20 mg d-amph in normal male subjects (Jacobs and Silverstone, in preparation).

and Goodall, in preparation), Fig. 27.7. But in this second study, food intake was measured two hours after the drug had been given whereas the most marked effect of TMX in the first study had not occurred until some three to four hours after it had been given. Thus the lack of agreement in the two studies may well be more of a reflection of the methodological differences between them than a true pharmacological inconsistency.

(b) Beta receptors

We found Propanolol (PPL) a centrally active β-NA-receptor blocking drug (Patel and Turner 1981), to be completely without effect on either d-amph-induced arousal or anorexia in normal female volunteers. Nor did it influence the reduction of food intake brought about by d-amph, Fig. 27.8. Such a complete lack of interaction between d-amph and PPL argues strongly against a primary involvement of β-NA-receptors in d-amph-induced arousal or anorexia.

5-HYDROXYTRYPTAMINE RECEPTOR BLOCKADE

Although 5-hydroxytryptamine (5-HT) is not thought to be directly involved in the mediation of d-amph anorexia or arousal, there is good evidence from animal studies that 5-HT neurotransmission is concerned in the regulation of

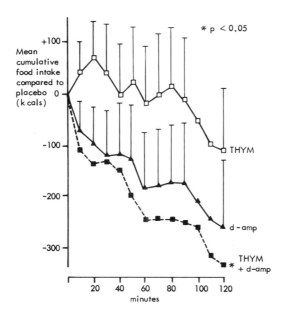

Fig. 27.7. Mean cumulative food intake (m ± SE) for eight normal female volunteers following d-amph alone, thymoxamine (THYM) alone and d-amph preceded by THYM, less the amount eaten in each subject following placebo; the means of these differences are presented.

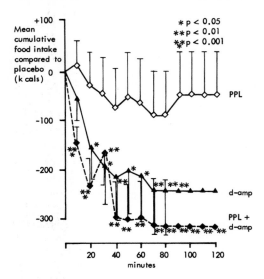

Fig. 27.8. Mean cumulative food intake (m ± SE) for eight normal female volunteers following d-amph alone, propanolol (PPL) alone, and d-amph given with PPL, less the amount eaten in each subject following placebo; the means of these differences are presented.

food intake (Blundell 1977). We therefore examined the interaction of the 5-HT receptor-blocking compound metergoline (MTG) with d-amph. In this study a single dose of 4 mg MTG or matching placebo was administered together with a single oral dose of 10 mg d-amph to healthy female subjects two hours before access to the automated solid food dispenser. MTG by itself increased food intake, whereas d-amph decreased it. The combination produced a net effect little different from placebo, Fig. 27.9. The fact that MTG has an intrinsic orectic action of its own argues more for a summation effect, occurring when the two active drugs are given, than a true drug interaction. That is, MTG is producing its orectic action through a mechanism independent from that by which d-amph is producing its anorectic action. If this interpretation is correct, then d-amph anorexia is not 5-HT-mediated.

CLINICAL IMPLICATIONS

From the results we have obtained in our series of experiments in human volunteers we can be reasonably confident that the stimulant activity of d-amph, and probably its euphoriant activity as well, is mediated through central DA pathways.

As manic illness also appears to be at least partly DA-mediated (Silverstone 1978) d-amph-induced arousal in normal subjects might provide a useful model for mania. Further evaluation of this possibility has yielded some striking

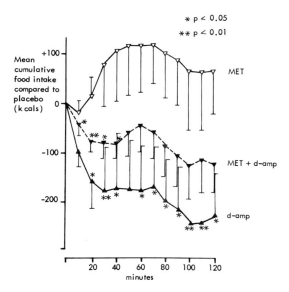

Fig. 27.9. Mean cumulative food intake (m ± SE) for eight normal female volunteers following d-amph alone, metergoline (MET) alone, and d-amph given with MET, less the amount eaten in each subject following placebo; the means of these differences are presented.

similarities in symptomatology, endocrine changes and pharmacological response between the model and the clinical correlation (Jacobs and Silverstone, in preparation).

The situation with regard to the mediation of d-amph-anorexia is less clear than that of arousal; certainly neither DA nor β-NA-receptors appear to be primarily involved. 5-HT pathways, while having a definite role in the overall regulation of human food intake, are probably not directly concerned in d-amph-mediated anorexia. Whether α-NA-receptors are, remains unresolved; in one study there did appear to be a definite interaction between the α-NA-receptor blocking drug TMX and d-amph anorexia. If it turns out to be confirmed that d-amph anorexia is NA-mediated then the possibility arises that other anorectic states, such as that which occurs in depressive illness may be a consequence of an abnormality in central NA neurotransmission. To this end we have examined the effect of a single intravenous injection of 15 mg methylamphetamine (m-amph) as compared to sterile water under strict double-blind conditions in twenty-one depressed subjects (Silverstone and Cookson, submitted for publication).

The question we were asking was: if methylamphetamine improved the mood of any of our depressed patients was there an associated improvement in appetite, such as occurs during recovery from a depressive illness, or was any such improvement in appetite suppressed by the direct anorectic action of the drug? Two intriguing findings emerged. First, as was expected from uncontrolled studies (Checkley 1978), only seven of the twenty-one patients responded to m-amph (but not to placebo) with an unequivocal improvement in mood. This suggests some impairment of the responsiveness of central DA pathways in the majority of severely depressed patients, but not in all. While the essential differences between m-amph responders and non-responders remains to be elucidated the possibility of delineating different categories of depressive illness on pharmacological grounds would appear to be a real one.

The other intriguing finding which emerged from this study in depressed patients was that of the seven who responded to m-amph with a marked improvement in mood, six experienced a concomitant increase in hunger. If d-amph-anorexia is in fact NA-mediated, then in these m-amph-responders the absence of m-amph-induced anorexia may reflect a reduction in central NA neurotransmission in at least some depressed patients, a hypothesis which has also been proposed by others on neuroendocrinological grounds (Checkley 1980).

CONCLUSION

Our quest for a greater understanding of how amphetamine works in human subjects which began as an exercise in academic psychopharmacology has led us into the very heartlands of clinical psychiatry. It is a sobering thought that the mysteries of human moods are now being explored with the aid of a drug which was synthesized as a cheaper substitute for ephedrine as a nasal decongestant: a drug which was only serendipitously noted to have central actions, and which on account of these central actions has been virtually completely banished from clinical use.

REFERENCES

Ahlskog, J. E. (1974). Food intake and amphetamine anorexia after selective forebrain norepinephrine loss. *Brain Res.* **82**, 211–40.

Anden, N. E., Butcher, S. G., Corrodi, H., Fuxe, F., and Ungerstedt, U. (1979). Receptor activity and turnover of dopamine nor-adrenaline after neuroleptics. *Eur. J. Pharmac.* **11**, 303–14.

Besser, G. M., Butler, P. W. P., Ratcliffe, J. G., Rees, L., and Young, P. (1968). Release by amphetamine in man of growth hormone and corticosteroids: the effects of thymoxamine and propanolol. *Br. J. Pharmac.* **39**, 196–7.

Blundell, J. E. (1977). Is there a role for serotonin (5-hydroxytryptamine) in feeding? *Int. J. Obesity* **1**, 15–42.

Carlsson, A. (1970). Amphetamine and brain catecholamines. In *Amphetamines and related compounds* (ed. E. Costa and S. Garattini), pp. 289–300. Raven Press, New York.

Checkley, S. A. (1978). A new distinction between the euphoric and the antidepressant effects of methylamphetamine. *Br. J. Psychiat.* **133**, 416–23.

—— (1980). Neuroendocrine tests of monoamine function in man: a review of basic theory and its application to the study of depressive illness. *Psychol. Med.* **10**, 35–53.

Davidoff, E. and Reifenstein, E. C. (1937). The stimulating action of benzedrine sulphate. *J. Am. med. Assoc.* **108**, 1770.

Jonsson, L. E. (1972). Pharmacological blockade of amphetamine effects in amphetamine dependent subjects. *Eur. J. clin. Pharmac.* **4**, 206–11.

Lader, M. H. (1975). *The psychophysiology of mental illness*. Routledge and Kegan Paul, London.

Lesses, M. F. and Myerson, A. (1938). Benzedrine sulphate as an aid to the treatment of obesity. *New Engl. J. Med.* **218**, 119–24.

Patel, L. and Turner, P. (1981). Central actions of beta-adrenoceptor blocking drugs in man. *Res. Rev.* **1**, 387–410.

Silverstone, T. (1978). Dopamine, mood and manic depressive psychosis. In *Depressive disorders* (ed. S. Garattini), pp. 419–30. Schattauer Verlag, Stuttgart.

Silverstone, T., Fincham, J., and Brydon, J. (1980). A new technique for the continuous measurement of food intake in man. *Am. J. clin. Nutr.* **3**, 1852–5.

—, Wells, B., and Trenchard, E. (1983). Differential dose-response effects of dexamphetamine sulphate on hunger, arousal and mood in human volunteers. *Psychopharmacology* **79**, 242–5.

Silverstone, J. T. and Stunkard, A. J. (1978). The anorectic effect of dexamphetamine sulphate. *Br. J. Pharmac. Chemother.* **33**, 513–22.

Index